fourth edition

Financial Management
for Nurse Managers

Merging the Heart with the Dollar

Edited by

J. Michael Leger, PhD, MBA, RN

Director, Department of System Quality,
Healthcare Safety, and Accreditation
Adjunct Professor, School of Nursing
University of Texas Medical Branch

Janne Dunham-Taylor, PhD, RN

Professor Emerita
East Tennessee State University

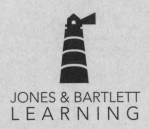

JONES & BARTLETT
LEARNING

World Headquarters
Jones & Bartlett Learning
5 Wall Street
Burlington, MA 01803
978-443-5000
info@jblearning.com
www.jblearning.com

Jones & Bartlett Learning books and products are available through most bookstores and online booksellers. To contact Jones & Bartlett Learning directly, call 800-832-0034, fax 978-443-8000, or visit our website, www.jblearning.com.

Production Credits
VP, Executive Publisher: David D. Cella
Executive Editor: Amanda Martin
Acquisitions Editor: Rebecca Stephenson
Editorial Assistant: Kirsten Haley
Senior Vendor Manager: Sara Kelly
Marketing Communications Manager: Katie Hennessy
Product Fulfillment Manager: Wendy Kilborn
Composition and Project Management: S4Carlisle Publishing Services

Cover Design: Theresa Manley
Rights & Media Specialist: Wes DeShano
Media Development Editor: Troy Liston
Cover Image (Title Page, Part Opener, Chapter Opener):
    © Spectral-Design/Shutterstock
Printing and Binding: Edwards Brothers Malloy
Cover Printing: Edwards Brothers Malloy

Library of Congress Cataloging-in-Publication Data
Names: Leger, J. Michael (John Michael), editor.
Title: Financial management for nurse managers : merging the heart with the
    dollar / [edited by] J. Michael Leger.
Other titles: Financial management for nurse managers (Dunham-Taylor)
Description: Fourth edition. | Burlington, Massachusetts : Jones & Bartlett
    Learning, [2018] | Includes bibliographical references and index.
Identifiers: LCCN 2017025739 | ISBN 9781284127256 (pbk. : alk. paper)
Subjects: | MESH: Economics, Nursing | Nursing Services--economics | Nursing
    Services--organization & administration | Financial Management--methods
Classification: LCC RT86.7 | NLM WY 77 | DDC 362.1068/1--dc23 LC record available at https://lccn.loc.gov/2017025739

6048

Printed in the United States of America
21 20 19 18 17   10 9 8 7 6 5 4 3 2 1

Brief Contents

Contents

PART II Budget Principles 107

Chapter 5 Budgeting 109

*Paul Brown, MSN, RN, Gary Eubank MSN, RN,
and J. Michael Leger, PhD, MBA, RN*

Chapter 6 Budget Development and
Evaluation 131

*Paul Brown, MSN, RN, and Gary Eubank MSN, RN,
and J. Michael Leger, PhD, MBA, RN*

Chapter 11   Accounting for Healthcare Entities 253

J. Michael Leger, PhD, MBA, RN, and *Paul Bayes,*
DBA Accounting, MS Economics, BS Accounting

Chapter 12   Financial Analysis: Improving Your Decision Making 279

J. Michael Leger, PhD, MBA, RN, and Paul Bayes,
DBA Accounting, MS Economics, BS Accounting

Index 305

Contributors

Paul Bayes, DBA, MS, BS
Former Chair and Professor of Accountancy
East Tennessee State University

Paul Brown, MSN, RN
Regional Director of Nursing
University of Texas Medical Branch, School of
  Nursing

Sandy K. Diffenderfer, PhD, MSN, RN, CPHQ
Assistant Professor, Graduate Program
East Tennessee State University, College of
  Nursing

Janne Dunham-Taylor, PhD, RN
Professor and Graduate Coordinator of
  Nursing Administration
East Tennessee State University, College of
  Nursing.

Joellen Edwards, PhD, RN, FAAN
Associate Dean for Research and Professor
East Tennessee State University, College of
  Nursing

Gary Eubank, MSN, RN
1999 Fellow, Johnson and Johnson Wharton
  Fellows Program in Management for Nurse
  Executives
The Wharton School, University of Pennsylvania

Dru Malcolm, DNP, MSN, RN, NEA-BC, CPHRM
Chief Nursing Officer and Assistant
  Administrator
Johnston Memorial Hospital, a facility of
  Mountain States Health Alliance

Mary Anne Schultz, PhD, MBA, MSN, RN
Former Faculty Member
California State University, Los Angeles,
  Department of Nursing

Karen W. Snyder, MSN, RN
Quality Improvement Specialist
Integrated Solutions Health Network

Norma Tomlinson, MSN, RN, NE-BC, FACHE
Associate Vice-President, Associate
  Executive Director
University of Toledo Medical Center

Patricia M. VanHook, PhD, MSN, RN, FNP-BC
Associate Dean of Practice
East Tennessee State University, College of
  Nursing

Preface

After working for more than 15 years as a nurse leader—Director, CNO, and VP of Nursing—I made the decision to follow my passion for teaching. During my first semester as faculty in a graduate nursing program, I was assigned to teach a financial management course because of my extensive experience in healthcare operations. It was then that I realized the gap of knowledge that many graduate-level nurses have with regard to healthcare financial management.

The class was composed of professional nurses with various levels of understanding of healthcare financial management, ranging from novice to expert. I also recognized that many of my students were serving in nursing leadership roles but not in inpatient settings. While the majority of the students had a basic knowledge of many of the financial terms presented in the course textbook, application of those terms and the actual process of budgeting were elusive to the majority of the students. The reason for this is that healthcare financial management continues to be driven by financial professionals, often to the detriment of the nurse leader truly understanding his/her role in healthcare finance.

When asked about my interest in serving as editor for the next edition of *Financial Management for Nurse Managers: Merging the Heart with the Dollar,* I saw an opportunity to take the fourth edition along a different sort of path. My vision was to provide a tool for nurse leaders at all levels of understanding, working in different areas along the healthcare continuum—inpatient, outpatient, acute, and subacute—to empower them with the knowledge they need, both theoretical and practical, to be more effective in their leadership roles and have a greater impact in financial management. While the information provided in the third edition serves students well, I recognized the need to provide students with practical examples of the material in an effort to promote their learning through application. Therefore, in editing material for the fourth edition, I made a conscious decision to remove some topics that I believe will serve students better in nonfinancial courses: ethics in nursing administration and contemporary legal issues for the nurse administrator, as examples.

I sincerely appreciate all of the contributing authors for their expertise and time in putting this book into the hands of nurse leaders, both current and future, who play such a large role in health care.

Acknowledgments

We would like to thank the author contributors in this book for sharing their time and expertise for this very worthwhile project.

▶ Dedications

This book is dedicated to the many nursing administration students and nurse administrators who have touched our lives and those who supported us by using this book. We learned a lot from you and we salute you.

—JDT & JML

Thanks to Mom, Dad, and the family for all your support and encouragement in completing this venture.

—JDT

I want to thank Charles, my spouse and best friend, for supporting me in, yet, another opportunity in my ever-evolving career path. And a special thanks to Kathleen, Carolyn, and Yolie for your unyielding support of me as your colleague.

—JML

Introduction

Every Management Decision Has Financial Implications—Every Financial Decision Has Management Implications!

Janne Dunham-Taylor, PhD, RN, and **J. Michael Leger**, PhD, MBA, RN

This text addresses healthcare financial management issues for nurse leaders in a variety of positions and settings: hospitals, ambulatory/outpatient clinics, long-term care facilities, and home care. This text is written to provide helpful, evidence-based information that pertains to each of these settings.

To be successful in financial management, nurse administrators must understand, regardless of setting, what affects the healthcare environment and the financial implications that result from these forces. The nurse administrator must express what needs to happen for good nursing practice and also must be able to articulate the financial aspects involved. Understanding the organization's finances is not sufficient. A nurse administrator must be able to anticipate actions in response to a changing financial environment and to encourage staff to do the same.

This text covers a wide range of financial information, including evidence, in healthcare finance, economics, budgeting, comparing reimbursements with cost of services provided, accounting, and financial strategies. Concepts are presented, followed by examples. At times, we make suggestions for actions that we have found to be helpful. Although many of the examples have an inpatient focus, a great number are provided from other healthcare settings, such as ambulatory care, home care, and long-term care.

Even though this book has a financial title, there is more included here than just the financial part of health care. This is because everything in health care is *interrelated/interconnected/interwoven* with finances. For example, when nurse administrators discuss budgeting, they must also be concerned with staffing, patient acuity, and the productivity of staff, as well as quality standards. We cannot ignore leadership in an organization, because if that is broken, everything else is.

It is important to note here that every financial decision we make has management implications. The same is true in reverse: Every management decision has financial implications. So, we cannot ignore the additional aspects we have included in this book because they are all interwoven and, if one is ignored, such oversight can negatively affect the bottom line.

The bottom line should *never* be the primary focus in a healthcare organization. *When the bottom line is most important, the organization will lose money.* Many in the organization will have forgotten that our reason for existence is to *serve patients.* That is our primary focus. As long as we stay in touch with this truth, we will thrive.

This is not to say that we can ignore the financial implications. As mentioned later: no margin, no mission. We cannot exceed the budget we have—if we do, we must have another area in the budget that we can draw from to counter the overspending. The bottom line must remain solvent. However, the patient *always* comes first.

We have entered into a new *value-based reimbursement environment* that demands different approaches for healthcare organizations to stay solvent. Our old volume-based reimbursement environment of the previous century is outdated. Healthcare organizations cannot continue to survive unless we change and create a value-based environment. This text outlines what is needed to achieve this objective.

We emphasize the importance of *giving the patient what is valued.* Many in health care do not fully understand this concept. Whereas we have been good about measuring patient satisfaction (although these data are often collected only after the experience), many times we miss the most important point: We have not *listened* to the patient. We have not involved the patient in making the decisions about care. To do this, we need to stay updated on the evidence and pay attention to individual patient differences. Many times, after care has been given, we find that the patient did not receive what he or she actually wanted! Sadly, often we do not realize this is the case.

How do we turn this situation around? For value-based reimbursement, the American Hospital Association advocates nurse and physician leadership at the point of care and making decisions with the patient about that care within the available finances. Administrators' roles need to change to support the point-of-care leaders.

Teamwork and interdisciplinary shared governance are necessities. Everyone—from the board/CEO/CNO/CFO to nurse aides/housekeepers—needs to be doing regular rounds listening to patients. This needs to replace some of the meetings, especially ones where administrators have no perception of what is going on at the bedside. Patients are more likely to get what they value when the whole thrust of the organization is toward finding out this information, and then providing it as much as possible. This creates messy communication, conflicts that lead to better solutions, and messy flat structures as well as better reimbursement.

In the value-based environment, we need to examine current practices. For instance, we burden RNs with a lot of paperwork and non-valued-added activities that take them away from the bedside for more than 50% of their time. We understaff units, which creates negative environments for everyone, yet we expect staff will do the care to achieve reimbursement. Evidence shows that missed care is occurring, which may cause side effects for the patient, such as pressure sores and infections requiring care that will not be reimbursed. Yet we do not pay attention to these issues. Instead, we allow these issues to continue and fester. We need to start valuing the staff nurse at the bedside, encouraging staff to lead and make changes as they do their work. In fact, 90% of the decisions about their work needs to be made by staff as they take care of patients each day.

An enormous challenge in the current healthcare climate is achieving quality care and safety while keeping expenses down. This is especially important now that reimbursement depends on appropriate, timely care and does not cover errors. The patient has always suffered from poor care, but now with value-based reimbursement, healthcare organizations are penalized as well with lower reimbursement.

The healthcare environment is complex and continues to increase in complexity. This causes increased bureaucracy, more errors, and more expense. Complexity and chaos are constantly changing the environment and affecting our work organizationally. We need to strive to involve all stakeholders, including those at the bedside—physicians, patients, and families—to simplify the environment. What we do today will be outdated tomorrow, so we need to continually stay tuned in to new evidence. This is interwoven with ethical and legal implications that cannot be ignored.

Finally, the financial aspects of health care cannot be ignored. To respond effectively in this complex healthcare environment and to work successfully with the financial arm of the healthcare entity, nurse managers must understand financial concepts, such as staffing, budgeting, identifying and analyzing variances, measuring productivity, costing, accounting, and forecasting, as well as the strategies that achieve a positive bottom line. Although finance and accounting terminology is used throughout the chapters, chapters focused specifically on accounting and assessing financial performance are included.

This text provides nurse leaders with an interconnected view of the nursing and financial sides of health care and suggests methods nurses can use to successfully integrate these viewpoints. This realistic integration of nursing and finance (along with all the other departments and professions) enhances nurse manager effectiveness.

A critical element for success is the ability of nurse managers to interface effectively with finance department personnel. An unusual feature of this book is that it contains both typical nursing administration terminology and financial accounting terminology. Suggestions are made for nurse leaders about how to communicate with and maximize the understanding of concepts and issues by financial personnel, who may come from different backgrounds and attach different meanings to the same terms.

The problem with the financial aspect of health care is that it is often viewed as a separate silo—a silo where nurses do not enter and where financial personnel reside. Meanwhile, nurses are in their own silo, and financial personnel are not found there. As coauthors of this book, we believe it is time to end this silo mentality. Our effectiveness in healthcare demands that *nursing and finance interface regularly* and conduct a healthy ongoing dialogue about every issue. We are most effective if we can face these issues *together*.

Nurses need to express themselves more effectively using financial principles and data; financial personnel need to more effectively understand the care side of health care. Because this book is written for the nurse administrator, we emphasize the first part. We hope this book will be helpful for finance personnel as well.

A problem that occurs when nurses and financial people try to talk together is that financial officers often think in a linear way. When they talk to each other, they talk about numbers, ratios, and stats. Nurses, however, tend to think in an abstract, interpersonal way. When nurses talk to each other, they talk about how someone feels, how someone will be affected by a certain treatment, or whether particular tasks have been accomplished.

The breakdown in communication occurs when nurses talk to financial people using abstract language, while financial people talk to nurses using linear language. The conversations run parallel to each other, with both sides not understanding what the other is talking about. Nurses complain that financial people never think about anything but the bottom line, while financial people complain that all nurses do is whine about quality. Thus, true dialogue and communication do not occur.

This book gives examples that nurses can use to better communicate with financial personnel, as well as with other linear-thinking administrators. In addition, we recommend that if a nurse administrator really wants to talk effectively with financial administrators, he or she should be able to *express/communicate the abstract information using linear language* (i.e., numbers that will be affected by something that has or has not occurred or that is being planned, including specific amounts of money needed to implement a project, and so forth).

Abstract thinking is effective in communication between nurses and physicians. However, it is often ineffective when communicating with the finance department. For example, concepts such as "care" might not have meaning to a finance officer. *Caring* is an abstract term. Exceptions occur when a financial person experiences a serious illness or when the financial officer previously worked as a healthcare professional.

At times, this communication problem can be compounded by simple differences in male and female communication techniques (remember *Men Are from Mars, Women Are from Venus* [Gray, 1992]), especially if the chief financial officer is male and the chief nursing officer is female. This is changing with less gender-specific roles in the workplace. In the past, a male chief nursing officer often had an edge because he could be "one of the boys." This is also slowly changing with more males in nursing and more females in finance.

Properly prepared nurse managers and nurse administrators can successfully provide an interface between finance and nursing, making decisions based on *both* clinical and financial perspectives. A nurse manager, as well as financial personnel, cannot make the mistake of ignoring the whole while dealing with the individual parts.

This interconnection goes beyond just nursing and finance. In this book, we strongly encourage every person and every department and profession to collaborate as they provide what the patient values. Because of this interconnection, there is a ripple effect. What one person or department does affect all the others. Nevertheless, some of us cling to the old silo mentality.

Another financial silo exists when the organization's mentality is that staff are not leaders and should not be involved with financial information. We are in the Information Age. Transparency is best. Because we are all interconnected, every task a staff member performs has financial implications. It is critical to *involve all staff and nurse managers with the finances,* such as the following: payment structures and how much is actually received; reimbursement that is lost when timely, appropriate care is not given; costs of technology and supplies; staffing costs; quality and safety costs; costs incurred with safety or quality issues; and legal costs. They should understand the impact their actions have on the bottom line.

Staff members need to be making 90% of the care decisions right at the bedside. We administrators only *serve* the staff and help them do their best work for the patients. We need to create positive environments because evidence shows that such environments generate the best outcomes—even regarding the bottom line. We need to empower staff, but more than that, we need to support them as being leaders in their work and also support patients being leaders in what care they choose to receive.

Solutions are always better when the people directly involved are involved in the process of devising the solutions. Therefore, we advocate that *staff and patients, as well as administrators, come to the table on issues and decide on the best way to accomplish the work through* **interdisciplinary** *shared governance.* This gets rid of another silo—the one where administrators make all the decisions and do not delegate to others—which is a leftover from the previous century.

We will have small successes we can celebrate, and we will have failures. Failures are natural, a fact of life. As they occur, we need to learn from each one and adapt and implement changes to simplify the environment. Many errors are actually caused by a series of events—because we are all interconnected. Dealing with failures goes beyond being blame-free. We must make incremental changes that will simplify processes that have become cumbersome.

We have written this book in interesting times. The U.S. economy has slowed down as many jobs were outsourced to other countries.

Weather events are getting more severe. Can you imagine experiencing no electricity—or worse yet, no home, and yet still taking care of patients? This has happened in a number of places right here in our country. We have pulled together in such times of crisis, and hopefully, we can pull together in fixing our healthcare system. It takes each of us. We are all interconnected.

Discussion Questions

1. How does understanding complexity break down silos?
2. What silos exist in your workplace? In your own thinking? How will you contribute to breaking down these silos?
3. What actions further the silo concept?
4. Give an example where a nurse administrator effectively expresses a need to the finance department using numbers and dollars.
5. State an administrative decision and explain its financial implications.
6. Describe a financial decision, giving the administrative implications of this decision.
7. Describe an administrative or financial decision and map out the ripple effect of this decision.

Reference

Gray, J. (1992). *Men are from Mars, women are from Venus.* New York, NY: HarperCollins.

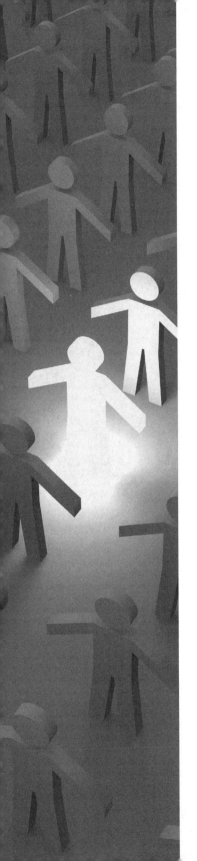

PART I

Health Care, the Economy and Value-Based Purchasing

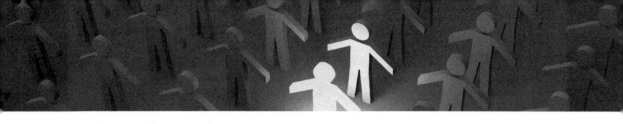

CHAPTER 1

How We Got to Where We Are!

J. Michael Leger, PhD, MBA, RN, **Janne Dunham-Taylor**, PhD, RN, and
Joellen Edwards, PhD, RN, FAAN

▶ How Did We Get into This Mess?

Presently, health care is a wonderful, complicated economic and quality quagmire with many issues requiring our attention. The term *health care* is a misnomer; in the United States, we most frequently address "illness care." We use the term *health care* in this book only because it is the common nomenclature for our illness system. Historically in this country, we have focused on the treatment of illness rather than studying and implementing what brings about good health.

We know that our present piecemeal, *tertiary approach* to illness care has many serious problems. (This is in contrast to an emphasis on *primary care*, as found in Australia, where the majority of healthcare dollars is spent on home visits and keeping individuals well.) Our dubious position as the only highly developed nation that still fails to provide basic health services to all its citizens creates unacceptable disparities in the health of our population, and persistently maintains a fragmented approach to provision of health care. Research on promoting and achieving health is happening, but much larger amounts of money are spent on such pursuits as treating cancer, heart problems, and strokes—the leading causes of death—*after* they occur rather than on learning *how we can achieve health and promote wellness*.

So, how did we get into this quagmire? Examining our path can give us a better understanding of the present situation and unresolved dilemmas and offers us some idea of what may come next.

Collectively, the rules and regulations that define who gets which healthcare services, who can deliver them, and how those services are paid for are the core of the health policies that continuously affect every citizen's well-being. The World Health Organization (WHO) defines health policy as

> "...decisions, plans, and actions that are undertaken to achieve specific health care goals within a society. An explicit

health policy can achieve several things: it defines a vision for the future which in turn helps to establish targets and points of reference for the short and medium term. It outlines priorities and the expected roles of different groups; and it builds consensus and informs people."

These decisions include those of the executive, legislative, and judicial branches of government. Over time, a number of partially successful attempts to repair the healthcare system in our country have occurred through the development of policies at all levels of government. However, they often address specific, isolated problems rather than creating a well-coordinated system that makes health care accessible and affordable to everyone.

Healthcare policies in the United States attempt to address three specific aspects related to public health concerns: (1) *access* to healthcare services, (2) *cost and cost control* of healthcare services, and (3) *quality of care* available to the population. The remainder of this chapter examines the development of healthcare policies that address these three concerns.

▶ Foundations of Health Care: The Early Days of Our Country

Early in this country's history, care was provided by women in the family who tended to the health needs of relatives in the home. There was no formal education or training for these women. Instead, they relied on their personal knowledge and experience. If they received any education or training at all, it was from other family members or neighbors who were "healers," or if they could read, they learned about it from books.

Physicians, if available, were consulted in more complicated or extreme medical situations, and home visits were the norm. Formal medical education was not accessible until the

1800s. A person could become a physician by apprenticing with another practitioner, and little scientific basis for the profession existed. There was no mechanism for testing competence, and licensure was not a requirement to practice.

Health care was a private matter, paid for by patients or their families with cash or barter. There was no regulatory interference or supportive services from federal, state, or local governments to protect and improve people's health. As our nation matured, governmental regulation of many aspects of health-related issues occurred. Over time, our governments became more and more involved in ensuring public well-being through the following:

- Regulations about the direct provision of health care through agencies and hospitals
- The promotion of sanitation and the prevention of epidemics through formal public health departments
- Health professions education and licensing, especially for physicians and nurses

Eventually, as presented in the following sections, governments became involved not only in the regulation of, but the actual payments for, healthcare services.

The development of the public health system serves as a good example of the gradually increasing governmental regulation of health-related issues. The origins of the Public Health Service date back to 1798 when Congress passed An Act for the Relief of Sick and Disabled Seamen. Public health activities first began in larger cities in the early 1800s with the dramatic increase in immigration into the United States. The main focus was sanitation and prevention of epidemics of smallpox, typhoid fever, tuberculosis, and diphtheria, among other highly contagious diseases. Regulations were concerned with waste removal, swamp drainage, and street drainage. If epidemics occurred, homes or ships would be quarantined. As immunizations were developed, public health officials got involved with administering them. The first state board of health was formed in 1869 in Massachusetts. By 1900, each state had a board of health that worked on the preceding issues with local boards of health. Today, myriad public laws and regulations affect people's health, and departments of health at the national, state, and local levels assess health needs, monitor compliance with health regulations, and implement programs to improve the public's health.

▶ Policies Addressing Access to Care

Access, or the *availability of care*, is a huge issue in the U.S. healthcare system. And, while legislation has been enacted to improve access of care, the problem is one that is growing rather than shrinking. The Institute of Medicine (IOM) (1993) defined access as the timely use of personal health services to achieve the best health outcomes. Access is not just about the ability to pay, however. Access also includes effective and efficient delivery of healthcare services, meaning that the services need to be culturally appropriate and geographically available, as well as delivered at a cost the user can afford.

Our system is unique in the developed world in that we do *not* systematically provide access to basic healthcare services for the entire population (*primary care*). One key factor in gaining access to services in this country is the ability to pay for them. The greatest contributing factor for access to healthcare services and getting recommended care is the availability of health insurance.

As of 2012, Medicare and Medicaid, federal and state policies that provide health programs, pay for various kinds of care for 32.2% of our citizens. The Indian Health Service offers basic health care to Native Americans living on reservations. Private insurance, most commonly obtained through employers with costs shared between employers and employees, covers 55.1% of the U.S. population, although many find themselves "underinsured" when it is time to pay the healthcare bills. Those individuals who have no healthcare coverage at all are left to pay healthcare bills directly, from their own pockets, or to seek care through safety net providers such as free clinics, rural health clinics (RHC), or federally qualified health centers (DeNavas-Walt, Proctor, & Smith, 2012). However, since the implementation of the Affordable Care Act, known as ACA and "Obamacare," the rate of uninsured citizens has dropped from 15.7%, or 48.6 million individuals in 2010, to 10%, or 32.9 million individuals in 2014.

Access to Direct Services: Hospitals and Beyond

Access to care beyond that available in the home was addressed by:

- Creating hospitals, nursing homes, and in-home care programs by trained nurses. Hospitals and nursing homes existed in the early 1800s, but in those days they existed on voluntary charitable contributions and served the indigent.
- Quarantine hospitals, opened and closed sporadically by public health officials to deal with epidemic diseases such as smallpox, yellow fever, or, later, tuberculosis.
- Access to health care for the wealthy who could pay for the services (i.e., hiding a family member with a psychiatric illness in an insane asylum).

By the mid-1800s, hospitals, for better or worse, became accepted as tertiary treatment centers for all types of diseases. Instruments such as the stethoscope, thermometer, sphygmomanometer, and microscope were introduced; air was viewed as a disinfectant, so good ventilation became important; antiseptic and sterile procedures were gradually introduced; better ways had been discovered to manage pain in surgery; and, later, the x-ray was invented.

In the early 1900s, visiting nurse agencies were started, especially in larger cities, to make health care more accessible for primarily poor residents. If able, clients paid a small fee for services provided. These services were financed, in part, through raised funds to support their work with the poor. Public health departments broadened to include maternal and child services and, in the slums of large cities, to detect tuberculosis (which had become the leading cause of death) and to control then-named venereal disease. In 1935, federal monies were made available to strengthen the work performed by local and state public health departments.

The Social Security Act

A major societal shift occurred in 1935 with the passage of the Social Security Act, which dramatically affected health care in the midst of the Depression. Until this event, local and state governments, individuals, and families had been responsible for providing healthcare services for the poor. In a landmark legislative effort, the Social Security Act shifted that responsibility to the federal government. Although not specifically intended to provide healthcare services, the Social Security Act provided funds for health-related programs for the poor in areas such as public health, maternal and child health, crippled children's programs, and benefits for elderly adults and disabled individuals.

The Social Security Act also dramatically affected the nursing home industry. This Act specified that money be given to private nursing homes but excluded public institutions (this latter exception was later repealed). Thus, for-profit and proprietary nursing homes (those privately owned) proliferated to serve the welfare patient. These homes gave first priority to paying patients because the government reimbursement was substantially lower than fees for services. (Sound familiar?)

Healthcare Access Changes Post–World War II

Our healthcare system, as we know it today, emerged after World War II. Through funding from the 1946 Hill-Burton Act, government money was made available to build hospitals, as more medicines, anesthesia agents, and technologies became available. National legislation emphasized *secondary/tertiary care*—highly technical hospital-based care, rather than *primary care*—defined as preventive, restorative, or medical treatment given while the patient lives at home. Hill-Burton funds focused especially on building hospitals in rural areas, creating geographical access to services that had not previously been available. Hill-Burton also required state-level planning for healthcare services.

Psychiatric treatment also changed dramatically. With the advent of psychotropic medications, more psychiatric patients could be treated in outpatient settings. In 1963, the federal government established community mental health centers for this purpose. Thus, many psychiatric patients who had been hospitalized for years were able to leave the hospitals and function in the community setting. Unfortunately, those who were more severely mentally ill suffered greatly because less money was available for their care.

Medicare and Medicaid: New Forms of Access

Until 1965, the federal government financed little in the way of direct healthcare services, concentrating only on public health issues and providing services for military personnel and Native Americans. Less than half of elderly adults and disabled Americans had health insurance. State and local governments established and supported special facilities for mental illness, mental retardation, and communicable diseases such as tuberculosis.

Then, in a wave of entitlement programming, the federal government became enmeshed in health care by establishing Medicare and Medicaid. Naturally, this Social Security Act Amendment (Titles XVIII and XIX) benefited elderly adults and poor persons and gave them more access to health care, but providers—hospitals, other healthcare organizations, physicians, and even suppliers and the building industry—benefited as well. Medicare often became *the largest source* of revenue for healthcare providers, resulting in the building of more hospitals and the expansion of long-term care programs. As more personnel were needed for the expansions and new buildings, additional federal programs were funded to supply more physicians, nurses, and allied health professionals.

Although Medicaid was (and is) particularly fraught with tension between federal regulators and states where the plan is administered, both Medicare and Medicaid opened previously unavailable access to elderly, disabled, and poor individuals. Both Medicare and Medicaid pay for hospital and long-term care, primary care, and some preventive services.

Medicare induced significant changes in long-term care. The federal government redefined who was eligible to care for Medicare patients by establishing care standards and requirements for skilled nursing facilities (SNF) and intermediate care facilities (ICF) that raised the level of care available to the public.

Medicare and Medicaid also infused the home health industry with money to expand agencies and services. Whereas there were approximately 250 home health agencies in 1960, by 1968 there were 1,328 official agencies providing home health services. Federal funding over the next 20 years gradually refocused home health on postacute services. Unfortunately, money became less available for the chronically ill client who needed longer-term services. Services also changed in the home health industry as home health funding began to include rehabilitative services—physical therapy, occupational therapy, speech therapy, and social work services. This continues today.

In 1965, the Older Americans Act mandated and funded Area Agencies on Aging (AAA). These agencies fund a wide array of services for elderly adults including:

- Senior centers with nutrition and recreation programs
- Health promotion and screening programs
- Mental health evaluation and treatment
- Respite care
- Case managers to plan care for elders so that they can stay in their homes rather than be institutionalized
- Services to the homebound, such as meals, homemaker services, chore services, and transportation

In 1980, the Omnibus Budget Reconciliation Act aided home care by expanding Medicare benefits to 100 visits per year and lifting a 3-day hospitalization requirement. For the first time, for-profit home care agencies could become Medicare-certified providers. In addition, advanced technology, such as ventilators, renal hemodialysis, and infusion therapy—originally found only in hospitals—all moved into the home, expanding the need for a home care nurse. This need was coupled with prospective payment for hospitals and resulted in earlier discharges and greater use of home care. The number of home care agencies increased exponentially. Battles ensued in response to the escalating cost of home care, and in 1984, visits were restricted to the homebound client. Later, after a 1989 court ruling (*Duggen v. Bowen*), eligibility requirements were eased once again.

Because Medicare standards required hospitals to renovate and rebuild in the 1970s, for-profit hospitals, like many other businesses, began to offer publicly traded stocks. Stockholders expected these hospitals to make a profit so stocks would increase in value and provide good dividends. In this arrangement, hospitals had to pay attention to stockholder interests. The profit-making motive applied to not-for-profit hospitals as well. They had to make profits too—using the money for pay increases, new equipment or building projects, and investments—but called it *excess of revenue over expenses* rather than profit. Investor-owned nursing homes and home care facilities also increased, creating access for those with private or public insurance.

The Medicare Pharmacy and Modernization Act of 2003 provides Medicare participants with access to coverage for prescription drugs. Coverage, which started in 2006, is provided through private standalone prescription drug plans or Medicare Advantage prescription drug plans administered by approved insurance companies. Prior to this act, Medicare beneficiaries had no prescription drug coverage.

Since that time, beneficiaries have seen their premiums and copays rise and have experienced closer monitoring of their utilization management. Although Medicare drug legislation has certainly provided relief for the costs of drugs, especially for lower-income beneficiaries, all beneficiaries experience a gap in coverage, often called the "doughnut hole." When Medicare recipients reach a level of spending on prescriptions (adjusted yearly), coverage stops completely and resumes when the individual spends a ceiling amount (also adjusted yearly). This means that beneficiaries with a limited income or no *gap insurance* may have limited access to needed drugs for a substantial portion of the year, with higher-spending (sicker) beneficiaries reaching their spending cap earlier (Stuart, Simoni-Wastila, & Chauncey, 2005).

This spending gap resulted in serious health consequences for Medicare beneficiaries, along with costs of more than $100 million a year in preventable hospitalizations (Morrison et al., 2012). The Affordable Care and Patient Protection Act (ACA), signed into law in March 2010, includes provisions to address the coverage gap and maintain quality outcomes for chronic illness. The U.S. Department of Health and Human Services (DHHS) reports that, as of 2012, seniors had already saved more than $4 billion in prescription drug costs as a result of the coverage assistance provided by the ACA (U.S. DHHS, 2012).

Safety Net Providers

Safety net healthcare services have gradually emerged in an effort to fill the care gaps in our system. These include services for underserved and uninsured rural and inner-city populations, non-English-speaking immigrants, homeless persons, and migrant workers. Two examples of legislated support for the poor and uninsured can be found in the clinics and services targeted toward these populations.

The Community Health Center (CHC) Act, passed in 1965, provided funds for comprehensive health and supportive social services to be provided through clinics established to make primary care available to specific types of populations in the clinic's service area. CHC are funded through federal grants available through the U.S. DHHS and operate under specific rules and conditions. They are required to provide services to anyone who needs access, regardless of the person's ability to pay.

The Rural Health Clinic (RHC) Act, passed in 1971, established higher rates of Medicare and Medicaid payments to rural primary care practices, provided that they employ a nurse practitioner (NP) or physician assistant and meet the qualifications for federal approval as a RHC. RHCs can be free-standing clinics or can be associated with a rural hospital or nursing home. Although there are no specific requirements to provide care to the uninsured, most RHCs do strengthen the rural safety net beyond just Medicare and Medicaid patients.

As the movement toward advanced nursing practice gained momentum, schools and colleges of nursing established primary care and nursing practice centers and community health services, collectively known as *nurse-managed care*. Community nursing centers (CNCs), community nursing organizations (CNOs), and nursing health maintenance organizations (HMOs) have been sponsored by local communities, community groups, and churches, and also by university schools and colleges of nursing that provide the majority of these access points. Most nursing centers provide care to poor and underserved population groups (Harris, 2009). Many of these centers are also partially supported on the federal level by the Division of Nursing located within the DHHS, Health Resources and Services Administration, Bureau of Health Professions. Nursing centers are specifically targeted for funding in the ACA and should see the benefit of this funding in coming years.

▶ Policies Addressing Cost

Cost, and controlling the cost of providing care, is one of the most perplexing issues facing the U.S. healthcare system today. The *cost* of health care can be defined as *the value of all the resources used to produce the services and expenditures* and refers to the amount spent on a particular item or service (Andersen & Davidson, 2007). Both cost and controlling cost are important concepts, but expenditures are more easily measured and tracked and thus are more commonly used to analyze financial aspects of the healthcare system.

Consumers and third-party payers have seen consistently higher rises in healthcare costs and expenditures than in other segments of the economy, with rates of increase slowing slightly for the past few years but continuing to rise (Rice & Kominski, 2007; Rice, 2007). Given that U.S. healthcare spending grew 5.3% in 2014, reaching $9,523 per person, insurance companies, employers, federal and state governments, and users of direct healthcare services are all vitally interested in payment systems and cost control.

Blue Cross/Blue Shield: Setting Trends in Paying for Care

The emergence of health insurance was a significant change in healthcare financing, moving payment for health care from personal business transactions to a third-party mediator. Initially, insurance coverage was created either to provide health care for people involved in rail or steamboat accidents or for mutual aid where small amounts of disability cash benefited members experiencing an accident or illness, including typhus, typhoid, scarlet fever, smallpox, diphtheria, and diabetes.

Then, in 1929, Justin Ford Kimball established a hospital insurance plan at Baylor University in Dallas, Texas. He had been a superintendent of schools and noticed that teachers often had unpaid bills at the hospital. By examining hospital records, he calculated that "the schoolteachers as a group 'incurred an average of 15 cents a month in hospital bills. To assure a safe margin, he established a rate of 50 cents a month.' In return, the school teachers were assured of 21 days of hospitalization in a semiprivate room" (Raffel & Raffel, 1994, p. 211). This was the beginning of the Blue Cross plans that developed across the country. Blue Cross offered *service benefits* rather than a *lump-sum payment*—also called *indemnity*, the type of benefits offered by previous insurance plans.

Following the success of Blue Cross, in 1939 the California Medical Association started the California Physicians Service to pay physician services. This became known as Blue Shield. In this plan, doctors were obligated to provide treatment at the fee established by Blue Shield, even though the doctor might charge more to patients not covered by Blue Shield. Blue Shield was, in effect, for people who earned less than $3,000 a year. In one of many unsuccessful attempts at national healthcare reform, physicians designed and agreed to this plan to *prevent the establishment of a national health insurance plan.*

While Blue Cross was quite successful, Blue Shield was not. As inflation occurred and patients made more money, the base rate was not changed, so fewer people were eligible for the Blue Shield rates. "Blue Shield made the same dollar payment for services rendered, but because the patient was above the service-benefit income level, the patient frequently had to pay an additional amount to the physician" (Raffel & Raffel, 1994, p. 213).

After World War II, private insurance companies proliferated and offered health insurance policies both to individuals and to employers. Large employers were expected to offer employees healthcare benefits due in large part to unionization. Health insurance became an *entitlement.* Soon private insurance companies (third-party payers) enrolled more than half the U.S. population. The McCarren-Ferguson Act of 1945 "gave states the exclusive right to regulate health insurance plans. . . . As a result the federal government has no agency that is solely responsible for monitoring insurance" (Finkelman, 2001, p. 188).

The Federal Role in Cost Containment

To administer the complex Medicare and Medicaid programs that had been established, the federal government initiated the HCFA, now called the Centers for Medicare and Medicaid Services (CMS), within the DHHS. Payment for Medicare and Medicaid services was based on the *retrospective* cost of the care—figured and billed to the government by healthcare organizations and by physicians seeing patients. This fee-for-service system did not limit what providers could charge for their services, and initially there was no systematic approach to fees: Providers charged what the market would bear. In the 1970s, faced with escalating healthcare expenditures, states began controlling the amount they would pay to a provider for a particular service. The rationale for setting rates that would be paid was to encourage providers to voluntarily control the costs of the care they delivered.

The federal government, along with states, was spending a tremendous amount of money on health care. In fact, the gross domestic product (GDP) for health care has grown from 6%, when Medicare and Medicaid were introduced, to 17.8% as of December 2016. To find money to support these programs, the government was faced with increasing taxes, shifting money from other services such as defense or education, or curbing hospital and physician costs. Curbing costs was the first choice for policymakers.

Hospital Prospective Payment: A New World for Hospitals and Providers

The next direct step by the federal government to control healthcare costs, particularly those generated in hospital settings, was the implementation of a *prospective* pricing system for Medicare patients. As previously noted, prior to this hospitals and providers simply billed Medicare for their services and were paid in full. In 1983, the Health Care Financing Administration (HCFA) implemented a plan to pay a set price to each hospital for each diagnosis regardless of how much the facility actually spent to provide the care. This payment strategy was called *diagnosis-related groups (DRGs).* If hospital staff could provide care for a patient with a hip fracture, for example, at less than the DRG payment, they could keep the money and, in a sense, make a profit. If the cost of care for the patient went above the DRG payment, the hospital lost money. DRGs required hospitals to become more efficient and aware of costs. Yet, the requirements of the DRG policy induced providers to release patients from the hospital as quickly as they could and to shift costs to other third-party payers who did not engage in prospective payment (e.g., home health agencies, SNF), leaving doubt as to the "bottom line" in cost savings to the healthcare system overall.

Prospective payment was expanded in 1989 to include physician services outside the hospital with the introduction of the *resource-based relative value system* (*RBRVS*). This policy, through Medicare Part B legislation, applied the same concept as hospital DRGs to the outpatient setting. Two goals of RBRVS were to control costs and to put more emphasis on primary care and prevention.

Health Maintenance Organizations

In another attempt to hold down healthcare costs, the Health Maintenance Organization Act of 1973 provided federal grants to develop *HMOs*. This act required employers with more than 25 employees to offer an HMO health insurance option to employees. HMOs had a good track record of bringing down healthcare costs because they had traditionally been serving younger, healthier populations. Thus, starting more HMOs sounded like a way to cut healthcare costs. This act provided a specific definition of what an HMO was and gave the states oversight (or licensing) responsibility.

The concept of *managed care*, as delivered by HMOs, has taken hold in the public sector as well. Both Medicare and Medicaid (in many states) have taken their own steps to promote managed care by contracting with private insurers or HMOs to take on the primary care of groups of people enrolled for healthcare coverage and to serve as gatekeepers to specialty services. These measures were intended to control healthcare costs for federal and state governments and to improve the quality of care. In actual practice, results have been mixed as the costs of health care continue to climb.

The Health Insurance Portability and Accountability Act of 1996

The *Health Insurance Portability and Accountability Act* (*HIPAA*) addresses several significant issues including access, quality, and cost. Major portions of HIPAA address the financing of health care. This act "establishes that insurers cannot set limits on coverage for preexisting conditions, . . . guarantees access and renewability [of health insurance], . . . [and] addresses issues of excluding small employers from insurance contracts on the basis of employee health status. In addition the law provided for greater tax deductibility of health insurance for the self-employed" (Finkelman, 2001, p. 192).

HIPAA started the *medical savings accounts,* a tax-free account provided by employers. Here the employee can annually set up an account and pay in the amount of money the employee expects to have to pay for health coverage for the year. The money paid into the account takes place before taxes are taken out by the employer. At the end of the year, if the money is not spent, it goes back to the employer.

The Balanced Budget Act of 1997

The *Balanced Budget Act* (*BBA*) significantly lowered payments for psychiatric care, rehabilitation services, and long-term care. Because ambulatory services, SNFs, and home care services were rapidly expanding and costing more healthcare dollars, the idea was to curb spending by placing these services under prospective payment. *Prospective payment* means that the payer (led by Medicare and Medicaid) determines the cost of care before the care is given:

- The provider is told how much will be paid for the given care.
- An *ambulatory payment classification system* was created, establishing a fixed dollar amount for outpatient services diagnoses.

- SNF experienced prospective payment through the *resource utilization group (RUG)* system.
- Home care was regulated by the *Outcome and Assessment Information Set (OASIS)* system.

BBA mandated payment reductions limiting DRG and RBRVS payment rates (as described previously), as well as reduced capital expenditures, graduate medical education, established open enrollment periods and medical savings accounts for Medicare recipients. Benefits for children's health care were increased through the creation of the Children's Health Insurance Program, more commonly known as CHIP, that "expands block grants to states increasing Medicaid eligibility for low-income and un-insured children, establishing a new program that subsidizes private insurance for children or combining Medicaid with private insurance" (Finkelman, 2001, p. 398). BBA also created new penalties for fraud.

BBA had a major impact on health care, causing a number of hospitals, long-term care facilities, and home care companies to fold. Profit margins were drastically reduced, and rural hospitals were disproportionately affected. This act encouraged *outsourcing*, the act of ob-taining services (contract labor) from outside of the organization, a practice that continues today (Roberts, 2001). BBA had such profound cost-cutting effects that in December 2000, Congress passed relief legislation providing additional money for hospitals and managed care plans.

Another positive aspect of the BBA was a major impact on recognition of the nursing profession. Under BBA, NPs and clinical nurse specialists (CNSs) practicing in any setting could be directly reimbursed for services provided to Medicare patients at 85% of physician fees. This occurred to both better serve populations not receiving medical care and to save costs because studies had determined that NPs could deliver as much as 80% of the medical care at less cost than primary care physicians could

with comparable, and sometimes better, clinical outcomes. This federal legislation overrode state legislation that, in some cases, required NPs to work under direct physician supervision, with reimbursement made only to physicians. This act was reauthorized in 2009, after a long battle in Congress.

▶ Policies Addressing Quality

Quality in health care can be defined as "the degree to which health services for individuals and populations increase the likelihood of desired health outcomes" (Andersen, Rice, Kominski, & Afifi, 2007, p. 185). Quality of care, measured in patient or population outcomes, is now con-sidered to be the result of the entire system of care. In many cases, aggregate results of care are public information and are readily available on the Internet (see, for instance, www.medicare .gov/hospitalcompare).

Throughout the development of our health-care system, the quality of care has been assumed to be the business of individual providers, such as physicians and nurses, and specific delivery institutions, such as hospitals, long-term care facilities, and home health agencies. The blame for errors and the praise for cures were held to be between the provider or agency and patient. Outcomes of care were not collected or measured by any external, governmental organization. This is not the case today, however.

The quality care movement began in the 1980s but took a strong hold in the 1990s. In 1999, the Institute of Medicine released a shocking report, *To Err Is Human: Building a Safer Health System* (Kohn, Corrigan, & Donaldson, 2000; Richardson & Briere, 2001). This report identified multiple systematic failures in the process of de-livering care. It was followed in 2001 by a second hard-hitting report, *Crossing the Quality Chasm: A New Health System for the 21st Century*, that provided specific recommendations for improve-ment of quality and safety. These two documents confirmed what quality experts had been saying: *Despite the enormous cost of health care in the United States, tens of thousands of patients are injured or die as a result of errors in the course of receiving care.* Yet, despite the research and the number of patient safety initiatives intended to reduce the number of preventable deaths due to medical errors, researchers have suggested that as many as 400,000 patients die from medical errors each year while patients in our hospitals (Leger & Phillips, 2016).

In the case of quality, a mix of public policy-makers and private foundations and organizations is concerned with promoting and monitoring quality across the healthcare system. The quality movement goes much further than specific clinical outcomes, although these are critically important. Outcomes of personal, emotional, or social importance to patients are also developing, such as *patient satisfaction* or *quality of life* indices. Policy decisions at the federal level have shaped current efforts to ensure that the highest quality of care possible is provided in our healthcare system. Through ACA, these outcome measures are also used as key metrics in determining hospital reimbursement rates by CMS:

- Hospital Readmissions Reduction Program
- Hospital Value-Based Purchasing (VBP) Program
- Hospital-Acquired Condition (HAC) Reduction Program

Governmental Agencies Concerned with Quality

The DHHS is the overarching federal administrative agency concerned with monitoring the quality of health care in the United States. Several components of the DHHS infrastructure assume national leadership and focus on quality issues. For instance, the Agency for Healthcare Research and Quality (AHRQ) engages in testing and reporting safety improvement strategies and makes available significant research awards to determine the best evidence for safe and effective practice guidelines. Another activity of the AHRQ is reporting disparities in health services based on race, ethnicity, and socioeconomic status. AHRQ also houses the National Clearinghouse for Quality Measures, where standards and processes for measuring healthcare outcomes can be found. The AHRQ website (www.ahrq.gov/qual/measurix.htm) offers a wealth of information on measures used to assess quality in health care. AHRQ issues two reports annually to describe the quality of health care in the United States, the *National Healthcare Quality Report* and the *National Healthcare Disparities Report*, both available at the AHRQ website. AHRQ now focuses extensively on comparative effectiveness research to determine the effectiveness, benefits, and harms of different procedures, medications, and treatments in improving health outcomes. Existing and new data are examined to recommend best practices based on scientific evidence (AHRQ, 2013). Comparative effectiveness research will be increasingly important as issues of access, cost, and quality are debated.

The Centers for Disease Control and Prevention (CDC) is also concerned with safety and quality. One focus of the CDC is the promotion of health information technology systems to reduce human error. Another is the collection of disease surveillance data that track both chronic and acute infectious diseases in the private sector and in health departments. Much of the quality data is housed at the Division of Healthcare Quality Promotion, whose mission is to protect patients and healthcare personnel and to promote safety, quality, and value in the healthcare delivery system. This division has three branches that are directly linked to quality: the Epidemiology and Laboratory Branch, the Prevention and Evaluation Branch, and the Healthcare Outcomes Branch. The CDC website provides substantial information (www.cdc.gov).

The U.S. Food and Drug Administration (FDA) promotes quality and safety outcomes through improving regulations for packaging and labeling of drugs and by maintaining strict reporting requirements. In addition, the FDA is responsible for the regulation of biologics, cosmetics, medical devices, radiation-emitting electronic products, and veterinary products.

CMS plays a significant role in transforming healthcare delivery and financing from volume-based to value-based payments (American Hospital Association, 2011). CMS collects, monitors, and reports patient and process outcomes of the healthcare system. These performance measures are used by insurers to determine reimbursement. Hospitals technically volunteer to report critical quality outcomes. Financial incentives are offered through the Medicare program to hospitals that report their outcomes on quality measures on a public website (www.cms.gov). A financial disincentive is levied against eligible hospitals that choose not to participate and contribute data. CMS publishes hospital outcomes, as well as outcomes from nursing homes, on its website Hospital Compare (www.medicare.gov/hospitalcompare). Other agencies and organizations publish data on health plan outcomes, medical group outcomes, and selected outcomes by individual physicians.

CMS introduced what is commonly termed "pay for performance" strategies. For the fiscal year (FY) 2016 HAC Reduction Program, hospitals are expected to prevent the development of eight iatrogenic conditions, including:

- Pressure ulcer
- Iatrogenic pneumothorax
- Central venous catheter-related bloodstream infections
- Postoperative hip fracture (falls with injury)
- Perioperative pulmonary embolism or Deep vein thrombosis
- Postoperative sepsis
- Postoperative wound dehiscence
- Accidental puncture or laceration

These conditions are commonly called "never events," meaning they should never occur under any circumstances. Medicare no longer pays for extended hospital stays or treatment for preventable complications if they occur during the patient's hospital course. Several of these conditions (pressure ulcers, falls with injury, and vascular catheter infections) are presumed to be directly attributable to nursing care (Buerhaus, Donlan, DesRoches, & Hess, 2009). Therefore, nurses—especially nurse leaders—are in a key position to lead improvement in this quality endeavor.

▶ The Affordable Care and Patient Protection Act

The ACA, enacted on March 23, 2010, is the most sweeping healthcare legislation since the inception of Medicare and Medicaid in 1965. Numerous attempts have been made to reform U.S. health care, but the ACA is the first to attempt to accomplish this overarching objective. It was passed after a hard-fought battle that extended from the 2008 presidential campaign into President Barack Obama's first months in office. The political battle to repeal and replace ACA is ongoing as evidenced by the recent failure of the proposed American Health Care Act (https://www.congress.gov/bill/115th-congress/house-bill/1628) in March 2017.

The overall goals of the ACA are to strengthen and systematize U.S. health care and to provide near-universal coverage for American citizens and legal immigrants. The legislation is complex and multifaceted—a true attempt at system reform. The ACA seeks to strengthen patient rights and protections, make coverage more affordable and widespread, ensure access to care, and create a stronger Medicare system to care for the growing number of elderly adults in our country. **TABLE 1.1** provides a broad overview of the ACA; a useful, detailed summary of the ACA and its many components can be found at the Kaiser Family Foundation Health Reform website (http://kff.org/health-reform).

TABLE 1.1 Patient Protection and Affordable Care Act (P.L. 111–148)

Overall approach to expanding access to coverage	■ Requires most U.S. citizens and legal residents to have health insurance. Creates state-based American Health Benefit Exchanges through which individuals can purchase coverage, with premium and cost-sharing credits available to individuals/families with income between 133% and 400% of the federal poverty level (the poverty level is $19,530 for a family of three in 2013), and creates separate exchanges through which small businesses can purchase coverage. Requires employers to pay penalties for employees who receive tax credits for health insurance through an exchange, with exceptions for small employers. Imposes new regulations on health plans in the exchanges and in the individual and small group markets. Expands Medicaid to 133% of the federal poverty level.

Individual Mandate

Requirement to have coverage	■ Requires U.S. citizens and legal residents to have qualifying health coverage. Those without coverage pay a tax penalty that will be phased-in according to the following schedule: $95 in 2014, $325 in 2015, and $695 in 2016 for the flat fee or 1.0% of taxable income in 2014, 2.0% of taxable income in 2015, and 2.5% of taxable income in 2016. Beginning after 2016, the penalty will be increased annually by the cost-of-living adjustment. Exemptions will be granted for financial hardship, religious objections, American Indians, those without coverage for less than three months, undocumented immigrants, incarcerated individuals, those for whom the lowest cost plan option exceeds 8% of an individual's income, and those with incomes below the tax filing threshold (in 2009, the threshold for taxpayers under age 65 was $9,350 for singles and $18,700 for couples).

Employer Requirements

Requirement to offer coverage	■ Assess employers with 50 or more full-time employees that do not offer coverage and have at least one full-time employee who receives a premium tax credit fee of $2,000 per full-time employee, excluding the first 30 employees from the assessment. Employers with 50 or more full-time employees that offer coverage, but have at least one full-time employee receiving a premium tax credit, will pay the lesser of $3,000 for each employee receiving a premium credit, or $2,000 for each full-time employee, excluding the first 30 employees from the assessment. (Effective January 1, 2014.) Employers with up to 50 full-time employees are exempt from any of the above penalties.
Other requirements	■ Requires employers with more than 200 employees to automatically enroll employees into health insurance plans offered by the employer. Employees may opt out of coverage.

(continues)

TABLE 1.1 Patient Protection and Affordable Care Act (P.L. 111-148)   *(continued)*

Expansion of Public Programs

Treatment of Medicaid	■ Expands Medicaid to all non-Medicare-eligible individuals under age 65 (children, pregnant women, parents, and adults without dependent children) with incomes up to 133% FPL, based on their modified adjusted gross income (under current law, undocumented immigrants are not eligible for Medicaid).
Treatment of CHIP	■ Requires states to maintain current income eligibility levels for children in Medicaid and the Children's Health Insurance Program (CHIP) until 2019 and extends funding for CHIP through 2015.

Health Insurance Exchanges

Creation and structure of health insurance exchanges	■ Creates state-based American Health Benefit Exchanges and Small Business Health Options Program (SHOP) Exchanges, administered by a governmental agency or non-profit organization, through which individuals and small businesses with up to 100 employees can purchase qualified coverage.
Eligibility to purchase in the exchanges	■ Restricts access to coverage through the exchanges to U.S. citizens and legal immigrants who are not incarcerated.
Qualifications of participating health plans	■ Requires qualified health plans to report information on claims payment policies, enrollment, disenrollment, number of claims denied, cost-sharing requirements, out-of-network policies, and enrollee rights in plain language.
Basic health plan	■ Permits states the option to create a Basic Health Plan for uninsured individuals with incomes between 133–200% FPL who would otherwise be eligible to receive premium subsidies in the exchange. Individuals with incomes between 133–200% FPL in states creating Basic Health Plans are not eligible for subsidies in the exchanges.
Abortion coverage	■ Permits states to prohibit plans participating in the exchanges from providing coverage for abortions. ■ Prohibits plans participating in the exchanges from discriminating against any provider because of an unwillingness to provide, pay for, provide coverage of, or refer for abortions.

Changes to Private Insurance

Temporary high-risk pool	■ Establishes a temporary national high-risk pool to provide health coverage to individuals with preexisting medical conditions. U.S. citizens and legal immigrants who have a preexisting medical condition and who have been uninsured for at least 6 months will be eligible to enroll in the high-risk pool and receive subsidized premiums.
Medical loss ratio and premium rate reviews	■ Requires health plans to report the proportion of premium dollars spent on clinical services, quality, and other costs, and provide rebates to consumers for the amount of the premium spent on clinical services and quality that is less than 85% for plans in the large group market and 80% for plans in the individual and small group markets. (Requirement to report medical loss ratio effective plan year 2010; requirement to provide rebates effective January 1, 2011.) ■ Establish a process for reviewing increases in health plan premiums and require plans to justify increases. Require states to report on trends in premium increases and recommend whether certain plans should be excluded from the exchanges based on unjustified premium increases. Provides grants to states to support efforts to review and approve premium increases. (Effective beginning plan year 2010.)
Dependent coverage	■ Provides dependent coverage for children up to age 26 for all individual and group policies. (Effective six months following enactment.)
Consumer protections	■ Develops standards for insurers to use in providing information on benefits and coverage. (Standards developed within 12 months following enactment; insurer must comply with standards within 24 months following enactment.)

State Role

State role	■ Enrolls newly eligible Medicaid beneficiaries into the Medicaid program no later than January 2014 (states have the option to expand enrollment beginning in 2011), coordinates enrollment with the new exchanges, and implements other specified changes to the Medicaid program. Maintains current Medicaid and CHIP eligibility levels for children until 2019 and maintains current Medicaid eligibility levels for adults until the exchange is fully operational. Permits states to create a Basic Health Plan for uninsured individuals with incomes between 133% and 200% FPL in lieu of these individuals receiving premium subsidies to purchase coverage in the exchanges. (Effective January 1, 2014.)

(continues)

TABLE 1.1 Patient Protection and Affordable Care Act (P.L. 111-148) *(continued)*

Cost Containment	
Medicare	■ Restructures payments to Medicare Advantage (MA) plans by setting payments to different percentages of Medicare fee-for-service (FFS) rates, with higher payments for areas with low FFS rates and lower payments (95% of FFS) for areas with high FFS rates. Phases-in revised payments over 3 years beginning in 2011, for plans in most areas, with payments phased-in over longer periods (4 years and 6 years) for plans in other areas. Provides bonuses to plans receiving 4 or more stars, based on the current 5-star quality rating system for MA plans, beginning in 2012; qualifying plans in qualifying areas receive double bonuses. Modifies rebate system with rebates allocated based on a plan's quality rating. Phases-in adjustments to plan payments for coding practices related to the health status of enrollees, with adjustments equaling 5.7% by 2019. Caps total payments, including bonuses, at current payment levels. Requires MA plans to remit partial payments to the Secretary if the plan has a medical loss ratio of less than 85%, beginning in 2014. Requires the Secretary to suspend plan enrollment for 3 years if the medical loss ratio is less than 85% for 2 consecutive years and to terminate the plan contract if the medical loss ratio is less than 85% for 5 consecutive years.
	■ Reduces annual market basket updates for inpatient hospitals, home health, skilled nursing facilities SNF, hospices, and other Medicare providers and adjusts for productivity. (Effective dates vary.)
	■ Reduces Medicare Disproportionate Share Hospital (DSH) payments initially by 75% and subsequently increases payments based on the percent of the population uninsured and the amount of uncompensated care provided. (Effective fiscal year (FY) 2014.)
	■ Allows providers organized as accountable care organizations (ACOs) that voluntarily meet quality thresholds to share in the cost savings they achieve for the Medicare program. To qualify as an ACO, organizations must agree to be accountable for the overall care of their Medicare beneficiaries, have adequate participation of primary care physicians, define processes to promote evidence-based medicine, report on quality and costs, and coordinate care. (Shared savings program established January 1, 2012.)
	■ Creates an Innovation Center within the Centers for Medicare and Medicaid Services to test, evaluate, and expand in Medicare, Medicaid, and CHIP different payment structures and methodologies to reduce program expenditures while maintaining or improving quality of care. Payment reform models that improve quality and reduce the rate of cost growth could be expanded throughout the Medicare, Medicaid, and CHIP programs. (Effective January 1, 2011.)
	■ Reduces Medicare payments that would otherwise be made to hospitals by specified percentages to account for excess (preventable) hospital readmissions. (Effective October 1, 2012.)
	■ Reduces Medicare payments to certain hospitals for hospital-acquired conditions by 1%. (Effective FY 2015.)
Medicaid	■ Extends the drug rebate to Medicaid managed care plans. (Effective upon enactment.)
	■ Prohibits federal payments to states for Medicaid services related to healthcare acquired conditions. (Effective July 1, 2011.)

Waste, fraud, and abuse	■ Reduces waste, fraud, and abuse in public programs by allowing provider screenings, enhanced oversight periods for new providers and suppliers, including a 90-day period of enhanced oversight for initial claims of durable medical equipment (DME) suppliers, and enrollment moratoria in areas identified as having an elevated risk of fraud in all public programs, and by requiring Medicare and Medicaid program providers and suppliers to establish compliance programs. Develops a database to capture and share data across federal and state programs, increases penalties for submitting false claims, strengthens standards for community mental health centers, and increases funding for anti-fraud activities. (Effective dates vary.)

Improving Quality/Health System Performance

Medicare	■ Establishes a national Medicare pilot program to develop and evaluate paying a bundled payment for acute, inpatient hospital services, physician services, outpatient hospital services, and post-acute care services for an episode of care that begins three days prior to a hospitalization and spans 30 days following discharge. If the pilot program achieves the stated goals of improving or not reducing quality and reducing spending, it develops a plan for expanding the pilot program. (Establish pilot program by January 1, 2013; expand program, if appropriate, by January 1, 2016.)
	■ Creates the Independence at Home demonstration program to provide high-need Medicare beneficiaries with primary care services in their home and allow participating teams of health professionals to share in any savings if they reduce preventable hospitalizations, prevent hospital readmissions, improve health outcomes, improve the efficiency of care, reduce the cost of healthcare services, and achieve patient satisfaction. (Effective January 1, 2012.)
	■ Establishes a hospital value-based purchasing (VBP) program in Medicare to pay hospitals based on performance on quality measures and extends the Medicare physician quality reporting initiative beyond 2010. (Effective October 1, 2012) Develops plans to implement VBP programs for SNF, home health agencies, and ambulatory surgical centers. (Reports to Congress were due January 1, 2011.)
Primary care	■ Increases Medicaid payments in FSS and managed care for primary care services provided by primary care doctors (family medicine, general internal medicine or pediatric medicine) to 100% of the Medicare payment rates for 2013 and 2014. States will receive 100% federal financing for the increased payment rates. (Effective January 1, 2013.)
National quality strategy	■ Develops a national quality improvement strategy that includes priorities to improve the delivery of healthcare services, patient health outcomes, and population health. Creates processes for the development of quality measures involving input from multiple stakeholders and for selecting quality measures to be used in reporting to, and payment under, federal health programs. (National strategy was due to Congress by January 1, 2011.)

(continues)

TABLE 1.1 Patient Protection and Affordable Care Act (P.L. 111-148) *(continued)*

Prevention/Wellness	
National strategy	▪ Develops a national strategy to improve the nation's health. (Strategy due one year following enactment.) Creates a Prevention and Public Health Fund to expand and sustain funding for prevention and public health programs. (Initial appropriation in FY 2010) Creates task forces on Preventive Services and Community Preventive Services to develop, update, and disseminate evidenced-based recommendations on the use of clinical and community prevention services. (Effective upon enactment.)
	▪ Establishes a grant program to support the delivery of evidence-based and community-based prevention and wellness services aimed at strengthening prevention activities, reducing chronic disease rates and addressing health disparities, especially in rural and frontier areas. (Funds appropriated for five years beginning in FY 2010.)
Coverage of preventive services	▪ Authorizes the Secretary to modify or eliminate Medicare coverage of preventive services, based on recommendations of the U.S. Preventive Services Task Force. (Effective January 1, 2011.)
	▪ Reimburses providers 100% of the physician fee schedule amount, with no adjustment for deductible or coinsurance for personalized prevention plan services when these services are provided in an outpatient setting. (Effective January 1, 2011.)
	▪ Provides incentives to Medicare and Medicaid beneficiaries to complete behavior modification programs. Requires Medicaid coverage for tobacco cessation services for pregnant women. Requires qualified health plans to provide recommended immunizations, preventive care for infants, children, and adolescents, and additional preventive care and screenings for women.
Wellness programs	▪ Provides grants for up to five years to small employers that establish wellness programs. Permits employers to offer employee rewards—in the form of premium discounts, waivers of cost-sharing requirements, or benefits that would otherwise not be provided—of up to 30% of the cost of coverage for participating in a wellness program and meeting certain health-related standards. Employers must offer an alternative standard for individuals for whom it is unreasonably difficult or inadvisable to meet the standard. The reward limit may be increased to 50% of the cost of coverage if deemed appropriate.
Nutritional information	▪ Requires chain restaurants and food sold from vending machines to disclose the nutritional content of each item.

Other Investments

Workforce

- Improves workforce training and development:
  - Increases the number of Graduate Medical Education (GME) training positions by redistributing currently unused slots, with priorities given to primary care and general surgery and to states with the lowest resident physician-to-population ratios to promote training in outpatient settings and ensure the availability of residency programs in rural and underserved areas. Increases workforce supply and the support training of health professionals through scholarships and loans; supports primary care training and capacity building; provides state grants to providers in medically underserved areas; trains and recruits providers to serve in rural areas; establishes a public health workforce loan repayment program; provides medical residents with training in preventive medicine and public health; promotes training of a diverse workforce; and promotes cultural competence training of healthcare professionals.
  - Addresses the projected shortage of nurses and the retention of nurses by increasing the capacity for education, supporting training programs, providing loan repayment and retention grants, and creating a career ladder to nursing. Offers grants for up to three years to employ and provide training to family nurse practitioners who provide primary care in federally qualified health centers and nurse-managed health clinics. Supports the development of training programs that focus on primary care models such as medical homes, team management of chronic disease, and those that integrate physical and mental health services.

Requirements for non-profit hospitals

- Imposes additional requirements on non-profit hospitals to conduct a community needs assessment every three years and adopt an implementation strategy to meet the identified needs, adopt and widely publicize a financial assistance policy that indicates whether free or discounted care is available and how to apply for the assistance, limits charges to patients who qualify for financial assistance to the amount generally billed to insured patients, and makes reasonable attempts to determine eligibility for financial assistance before undertaking extraordinary collection actions. Imposes a tax of $50,000 per year for failure to meet these requirements.

American Indians

- Reauthorizes and amends the Indian Health Care Improvement Act.

Data from Kaiser Family Foundation. (2013). Summary of the Affordable Care Act. Retrieved from http://www.kff.org/health-reform/fact-sheet/summary-of-the-affordable-care-act/

▶ A Look to the Future

Issues of access, cost, and quality will remain driving forces in the healthcare world for years to come, and perhaps forever. *Ever-tightening governmental funding and regulations*, such as the value-based reimbursement issues and the requirements of the ACA, force healthcare providers and institutional leaders to pay attention to patient outcomes in ways never before expected.

Our *aging population* of baby boomers, now rapidly retiring, will continue to strain our healthcare system in both private and public sectors. Shortages of healthcare professionals (such as nurses, physical therapists, and, in some parts of the United States, physicians) to care for them, as well as those who are newly insured through the provisions of the ACA, will continue to be a problem. Women especially feel the impact of this because they live longer and possibly face living at the poverty level in their older years. According to March 2015 data from The Kaiser Family Foundation, 91% of the nursing workforce are women and, in the general workforce, earn 77% of what their male counterparts make (Pew Research, 2015). Retirement incomes will continue to reflect this societal problem.

Economic issues continue to plague federal, state, and local budgets as all face major deficits. Increasing taxes has not been popular, although as of 2013 federal taxes have increased. Increased spending cuts are also not popular. ACA creates an additional burden for federal and state budgets, with many state governors working on ways to both cut Medicaid payments and not support ACA requirements for Medicaid (a states' rights issue as yet unresolved).

The effects of the ACA, particularly the impact of accountable care organization (ACOs) and provider payments, will bear watching, especially as they are implemented in safety net and rural areas. Hospital closures in the past have disproportionately affected safety net and rural areas, and it is possible that some provisions of the ACA may have unintended consequences for citizens. As more citizens become insured and seek primary care, a dedicated effort will need to be made to ensure there are enough primary care providers to meet the anticipated needs. Federal laws to ensure the full scope of practice for NPs and other advanced practice nurses may be required to adequately meet patient needs, especially because some states continue to artificially limit advanced practice.

Alternative therapies generally focus on health promotion. In the midst of all the cost-cutting in our illness care system, alternative therapies have been enjoying increased popularity with the American public, even though consumers most often pay out of pocket for the services. As patients visit physicians and receive medications for diseases, they frequently discover this does not cure the problem. In many cases, the medications cause other medical problems. Alternative therapies provide a way to stay healthy, as well as to treat disease, and bring comfort without producing as many side effects and as much pain. These are likely to assume even greater importance in health care in the future.

Another issue affecting our future in health care is the technology explosion. As telehealth capabilities increase, healthcare availability expands to meet the demand, opening the door for increased access to care for selected populations. *Electronic health records* (*EHRs*) have great potential for increasing patient safety and the efficiency of care, and yet present the ethical challenge of protecting patients' personal health information and the cost of implementation is burdensome on healthcare organizations. Facilities that have accepted federal monies for EHR systems will have to meet the federal "meaningful use" requirements (http://www .healthit.gov/providers-professionals/meaningful -use-definition-objectives). This is slowly being incorporated into practice settings of all kinds and has significant implications for nurse leaders and providers (Wilson & Newhouse, 2012). In addition, the Internet has vastly improved clinician information on *evidence-based practice*. Consumers continue to access the Internet to research their specific illnesses and determine which providers are most effective. They use this information to evaluate how effectively their provider is determining their care (Meadows, 2001) and will continue to do so with even more frequency in the future.

The science of *genomics* adds a new dimension to health care that looks to have an ever-increasing presence in the future. Currently, scientists have joined forces with private companies that supply enormous funds to map genes. With commercial enterprises involved, it has created great ethical implications because business leaders believe this information can produce future profits.

On one side of the U.S. healthcare landscape are people with excellent insurance, high levels of computer literacy, and life situations that allow them to seek the best care available, wherever it is available. These people will be able to obtain the "personalized medicine" offered by genetic breakthroughs. On the other side of the landscape are the uninsured and those who are losing benefits, such as retirees, who may lack access to such sophisticated technologies. The growing numbers of uninsured and underinsured people, as well as the documented health disparities in health status of racial and ethnic minority populations and all populations living in poverty, will eventually force our legislators to address the inequalities of access and quality of care in our system.

Another contributor to future changes in our healthcare system will be the effects of global warming, magnetic field fluctuations, solar flares, and the earth's poles changing directions. The impact of extreme weather events, including ice-age conditions, heat waves, fires, volcanic eruptions, earthquakes, floods, and storms, is predicted to lead to higher levels of insect- and water-borne illnesses and the reduction of food production and safe drinking water. Healthcare providers will need to address the physical and mental health needs that arise from these conditions (Blashki, McMichael, & Karoly, 2007). Hospitals and other institutional providers will need to be even more focused on disaster preparedness and be ready to deal with increasing numbers of patients needing care for illnesses related to heat exposure and poor air quality (Longstreth, 1999). Drug-resistant organisms are predicted to increase, bringing new challenges in the treatment of infectious diseases, such as with the fungal meningitis outbreak in 2013 and, more recently, the Zika virus outbreak of 2015–2016. These developments require significant adaptation in healthcare delivery and are likely to disproportionately affect children, elderly adults, and poor people.

The problem is that healthcare costs are still high, with many individuals and employers finding health care unaffordable. Recent health policy changes hold promise to better manage healthcare resources but are fraught with political and economic unknowns. This is a time in the development of our healthcare system when nursing leadership is of paramount importance. Nurses represent the lived reality of the system; they see and hear on a daily basis patients' stories of both healing and unnecessary complications. Nursing knowledge and leadership are critical to improving our healthcare system and ensuring access, cost, and quality care for all.

That which is, already has been; that which is to be, already is.

—*Ecclesiastes* 3:15

Summary

Chapter 1 shows how the United States became a tertiary care, illness-based system that often does not meet the needs of our population, even those who are lucky enough to have health insurance. Historically, when people were ill someone in the home cared for them. Amazingly, we are moving back toward that model again. Meanwhile, we can examine how insurance companies surfaced; how Social Security, Medicare, and Medicaid coverage emerged as the most prominent player in health care; how legislation like the Hill-Burton Act drove the healthcare industry to build hospitals and provided money for hospital (tertiary) care rather than for home care; and how value-based reimbursement and prospective payment have affected finances in health care. This has led to an ineffective healthcare system, which probably will not be able to pay for itself in a few years. With the present poor U.S. economy, health care is now at a crisis point. Hopefully, nurses using the knowledge presented here to understand how we got to our present situation in health care, we can more effectively deal with our current situation.

Discussion Questions

1. What implications does CMS pay for performance have for nurse administrators and managers? Why?
2. What changes might you anticipate in your employment setting as the effects of the ACA move forward?
3. What implications do the increasing number of elderly and frail elderly adults hold for nurse leaders across settings?
4. In your opinion, what health policy has had the greatest impact on health care in the United States? Why?

Glossary of Terms

Access the availability of health care to the population; the use of personal health services in the context of all factors that impede or facilitate getting needed care. This includes effective (culturally acceptable) and efficient (geographically accessible) delivery of healthcare services.

Ambulatory Payment Classification System prospective payment system for ambulatory settings giving a fixed dollar amount for outpatient services diagnoses.

Cost the value of all the resources used to produce services and expenditures.

Diagnosis-Related Groups (DRGs) prospective payment plan for hospitals where reimbursement is based on the diagnosis of the patient.

Entitlement what a population expects from government (started in 1935 with Social Security).

Gross Domestic Product (GDP) monetary value of all private or public sector goods and services produced in a country on an annual basis less imports.

Health Insurance Portability and Accountability Act (HIPAA) legislation that ensures that written, oral (telephone inquiries and oral conversations), and electronic (computer or fax) patient health information is kept confidential and private.

Health Maintenance Organizations (HMOs) type of health insurance that provides a full range of integrated care but limits coverage to providers who are employees of or contract with the insurance organization.

Health Policy the entire collection of authoritative decisions related to health that are made at any level of government through the public policymaking process.

Indemnity lump-sum payment for healthcare services based on the retrospective cost of the care.

Managed Care healthcare coverage where insurance companies and Medicare/Medicaid contract with private insurers or HMOs that assume the primary care of groups of people enrolled in a plan and serve as gatekeepers to specialty services. These measures were intended to control healthcare costs and to improve the quality of care.

Outcome and Assessment Information Set (OASIS) prospective payment system for home care.

Outsourcing where another organization that can provide services (such as housekeeping, food service, and groundskeeping) efficiently for a healthcare organization is hired to perform those services.

Primary Care basic healthcare services provided as the first and continuing point of contact for prevention and health promotion, diagnosis and treatment, and referral.

Prospective Payment where the payer determines the cost of care before the care is given; the provider is told how much will be paid to give the care.

Quality of Care extent to which the provided healthcare services achieve or improve desired health outcomes; these are based on the best clinical evidence, are provided in a culturally competent manner, and involve shared decision making.

Resource-Based Relative Value System (RBRVS) prospective payment system for physician services.

Resource Utilization Group (RUGs) prospective payment system for skilled nursing facilities.

Secondary/Tertiary Care highly technical hospital-based care or long-term care.

Utilization Review (UR) where providers are required to certify the necessity of admission, continued stay, and professional services rendered to Medicare and other insurance beneficiaries.

References

American Hospital Association. (2011, September). *Hospitals and care systems of the future*. Retrieved from www.aha.org/about/org/hospitals-care-systems-future.shtml

Andersen, R., Rice, T., Kominski, G., & Afifi, A. (Eds.). (2007). *Changing the U.S. healthcare system: Key issues in health services policy and management* (3rd ed.). San Francisco, CA: Jossey-Bass.

Andersen, R. M., & Davidson, P. L. (2007). Improving access to care in America. In R. Andersen, T. Rice, G. Kominski, & A. Afifi (Eds.), *Changing the U.S. health care system: Key issues in health services policy and management* (3rd ed., pp. 3–31). San Francisco, CA: Jossey-Bass.

Blashki, G., McMichael, T., & Karoly, D. J. (2007). Climate change and primary health care. *Australian Family Physician, 36*(12), 986.

Buerhaus, P. I., Donelan, K., DesRoches, C., & Hess, R. (2009). Registered nurses' perceptions of nurse staffing ratios and new hospital payment regulations. *Nursing Economic$, 27*(6), 372.

DeNavas-Walt, C., Proctor, B., & Smith, J. (2012). *Income, poverty, and health insurance coverage in the United States: 2006*. Washington, DC: U.S. Government Printing Office. U.S. Census Bureau Current Population Reports, P60–233. Retrieved from http://www.census.gov/prod/2012pubs/p60-243.pdf

Finkelman, A. W. (2001). *Managed care: A nursing perspective*. Upper Saddle River, NJ: Prentice Hall.

Gottlieb, S. (2001, March). One doctor: One patient. *Cost & Quality*, 23–24.

Harris, M. D. (2009). *Handbook of home healthcare administration* (5th ed.). Sudbury, MA: Jones and Bartlett.

Institute of Medicine. (1993). Committee on Monitoring Access to Personal Healthcare Services. *Access to Healthcare in America*. Washington, DC: National Academies Press.

Kohn, L. T., Corrigan, J. M., & Donaldson, M. S. (Eds.). (2000). *To err is human: Building a safer health system* (Vol. 627). Washington, DC: National Academies Press.

Leger, J. M. & Phillips, C.A. (2016). Exerting capacity: Bedside RNs talk about patient safety. Western Journal of Nursing Research, 1-14. doi:10.1177/0193945916664707.

Longstreth, J. (1999). Public health consequences of global climate change in the United States—some regions may suffer disproportionately. *Environmental Health Perspectives, 107*(Suppl. 1), 169.

Martin, A. B., Lassman, D., Washington, B., & Catlin, A. (2012). Growth in US health spending remained slow in 2010; health share of gross domestic product was unchanged from 2009. *Health Affairs, 31*(1), 208–219.

Meadows, G. (2001). The Internet promise: A new look at e-health opportunities. *Nursing Economic$, 19*(6), 294–295.

Morrison, C. M., Glove, D., Gilchrist, S. M., Casey, M. O., Lane, R. I., & Patanian, J. (2012). *A program guide for public health: Partnering with pharmacists in the prevention and control of chronic diseases*. Atlanta, GA: Centers for Disease Control and Prevention. Retrieved from http://www.cdc.gov/dhdsp/programs/nhdsp_program/docs/pharmacist_guide.pdf

Raffel, M. W., & Raffel, N. (1994). *The U.S. health system: Origins and functions* (4th ed.). New York, NY: Delmar.

Rice, T., & Kominski, G. (2007). Containing healthcare costs. In R. Andersen, T. Rice, G. Kominski, & A. Afifi (Eds.), *Changing the U.S. healthcare system: Key issues in health services policy and management* (3rd ed.). San Francisco, CA: Jossey-Bass.

Rice, T. H. (2007). Measuring healthcare costs and trends. In R. Andersen, T. Rice, G. Kominski, & A. Afifi (Eds.), *Changing the U.S. healthcare system: Key issues in health services policy and management* (3rd ed.). San Francisco, CA: Jossey-Bass.

Richardson, W., & Briere, R. (Eds.). (2001). *Crossing the quality chasm: A new health system for the 21st century*. Committee on Quality Health Care in America, Institute of Medicine. Washington, DC: National Academy Press.

Roberts, V. (2001). Managing strategic outsourcing in the healthcare industry. *Journal of Healthcare Management/American College of Healthcare Executives, 46*(4), 239.

Stuart, B., Simoni-Wastila, L., & Chauncey, D. (2005). Assessing the impact of coverage gaps in the Medicare Part D drug benefit. *Health Affairs, 24*, 167–179. Retrieved from http://www.ncbi.nlm.nih.gov/pubmed/15840626

U.S. Department of Health and Human Services. (2012). *News release: People with Medicare save more than $4.1 billion on prescription drugs*. Retrieved from http://www.hhs.gov/news/press/2012pres/08/20120820a.html

Wilson, M. L., & Newhouse, R. P. (2012). Meaningful use: Intersections with evidence-based practice and outcomes. *Journal of Nursing Administration, 42*(9), 395–398.

CHAPTER 2

Healthcare Stakeholders: Consumers, Providers, Payers, Suppliers, and Regulators

J. Michael Leger, PhD, MBA, RN, and **Janne Dunham-Taylor**, PhD, RN

OBJECTIVES

- Recognize the challenges that confront the healthcare industry.
- Define and identify where the healthcare costs are primarily used.
- Identify the major stakeholders within the healthcare system.
- Provide information on how the federal, state, and other regulatory agencies affect the industry.

Our current healthcare environment is a wonderful example of complexity—becoming more and more complex every year. Remember that complexity, if unchecked, grows exponentially and creates more problems and errors. This is evident in the healthcare environment, which has been complicated by a major recession in the U.S. economy, a major federal budget deficit (with the states not far behind), and a dwindling middle class. We, as a country, could benefit from working to simplify the entire healthcare environment in small increments. However, this is not the case today. Instead, we continue to create more complexity.

Health care has changed from a social good to a product. Healthcare delivery has become commercialized, and healthcare professionals, such as hospitals and physicians, have turned more toward using business techniques to survive. This pressure has led to economic problems, major quality and safety issues, spiraling costs, and new healthcare delivery approaches. Not all of these factors have been negative. For instance, technology has developed less invasive approaches in dealing with disease.

Healthcare expenditures are predominantly spent on illness care. One major issue in health care is that we are predominantly paying for tertiary illness care and spending little on prevention and primary care.

▶ Healthcare Dilemmas: Access, Cost and Quality

There are three major dilemmas in health care: universal coverage (*access*), paying for care (*cost*), and *quality*. According to economic theory, it is possible simultaneously to achieve any two of the three but not the third. For example, if you achieve universal coverage and can pay for it, costs will be very high. If you contain costs and pay for it, you will not be able to achieve coverage for everyone. As you can see from the quote at the beginning of this chapter, even though we are spending the most in the world, all we have achieved are third-world outcomes, and we certainly do not have universal access to care.

The United States has struggled for some time to determine the best way to achieve reasonable, equitable distribution of health care without losing control of total spending. This struggle continues today. Most industrialized countries have chosen to focus on equitable distribution of health care by providing universal coverage; however, the United States continues to vacillate between equity and containing costs. The result has been limited success on both issues.

A definite result of this struggle has been the development of the medical–industrial complex.

▶ Five Stakeholders: Consumers, Providers, Payers, Suppliers, and Regulators

To better understand this complicated healthcare system, it is necessary to examine the five key stakeholders, or players, in the healthcare arena: consumers, providers, payers, suppliers, and regulators. Simplistically, *consumers* receive the health care; *providers* give the care; *payers* finance the care; *suppliers* provide materials and supplies to the providers; and *regulators* set laws, rules, and regulations that must be followed for giving and paying for care.

Yet, realistically, these terms are more complicated. First, these players are integrated in a healthcare system where actions taken by one stakeholder affect the other stakeholders. So, when the federal government passes a law establishing a set of regulations, consumers are affected, providers must make sure they meet the regulations, payers may be involved in meeting or policing the regulations, and suppliers may have to change supplies to meet the regulations.

Second, at times stakeholders intermingle functions. For instance, (1) the consumer receives the care but is a payer when paying deductibles, (2) the federal government owns the Veterans Administration hospitals (is a provider) yet is a regulator through the Centers for Medicare and Medicaid Services (CMS), and (3) Kaiser Permanente provides insurance (is a payer) and owns healthcare organizations (is a provider).

Consumers

Consumers are patients in hospitals, residents in long-term care facilities, clients in home care, enrollees in insurance plans who receive health care, and people who pay out of pocket for health care. Consumers in health care are different from consumers in other industries because they are vulnerable. An insurance term for the consumer is *covered life*.

As the United States moves from a manufacturing-based economy to a service economy and employee work patterns continue to evolve, health insurance coverage becomes less stable. First, the service sector offers less access to health insurance than the manufacturing sector. Second, there is an increasing reliance on part-time and contract workers who have not historically been eligible for insurance, so fewer workers have access to employer-sponsored health insurance. The Patient Protection and Affordable Care Act (ACA) was passed with the intent to ensure that most people will have health insurance.

As the ACA evolves, all individuals will need to secure health insurance. Subsidies are built in presently for those earning up to 400% of the federal poverty level. In addition to paying for insurance, many people need more extensive medical care. Additional money is needed (tax dollars so far) to cover this expense unless something is cut back, and cuts in federal (and state) budgets are already happening to deal with present deficits. With ACA, small business owners are required to supply employees with health insurance and will get tax credits for this.

Will this force more small business owners to fail? No one can be denied insurance regardless of preexisting conditions, and there will be no financial limits on care for chronic, long-term conditions. *Does this mean that our insurance premium costs will spiral upward even more?*

So, who pays for health care? Some consumers pay cash for care. Examples include wealthy persons (sometimes) and Amish. Employers offer what has become known as *consumer-directed health plans* where consumers pay upfront in several ways:

- By sharing insurance premium costs. These continue to rise each year.
- By paying deductibles (the amount of money a consumer must pay before the insurance company will pay for healthcare services).
- By paying copayments (the amount of money a consumer must pay out of pocket for every healthcare service received). This amount can be fairly small, such as for a doctor's visit, but can be substantial—for example, 20% to 50%, for a procedure.
- By paying more if providers do not participate in the covered plan.
- By paying for any services not covered by the insurance plan, such as alternative therapies or plastic surgery.
- By paying the amount above what the payer has established as a reasonable and customary charge, such as for outpatient services.[1]
- By choosing to pay cash for a healthcare service so it will not be necessary to go through the insurance company.

As the price of health care rises, consumers are paying more and employers are paying less. Examples include the following:

- Insurers are starting to expect consumers to have healthier habits and participate in wellness activities to obtain better premium rates.
- A reduction in explicit coverage has occurred, most notably for pharmaceutical benefits.
- Greater de facto limitations are placed on covered care, especially by *health maintenance organizations* (HMOs).

- The consumer may have to change providers based on the insurance plan his or her employer chooses.
- The cost of "Medigap" coverage is rising. This is insurance purchased by elderly adults to cover the 20% of costs that Medicare does not cover.
- Some employer-based plans now have a *maximum out-of-pocket* limit on the amount the employee has to pay annually for actual medical costs. For instance, say an employee experiences a catastrophic illness that costs $500,000 during the year. If the plan has specified a maximum out-of-pocket limit, once the employee has paid that amount (reached the limit), the employer pays 100% of the medical expenses until the maximum out-of-pocket as set by the employer. *Other plans, including Medicare, do not have this limit. Note here that Medicare only pays 80% of expenses.*

In addition, employers offer *cafeteria plans* for employees. In this arrangement, an employee chooses the amount and type of healthcare coverage (and other benefits) needed, within certain limits set by the employer.

Most often, employers charge employees a *monthly fee* for the health insurance benefit. If spouses each have an insurance plan, it is necessary to *delineate which plan* would first cover family healthcare needs, with the other spouse's plan picking up uncovered expenses only. If the employee's spouse has a good insurance plan, it is possible the employee would not require health insurance at all. This saves employers and employees money.

Then, there is the problem of *uncompensated care* when uninsured or nonpaying patients do not pay for services. Even though more people are covered with ACA, there will continue to be some people, such as migrant workers, who will not have insurance coverage and who may not be able to pay for services. Even with insurance, people must pay a portion of the payment themselves. When they do not or cannot, it becomes bad debt and providers lose money. In a climate

where providers get less from insurers anyway, this becomes a burden and, as a result, drives up prices.

Safety-net hospitals serve indigent and uninsured persons. Often, federal and state governments give these hospitals additional payments for uncompensated care. With the advent of ACA and more people at the poverty level being served, will these hospitals get even more payments? Is the government going to continue to provide additional payments?

One enormous problem in our current payment system is the costs incurred in the last year of life. End-of-life care costs amount to as much as a quarter of U.S. healthcare spending (Kovner & Lusk, 2012). *Nursing Economic$* (May/June 2012) devoted a whole issue to this topic. This is an area being examined closely by insurers to make sure unnecessary costs are avoided.

As the middle class dwindles, many cannot afford needed home health care. This problem results in more *uncompensated, untrained caregivers*—most often relatives with no nursing training—caring for consumers. These caregivers need basic care information, such as turning the patient frequently to prevent bedsores, encouraging hydration, and providing better nutrition—education that a public health nurse could spearhead in the community if public health programs were more adequately funded.

Another consistent problem for consumers is *patient education and prevention* measures. Everyone seems to agree that more of this needs to be done, but in the past, we have funded tertiary care with very little money going to prevention and keeping people in their homes. The question is how to achieve this change yet keep costs down. Enter ACA, which mandates more prevention. This will create additional CMS expenditures right when present costs need to be cut. One obvious answer, used by other countries, is to have the public health department provide more population-based education and prevention programs. However, public health continues to be drastically underfunded in the United States.

Providers

Providers are the individuals (nurses, physicians, dietitians, social workers, pharmacists, physical or respiratory therapists, dentists, and other healthcare personnel) and organizations (hospitals, outpatient facilities, long-term care facilities, home care agencies, or other healthcare organizations) providing the healthcare services. Some common provider organizational terms are *managed care organization (MCO)* or *health services organization (HSO)*. Healthcare organizations are groups of people working within an organizational structure to provide healthcare services to consumers. Healthcare services can be provided across the continuum of care, from how to achieve health, such as through alternative or preventive care, to treating disease, such as through acute, chronic, restorative, or palliative care.

Providers generally have several payer contracts and are concerned with *payer mix*. The issue is that different payers actually pay different amounts for the same services. For example, if most of the patient population served has Medicaid or Medicare as a payer, it is probable that the provider will lose money because neither pay the full amount needed to care for patients. In fact, Medicare and Medicaid pay less than 50 cents for every dollar spent. Providers prefer having a majority of private-pay patients who provide better reimbursement. Even with private-pay patients, discounts are generally given to payers. Discounts can be just a flat discount on all services rendered or calculated on a sliding scale based on volume. The provider must know whether the true reimbursement amount can still provide a profit or at least cover costs.

Pay for performance (also called *value-based purchasing*) has affected providers. Here, providers are reimbursed based on performance data (certain core measures that must be met to receive full reimbursement) that examine patient outcomes—length of stay, readmission rates, adverse reactions (many have become nonpay events), complications, infections, deaths, number of medications per patient, and consumer satisfaction and complaints. Note that since 2009, payers have refused to pay for hospitals' mistakes and infections, called "never events," and now a hospital readmission within 30 days of the patient's most recent hospital discharge may not be reimbursed.

Payers use the performance data to compare providers' performance and determine who gives the best care for the best cost. This is called a *performance-based reimbursement* evaluation. Payers use this evaluation before contracting with providers for healthcare services. Better payments are given to hospitals that have good quality performance ratings, whereas hospitals that do not achieve as high a performance rating are penalized with lower payments the next year. The contract is for a specified time and for specified services.

With managed care, another provider issue emerged: *provider protection*. Physicians are expected to follow the rules of the HMO to continue working for that HMO. For example, they might agree not to order expensive or frequent diagnostic tests or authorize many patient hospitalizations. The idea behind the rules is to keep down expenses. Often, the HMO uses monetary incentives—withholds or bonuses—to ensure that costs do not skyrocket. *Withholds* are when the HMO holds part of the physician's or hospital's income until the end of the year and pays it back to the provider based on performance. Withholds may never be paid back to the provider and may be used instead to cover other expenses the HMO encounters. Year-end *bonuses* are another incentive method used by payers. Such practices have recently resulted in legislation aimed at either limiting the incentives or revealing the incentives to consumers. Providers need protection for due process in their relationship with payers in these matters because payers may expect that providers remain quiet about the incentives (*gag rules*).

Nurses are also providers, though at times they are not treated as such. Nurse practitioners and clinical nurse specialists can bill directly for some services provided in a healthcare organization. However, with the exception of private duty nursing, nursing costs have been bundled into room charges. Only a few organizations have broken away from this model.

Payers

Payers directly pay for healthcare services and can be individuals, employers, insurance companies, or the government. When insurers are the payers, they are not at the point of service. This is different from how payers operate in other businesses.

Employers are payers when they choose to provide healthcare benefits for employees. They can do this in one of two ways: (1) purchase (or make available) health insurance for employees, or (2) be self-insured (usually only larger employers are self-insured) and directly pay employee healthcare costs. In the latter case, the employer pays an insurance company (third-party administrator) to administer the insurance plan. The employer sets up the limitations of the plan, including annual limits per employee; provides claim forms for employees; verifies employee claims; and pays providers from the employer budget. This arrangement can confuse employees who might believe they have insurance such as through Blue Cross, when in actuality their employer is self-insured and Blue Cross is only the intermediary administering the insurance plan. For self-insured employers, healthcare costs are listed as a line item on their budget. This can create the need for huge midyear budget readjustments for unexpected large costs such as when an employee experiences a catastrophic illness that costs the employer $500,000. In this situation, the employer must find additional money to cover the healthcare line item in the budget.

Insurance companies provide individual or group insurance coverage for *covered lives*—the individuals included in the plan—for a contracted amount of time, often a year. The purchaser(s) pays a premium to the insurance company. In group plans, the premium payment is shared, or actually paid for, by employees. Generally, individuals, or even small business employers, pay more for insurance premiums than large employers.

A major change has been to have an *ambulatory-oriented patient care delivery system* that prevents hospitalization and to have more services available to *keep patients in their homes* such as what is provided by the Centers on Aging and Health. Another goal of current legislation is to make a more seamless provider system so there is better planning and less duplication in the continuum of care.

A second major shift in the area of payers is the move from a *volume-based reimbursement* environment to a *value-based payment system* (American Hospital Association, 2011). Whereas payment systems of the past were concerned with the number, or volume, of patients, the new value-based environment rewards providers for positive patient outcomes (providing what patients value). In this new value-based environment, providers are not reimbursed for never events, for not following designated protocols of care within the required and specified time, or for having patients who need to be readmitted to the hospital in less than a month. *The better the hospital's performance, the higher the value-based incentive payment.*

This move to a value-based reimbursement system requires major changes in the healthcare environment. The American Hospital Association (AHA) recommends 10 must-do strategies for hospitals to be successful in the new value-based environment:

1. Aligning hospitals, physicians, and other providers across the continuum of care.
2. Utilizing evidence-based practices to improve quality and patient safety.
3. Improving efficiency through productivity and financial management.
4. Developing integrated information systems.
5. Joining and growing integrated provider networks and care systems.
6. Educating and engaging employees and physicians to create leaders.
7. Strengthening finances to facilitate reinvestment and innovation.
8. Partnering with payers.

9. Advancing an organization through scenario-based strategic, financial, and operational planning.

10. Seeking population health improvement through pursuit of the "triple aim." (The triple aim is to simultaneously focus on population health, increased quality, and reduction in healthcare cost per capita, as identified by the Institute for Healthcare Improvement in 2007.)

Governments are the biggest force in the healthcare payer arena. The *federal government* is a major payer, covering more than 50% of total healthcare revenue. Federal government insurance programs include Medicare, part of Medicaid, the Federal Employees Health Benefit Program (FEHBP), Tri-Care, and the Civilian Health and Medical Program of the Uniform Services (CHAMPUS). *Thus, as the federal government implements a payment strategy, other insurers follow suit.* The state governments, often the largest employer in a state, have been responsible for health insurance for state employees in addition to sharing responsibilities for Medicaid programs with the federal government.

The term *third-party payers*, or *insurers*, refers to insurance companies, employers, or government agencies that provide healthcare insurance. The insurance company acts as an administrator of the pool of money collected from all its members, paying, or *underwriting*, the defined illness care coverage to a provider when the consumer has received healthcare services. With insurance, there is a risk to the insurance company. What if more people need coverage than anticipated? To determine the risk, the insurance company uses *actuarial data,* a statistical method that takes into account such factors as the age and sex of enrollees, past use, and cost of medical services, to determine both premium costs and definition of coverage. Obviously, it benefits the insurance company to serve a larger population, which reduces the risk and has the additional benefit of costing less to administer the plan. It is also better for the insurance company to have healthier people in the plan. This is especially an issue for the federal government, in Medicare, because it serves an older population that is more likely to need expensive illness care. The purchaser's perception of risk is also an issue. Insurance is only worth purchasing if people perceive that they may experience a risk, such as expensive surgery or other care.

Retrospective Payment

Historically, typical health insurance was *indemnity insurance*, where payment occurred after the care was given. This was called *retrospective payment*. The consumer chose the provider, the provider determined what was charged, and the insurance company paid it (*fee for service*). The insurance contract was with the individual or employer. Except for those who pay cash, true indemnity insurance is largely nonexistent today because health insurance plans use some form of managed care, or financial incentives, to be cost effective.

Prospective Payment

Like the name implies, *managed care* refers to any method of healthcare delivery that is designed to cut costs yet provide needed services (i.e., use the least expensive option for delivery of care, only pay for necessary services, control costs by contracting and telling providers what will be paid for services before the services are delivered, and involve consumers in paying for part of their care). In managed care, payers determine the amount they will reimburse for a medical service. Generally, the reimbursement strategy is *prospective payment*, where the payer determines the cost of care before the care is given. The provider is then told how much will be paid for the care. This is called the *prospective payment system* (PPS).

Service Benefit Plans

Service benefit plans, an example of both prospective payment and managed care, directly pay providers after negotiating and specifying the prices paid for each healthcare service. In service benefit plans, the patient pays part of the costs of care through deductibles and coinsurance. Medicare and preferred provider organizations (PPOs), such as Blue Cross, have service benefit plans. (This can be confusing because Blue Cross and Medicare also offer HMOs, a direct service delivery plan, discussed in the next section. In addition, Blue Cross and other insurance companies are the fiscal intermediaries for Medicare.) Because more than 50% of our country's population is covered by Medicare/Medicaid, this chapter provides more information on these two plans.

Medicare

Medicare, supported by payroll cash contributions placed in the Medicare Trust Fund, pays for healthcare services for Americans aged 65 years and older, for some people with disabilities who are younger than age 65, and for people with end-stage renal disease. Medicare covers approximately 80% of healthcare costs for these groups. There has been some debate as to whether there will be enough Medicare payroll cash contributions to cover health care as more baby boomers become eligible.

Medicare is administered by the CMS. Medicare usage is monitored by the Medicare Payment Advisory Commission (MedPAC) that independently advises Congress about more effective or less costly ways to manage Medicare. CMS pays an administrative fee to *fiscal intermediaries* to carry out the actual payment system for Medicare. Fiscal intermediaries are other insurance companies who already have experience with processing insurance claims—companies, such as Blue Cross.

TABLE 2.1 provides an overview of how Medicare divides defined services and payments into four parts.

Part A is an automatic coverage, for those who apply, on a person's 65th birthday. There are no premiums to pay because Medicare taxes were paid while the recipient, or their spouse, were working. However, there are deductibles and coinsurance costs for consumers. Additional information can be found at www.Medicareconsumerguide.com/medicare-part-a.html.

Part B coverage is a choice that is left up to the individual. Paying Medicare taxes before age 65 constitutes eligibility to participate. However, there is a monthly fee for Part B coverage in addition to deductibles and copayments. Go to www.Medicareconsumerguide.com/medicare-part-b.html for more information.

TABLE 2.1 Overview of Medicare Services	
Part A	**Part B**
Hospital inpatient services Blood transfusions in hospitals Skilled nursing (up to 100 days/benefit period) Home care/home durable medical equipment (DME) (limitations) Hospice care (less than 6 months to live)	Physician & outpatient services, tests and preventive treatments (not covered by Part A)
Part C	**Part D**
Medicare Advantage Plan (provided by private insurance companies) – combines Parts A & B	Prescription drug coverage (through private insurance companies approved by CMS)

Data from Centers for Medicare and Medicaid Services.

Part C was supposed to be a lower-cost alternative plan, a combination of Parts A and B, provided by private insurance companies approved by CMS. In reality, the cost for providing medical coverage to participants in Part C is more expensive. With ACA, there has been a significant cut in this plan, bringing it in line with Parts A and B. (See www.Medicare consumerguide.com/medicare-part-c.html.)

Part D is the most recent provision to the Medicare program. Part D generally is where the individual pays a separate premium or yearly deductible, along with copays, coinsurance, or a deductible, when s/he actually buys a prescription. The person must have another plan of equal value or pay a penalty. Originally, if a person exceeded the limit, the person would have to pay 100% for prescriptions (called a "donut hole") until s/he reached the catastrophic level where discounts were available. ACA attempts to fix this partially by offering gradually decreasing payments until a person reaches the limit, and then offers some drugs directly from drug companies at 50% of the cost.

Besides what the user is paying, federal tax dollars pay the rest of the costs. *Medicare only provides 80% coverage.* This means that additional insurance is needed. Consumers can purchase *Medigap* plans, sponsored by private insurance companies, in addition to paying for Medicare Parts A, B, C, and D. Medigap plans provide supplemental insurance for Medicare consumers. Plans vary. Some Medigap premiums are quite expensive, and many elderly adults cannot afford them.

Despite the prevalence of public and private supplemental coverage, Medicare beneficiaries face substantial out-of-pocket expenses. Medicare covers less than half of older adults' total health spending and is less generous than health plans that are typically offered by large employers. On average, older adults often spend at least 20% of their household income on health services and premiums.

Medicare's *service benefit plan uses prospective payment* mechanisms for care that set fixed rates for specific diagnoses (see **TABLE 2.2**). CMS sets the rates.

As CMS established these prospective payment mechanisms, other insurance companies have

TABLE 2.2 Medicare's Service Benefit Plan

Level of Care	Prospective Payment Mechanism
Inpatient/ hospitals	Diagnosis-related groups (DRGs)
Long-term care	Resource utilization groups (RUGs)
Ambulatory care	Ambulatory payment categories (APCs)
Physicians	Resource-based relative value scale (RBRVS)
Home care	Outcome and assessment information set (OASIS)

also adopted them. Here is how they work. With Diagnosis-related groups (DRGs), the physician is responsible for identifying the principal diagnosis upon discharge, which must be the reason for admission, using the International Classification of Diseases, Clinical Modification (ICD-10-CM 10th Revision). Up to four secondary diagnoses can be documented. If the physician does not adequately document all this, payment will not be forthcoming. When never events occur, when certain protocols are not met within the specified time, or when patients need to be re-admitted within 30 days of discharge, this will not be reimbursed. The never events are labeled MS-DRGs (which stands for medical severity DRGs). Hospitals are still required to report these events. Hospitals cannot charge patients for never events, but some reimbursement is provided for physician care and other services the patient requires upon discharge that only became needed because the never event occurred.

In long-term care, Medicare reimbursement has been based on Resource utilization groups (RUGs). RUGs measure resident characteristics and staff care time for various categories of patients.

RUGs have seven categories of patient severity. Caregivers derive the classifications from assessments recorded in the resident *Minimum Data Set* (*MDS*) assessment instrument required for days 5, 14, 30, 60, and 90 during a Part A stay. Facilities must also complete a comprehensive assessment if a patient's condition changes significantly. So, in long-term care, reimbursement is determined by how effectively staff complete the MDS data.

Ambulatory payment categories (APCs) have been developed for the whole range of ambulatory services. APCs group thousands of procedures and diagnoses costs into several hundred categories, with separate classifications for surgical, medical, and ancillary services. Each group includes clinically similar services that require comparable levels of resources. A relative weight based on median resource use is assigned to each classification. Payment for each APC is determined by multiplying the relative weight by a conversion factor, which is the average rate for all APC services.

The resource-based relative value scale (RBRVS) was started in an attempt to even out payments to specialty physicians (who were paid more) compared with family and general practice physicians (who received less). Presently, physicians are paid for each treatment, so there is an incentive to overuse services.

Home health care presently serves patients after acute care episodes where no money is allotted for chronic illness needs. The Outcome and Assessment Information Set (OASIS) is a tool, similar to that of the MDS in long-term care, used by staff to document their patients' healthcare needs and, thus, what drives the reimbursement through the number of approved home care visits.

The problem with all these payment changes is that patients are often discharged too soon. For example, patients might still be medically unstable at the time they leave the hospital or may not be able to care for themselves and need medical care but have used up their long-term care or home care allotment. With ACA, the plan is to develop better ways to provide care to patients with long-term chronic illnesses.

Overall, ACA initiated several delivery system reforms that are designed to promote coordinated, accountable, high-quality, and low-cost care. Mechanisms specified in the law to improve the delivery system include accountable care organizations (ACO), the patient-centered medical home, payment reforms (payment for care coordination, bundling of payment, and value-based purchasing), support for primary care, and reductions in hospital payments for preventable hospital readmissions (Trautman, 2011, p. 29).

Where the money will come from for all this is unclear. Taxes have been raised, but with governments cutting budgets because of deficits, it remains to be seen how the goals of ACA will be realized.

Medicaid

Medicaid, a cost-sharing program involving both state and federal funds, provides services for

- medically indigent people, including children, and
- for people with severe and permanent disabilities who are younger than age 65—although elderly adults older than age 65 who receive welfare are also covered by Medicaid.

The federal government mandates certain basic coverage:

- inpatient and outpatient hospital services;
- physician, midwife, and certified nurse practitioner services;
- laboratory and x-ray services;
- nursing facility and home health care;
- early and periodic screening, diagnosis, and treatment (EPSDT) for children younger than age 21;
- family planning; and
- rural health clinics/federally qualified health centers.

States can add coverage for such things as prescription drugs, clinic services, prosthetic devices, hearing aids, dental care, and intermediate care facilities for people with mental retardation. Services and reimbursements vary widely from state to state. Each state has designed a different version of Medicaid.

Medicaid predominantly pays for custodial long-term care of more than 100 days, which represents 48% of Medicaid expenses. If people need custodial long-term care, they must be at the poverty level, as established by each state, before Medicaid will pay. If people are not at the poverty level, they can pay cash for care or let their long-term care insurance (including Medigap insurance) pay.

If a person does not have one of these options and is above the poverty level, it is possible to receive Medicaid benefits for custodial long-term care by *spending down* all assets (income, property, and other assets) until the patient is below the poverty level. Then, Medicaid benefits will begin. (In this case, the spouse is allowed a house, car, and a specified amount of money, but the rest must be "spent down.") The other option, used by a significant number of elderly adults who need custodial care, is to be cared for by a relative in the home. This avoids spending down life savings.

ACA has changed Medicaid in several significant ways: It covers people at 133% of the poverty level, will specify essential benefits for newly eligible members, and will give increased funding to states *if states choose to accept this*. A number of states are resisting this by refusing to accept additional federal money for the ACA changes because then states will be mandated to add Medicaid services the way ACA outlines. Because ACA covers most of the U.S. population, this will enormously increase the money needed in federal and state budgets, right at a time when the country is recovering from a severe recession. The question is: Where will the money come from to pay for this? This question remains to be answered. So far, it seems that additional taxes will be the source for additional expenditures.

Medicaid is quickly becoming a federal-versus-state-rights issue. The federal government has mandated the states to support Medicaid, yet states struggle to continue to pay their share of Medicaid spending. This is nearing crisis proportions.

Direct Service Delivery Plans

A *direct service delivery plan* is another type of plan used by HMOs. This plan is different because it pays the provider in advance. Generally, there are five types of HMOs:

1. Staff HMOs that employ physicians individually.
2. Group model HMOs that contract with one multispecialty group of physicians. A per capita rate is paid to the physician, as specified in the contract.
3. Network model HMOs that operate just like group models, except that they contract with more than one group of physicians.
4. Individual practice association (IPA) members that include both individual and group practice physicians. The HMO contracts with the IPA for physician services. IPA physician members provide services for the HMO but also treat other patients.
5. Point-of-service HMOs. These came about more recently. Here, an HMO patient can go to a physician or hospital outside the HMO but pays more out-of-pocket expense.

HMOs use *capitation* as the reimbursement mechanism. The word *capitation* comes from the per capita (per person) fee the purchaser pays. To purchase HMO services, the employer (or individual purchaser) pays a monthly (capitated) fee to the HMO. The HMO agrees to provide healthcare services specified in the contract for no additional costs to the employer or the individual. The HMO either contracts with, or hires, providers who agree to be paid in advance a monthly or yearly fee in return for providing all services that enrollees will need for that period.

Under capitation, a provider could lose money if too many services are provided in the covered period, so providers want to provide only needed services. To better deal with this, consumers must first see a gatekeeper provider, such as a primary care physician or nurse practitioner, who determines whether care is necessary. If so, the gatekeeper makes the decision whether the patient should be referred to a specialist. The advantage to the patient is that there is no charge to see the gatekeeper and no insurance paperwork is necessary for reimbursement. In addition, there is no charge for specialty care, as long as the gatekeeper makes the specialty referral. The disadvantage to the consumer with an HMO is when the gatekeeper does not believe specialty care is needed. In this case, if the patient still wants specialty care, the patient has to pay for the specialty service or go without.

HMOs use *disease management* to manage chronic, long-term illnesses. Disease management identifies the best practices to achieve fewer poor outcomes or at least to slow down the degenerative aspects of chronic diseases. The physician or provider is given a mandated, systematic, population-based approach that defines the patient diagnosis or problem and the specific intervention(s) to take with all patients who meet this definition. The HMO then collects data on the physician practice patterns and the patient clinical outcomes to determine how effectively the physician followed these mandates.

Who Is the Bad Guy?

A common fallacy is to view third-party payers as the "bad guys"—the cause of our societal dilemmas: the inadequacy of healthcare coverage, limitations on healthcare coverage, the predominance of tertiary illness care, and the high cost of health care. However, who really is the bad guy? By reviewing the history of health care in this country, we can see a much larger societal problem. Employers spend large amounts of money on illness needs of employees, who expect the best tertiary care possible and want someone else to pay for and cure all their illnesses. Although the cost of care is shared with employees in the form of deductibles and copayments, the majority of the cost is passed on

to the public through the price of whatever widget or service the employer sells. When consumers purchase the widgets or services, they complain about the high costs. Who is really to blame for these high costs? It turns out that finding the bad guy is really a hunt for a much larger societal dysfunction with many implications. We are all a part of this dilemma—the general public, consumers, employers, payers, providers, suppliers, and regulators. We all contribute to this complex problem, and we all must be involved in finding the solution.

Suppliers

Suppliers—individuals or companies—provide the supplies, equipment, and services used by healthcare providers. In the late 1970s, in response to the importance of cutting costs, nationwide purchasing alliances were formed. The idea was that materials and supplies could be purchased at less cost (many touted a 10% savings) because of the higher volume that could be purchased at once by the alliance. This has caused other issues:

- Size brings big discounts, but not everyone wants to use the products.
- From a nursing perspective, it can be an issue when everyone is trained to use one supply, but the purchasing alliance gets a better deal on another similar supply that staff members have not been trained to use properly.
- The purchase itself may save money; however, staff education may cost the organization more on such purchases.

When healthcare organizations join a purchasing alliance, they still must rely on local companies for certain supplies and services such as waste removal, physician contractual services to staff the emergency room, and laundry facilities (if contracted outside the healthcare organization).

Regulators

Regulators are the organizations and agencies that set the rules, regulations, and/or standards that providers must meet to stay in business. This includes many groups, such as the federal, state, and local governments and judicial systems, accrediting bodies, regulators of professions such as medicine and nursing, and professional organizations. The standards used by regulators come from many sources, including consumers, providers, payers, professional organizations, and even state or federal laws or executive orders.

Federal Regulation

In health care, the federal government, as a regulator, has the overall responsibility for both achieving quality and holding down costs. The Constitution specifies that the federal government has the authority to regulate interstate commerce and provide for the general welfare of its citizens. The main federal healthcare regulator is the CMS, established to administer Medicare and Medicaid and enforce national healthcare regulations. For example, federal legislation, in a 1972 cost reduction strategy, mandated *utilization review*, which is still in force today to assess medical necessity, efficiency, and/or appropriateness of services and treatment plans. Utilization review is accomplished using several mechanisms:

- *Preadmission certification:* The insurer approves care in advance. If this is required and certification is not obtained, the insurer can refuse to pay for the care.
- *Concurrent review:* Some insurers monitor patients' lengths of stay to ensure the patients are discharged timely. If an insurer determines that the patient has received all the appropriate tests and treatments, the insurer will not authorize additional care and will refuse to pay for additional days.
- *Discharge planning:* Discharge planning has always been important and needs to begin at admission. It is important to keep lengths of stay as short as possible. However, now it is critical because if a patient is readmitted within 30 days, reimbursement will be lost for the readmission. The discharge

plan may include additional care needed in the home or by transferring the patient quickly to long-term care, home care, and/or ambulatory care, which is less expensive than the hospital stay.

- *Case management:* Case care plans are developed for complicated patients to provide the needed care in the least expensive way. For example, perhaps a hospitalization can be prevented by providing home care 7 days a week.
- *Second surgical opinions:* For elective surgeries, insurers often require that the patient see a second physician to determine whether the surgery is necessary. Additionally, the insurer wants the surgery to be done in the least expensive way—outpatient is preferred, but if hospitalization is needed, it needs to be specified.

To accomplish quality monitoring, the federal government delegates specific responsibilities to each state's licensure and certification agency. For a facility to participate in Medicare and Medicaid programs, it must undergo this licensure and certification process. States vary as to actual requirements. In addition, healthcare organizations must be accredited to be eligible for Medicare reimbursement.

Other federal regulators affect health care:

- The Department of Justice and Federal Trade Commission enforce antitrust issues, which prohibit anticompetitive practices.
- The National Labor Relations Board regulates union organizing and collective bargaining.
- The Food and Drug Administration regulates drugs and medical devices and dietary regulations and inspections.
- The Securities and Exchange Commission regulates how investor-owned healthcare organizations can market, sell, and trade stock.
- The Nuclear Regulatory Commission regulates hazards arising from storage, handling, and transportation of nuclear materials.
- The Equal Employment Opportunity Commission enforces equal employment

opportunities in hiring, equal pay, civil rights, and nondiscrimination regarding age.

■ The judicial system has determined many healthcare regulations.

State Regulation

When the states delegated certain powers to a federal government and ratified the U.S. Constitution, they retained a wide range of authority known as the police powers, defined as the powers to protect the health, safety, public order, and welfare of the public. Consistent with the police powers, states have enacted legislation to regulate and license a wide variety of healthcare organizations that are required to obtain and retain a license and must submit to inspections and other regulation (Longest, Rakich, & Darr, 2000, p. 69).

Health and safety issues include radiation safety, sanitation of food and water, and disposal of wastes. States may delegate some of the safety, sanitation, and waste disposal responsibilities to city and county governments. Therefore, the states regulate, inspect, and license healthcare organizations on physical plant safety issues and license and regulate various healthcare professionals and nursing education programs. In addition, each state has an insurance commission.

To be eligible for Medicare and Medicaid funding, a healthcare organization must be licensed by the state annually. Certification is needed each year to receive Medicare reimbursement. After the inspection, the states make recommendations to CMS for Medicare certification. Because about 50% of Medicaid funds are for long-term care, the federal government has mandated each state to do a more involved annual inspection of the long-term care given to each Medicaid-funded resident. As part of the inspection,

a multidisciplinary survey team must ensure that the care reimbursed with

Medicaid funds is necessary, available, adequate, appropriate and of acceptable quality to maximize the physical and mental potential and well-being of the resident. The review also includes an assessment of [each] resident's continued placement in the home and the feasibility of meeting his needs through alternative institutional or non-institutional services. The survey team looks for evidence that the resident's discharge potential was evaluated. (Mitty, 1998, p. 248)

If the facility meets all the federal requirements, the state, representing CMS, then certifies or recertifies the long-term care facility on the day of the survey.

Another important state responsibility concerns individual licensing and certification of various health occupations. Perhaps, as nurses, we are most aware of the *board of nursing*. Each state has a nurse practice act that defines nursing practice and establishes the board of nursing. In addition, there are other professional boards, such as the board of medicine or the board licensing long-term care administrators. The professional boards define professional practice, license caregivers and set standards. To become licensed, a person must show that he or she has achieved minimum competencies, and the board keeps an official roster of all who are licensed. Boards of nursing also license licensed practical nurses (LPNs) and nurse assistants for long-term care.

Generally, nurse practice acts specify that registered nurses can treat patients independently, whereas licensing for LPNs or nurse assistants specifies that licensees are dependent on the orders of a registered nurse or physician. In addition, the professional boards hold regular hearings, regulate practice, determine what is unprofessional conduct, take disciplinary actions when infractions occur, introduce legislation to better define professional practice, license new nursing education programs, and oversee the quality of current nursing education programs. Most states have mandated that nursing education programs achieve an 85% student pass rate on the National Council Licensing Exam (NCLEX).

Having representation on the board of nursing can be an important role in policymaking.

Although it is not a state regulatory body, it is important to note here that the purpose of the National Council of State Boards of Nursing (NCSBN) is to be a national organization where boards of nursing can "act and counsel together on matters of common interest and concern affecting the public health, safety and welfare, including the development of licensing examinations in nursing" (NCSBN, n.d.). NCSBN has been involved in several important issues. First, it has developed computerized licensure examinations, the NCLEX-RN and the NCLEX-PN, which are administered by a national test service to all individuals who want to be newly licensed as a registered nurse or LPN. Second, NCSBN has established a multistate Nurse Licensure Compact. Presently, nurse practice acts are not uniform in all states. A state legislature can pass a law to become a part of this compact. Once passed, nurses can practice across state lines of states in the compact without getting licensed in another state, as long as they follow the practice provisions in place in the states in which they practice. The list of states that currently belong to the Nurse Licensure Compact is on the NCSBN website (www.ncsbn.org/nlc.htm).

Credentialing

Credentialing of healthcare occupations takes place in several ways: through licensure, registration, certification, and competency. With *licensure*, a person must show the state licensing board, such as the board of nursing, that he or she has achieved minimum competencies. *Registration* is the official roster kept by the board of nursing that lists all who are licensed. *Certification* is awarded to individual providers by a nongovernmental organization/registry when the individual has met certain educational requirements and passed an examination. For example, family nurse practitioners or certified nurse assistants are certified.

A number of nursing specialty organizations certify nurses (listed at http://medi-smart.com/cert.htm). In turn, these professional certifying organizations are certified by the American Board of Nursing Specialties, a certifier of certifiers (Bernreuter, 2001). Boards of nursing, as well as employers, require that people in certain health occupations are certified (i.e., nurse practitioners).

Certification can also be given to organizations that meet specified qualifications, such as the requirements of Medicare and Medicaid certification. A component of organizational accreditation includes the standard that employees are properly *credentialed* to do their assigned work. The evaluation process for this standard examines licenses, certification, educational background, and competency (evidence of current, safe practice or performance quality) of personnel, as well as that of the physicians.

Accreditation

Accreditation is the process by which organizations are evaluated on their quality, based on established minimum standards. As purchasers and consumers are interested in cost and quality, there are two major reasons for healthcare organizations to seek an accreditation status:

1. The availability of objective data for healthcare purchasers to make informed decisions about health plans for their subscribers; and,

2. Consumers want the data to make more-informed decisions about the options they have among organizations from where they seek their health care (Finkelman, 2001, pp. 230–231).

Generally, accreditation involves two steps: reviewing written materials (self-study), and an on-site visit from the accrediting body to determine whether the minimum standards have been met. Personnel in healthcare organizations must have ongoing education about current/new standards to maintain accreditation. There are many healthcare accrediting bodies (https://www.cms.gov/Medicare/Provider-Enrollment-and-Certification/SurveyCertificationGenInfo/Downloads/Accrediting-Organization-Contacts-for-Prospective-Clients-.pdf).

Professional Organizations

Professional organizations, such as American Nurses Association (ANA) and American Organization of Nurse Executives (AONE), continually examine professional scope of practice and professional standards. AONE, ANA, the American Association of Colleges of Nursing (AACN), and the National League for Nursing (NLN) have formed a national tri-council on nursing. Together, they represent nursing on certain national issues. In long-term care, directors of nursing can belong to the American Association of Directors of Nursing Administration in Long-Term Care or to the National Conference of Gerontological Nurse Practitioners (NCGNP). The American Academy of Ambulatory Care Nursing (AAACN) focuses on ambulatory nursing practice. The National Association for Home Care (NAHC) represents home care professionals.

Nursing professional organizations are listed at http://www.nurse.org/orgs.shtml. The authors suggest that nurse managers belong to both clinical and administrative professional organizations that are appropriate for the area of practice in which they are working. In addition to nursing organizations, nurse administrators might want to consider other professional organizations that are pertinent to their work setting, such as the American College of Healthcare Executives (ACHE).

Note

1. As mentioned previously, this is true for coinsurance deductibles and what is above the reasonable and customary costs with regular insurance. However, with Medicare Part A and Medicaid, other than billing the deductible and coinsurance, it is illegal to bill the patient for the amount of reimbursement not paid by the government. In Medicare Part B, providers can bill up to 15% more for services than the cost covered by Medicare.

Summary

Chapter 2 is concerned with the five stakeholders in health care: consumers, providers, payers, suppliers, and regulators. All are interrelated and complex, and this chapter gives us a better understanding of each and the role they play in health care. Our current dilemma is that we have not figured out how to achieve all three healthcare needs at once: universal coverage, quality, and cost containment.

Discussion Questions

1. What are the characteristics of the consumers that you regularly see in your current work environment? What are some ways in that they are impacted by the other identified healthcare stakeholders?
2. What effect has ACA had on stakeholders? Explain what strategies a nurse leader might adopt that would make it more effective?
3. What is important for nurse leaders to share with their staff regarding payers? Why?
4. Who are the various regulators that affect your healthcare organization? What is your role in the respective regulatory process?

Glossary of Terms

Bonuses monetary incentives given to providers at the end of the year based on the providers' performance or the total plan performance.

Capitation a reimbursement mechanism. *Capitation* comes from the per capita (per person) fee the purchaser pays. To purchase HMO services, the employer (or individual purchaser) pays a monthly capitated fee to the HMO.

Concurrent Review a plan where health care is reviewed as it is provided. Some insurers will monitor patients' lengths of stay to ensure that the patients are discharged quickly. If an insurer determines that the patient has received all the appropriate tests and treatments, the insurer will not authorize additional care and will refuse to pay for additional days.

Covered Lives individuals included in an insurance plan.

Direct Service Delivery Plan a plan used by HMOs where the HMO pays the provider in advance and the provider agrees to provide certain services.

Disease Management a plan often used for chronic, long-term illnesses. The physician, or provider, is given a mandated, systematic, population-based approach that defines the patient diagnosis or problem and the specific intervention(s) to take with all patients who meet this definition.

Fee for Service when the provider is reimbursed a specific amount of money, reasonable and customary charges, for each service and/or product provided. A discounted fee for service reimburses the provider for the service and/or product but with a discount, either a fixed amount or a percentage, as specified in the payer–provider contract, subtracted from the fee.

Gag Rules providers need protection for due process in their relationship with payers because payers may expect that providers remain quiet about the incentives payers give providers.

Gatekeeper a primary care physician or nurse practitioner who determines whether care is necessary and, if so, makes the decision whether the patient should be referred to a specialist. In an HMO, when consumers need care, they must first see a gatekeeper. The advantage to the patient is that there is no charge to see the gatekeeper, and no insurance paperwork is necessary for reimbursement. In addition, there is no charge for specialty care, as long as the gatekeeper makes the referral and the contract specifies that specialty care is available.

Health Maintenance Organizations (HMOs) an insurance plan where the plan pays the provider in advance. The purchaser (an employer or an individual) pays a monthly fee to the HMO. The HMO agrees to provide healthcare services specified in the contract for no additional costs to the employer or the individual. The consumer sees a gatekeeper who determines what care the consumer needs.

Managed Care any method of healthcare delivery that is designed to cut costs yet provide needed services.

Payer Mix the percentage of different payers (i.e., Medicare, Blue Cross, self-pay) who paid for services to a healthcare organization over a year.

Performance-Based Reimbursement data collected on patient outcomes—length of stay, readmission rates, adverse reactions, deaths, etc.—within a healthcare organization (provider performance). Payers use this evaluation before contracting with providers for healthcare services.

Preferred Provider Organizations (PPOs) an example of a service benefit plan. It consists of a group of providers—such as physicians and hospitals—who have agreed to provide services at lower-than-usual rates to enrollees. The PPO acts as the intermediary between providers and consumers. The PPO pays prearranged fees for services provided. The enrollee incentive is to use the providers in the plan and not have to pay for many of the services provided. If an enrollee chooses to go to a physician not included in the PPO, the PPO only pays part—or none—of the fee, with the enrollee having to pay the remainder.

Practice Patterns where physicians are under scrutiny about their practice. Data are collected on such things as length of stay, and individual physician data are compared with other physician data.

Preadmission Certification the insurer approves care in advance. If this is required, and certification is not obtained, the insurer can refuse to pay for the care.

Prospective Payment the payer determines the cost of care before the care is given. The provider is then told how much will be paid to give the care.

Provider Protection legislation aimed at either limiting incentives offered to providers or revealing the incentives to patients.

Retrospective Payment indemnity insurance where payment occurs after the care is given.

Service Benefit Plan plans that directly pay providers after negotiating and specifying the prices paid for each healthcare service. In service benefit plans, the patient pays part of the costs through deductibles and coinsurance.

Underwriting when an insurance company acts as an administrator of the pool of money collected from all its members and pays the defined illness care coverage to a provider when the consumer receives healthcare services.

Value-Based Reimbursement when providers are reimbursed based on achieving positive patient outcomes (providing what patients value). In this new value-based environment, providers are not reimbursed for never events, for not following designated protocols of care within the required and specified time, or for having patients who need to be readmitted to the hospital in less than a month. The better the hospital's performance, the higher the value-based incentive payment.

Volume-Based Reimbursement when payment to providers is based on the volume of patients who receive care.

Withholds when an HMO, or payer, holds part of the physician or hospital income until the end of the year and pays it back to the physician or hospital based on performance.

References

American Hospital Association. (2011, September). *Hospitals and care systems of the future*. Retrieved from http://www.aha.org/about/org/hospitals-care-systems-future.shtml

Bernreuter, M. (2001). Spotlight on . . . the American Board of Nursing Specialties: Nursing's gold standard. *JONA's Healthcare Law, Ethics, and Regulation, 3*(1), 5–7.

Finkelman, A. (2001). *Managed care: A nursing perspective*. Upper Saddle River, NJ: Prentice Hall.

Kovner, C., & Lusk, E. (2012). Introduction: How can we afford to die? *Nursing Economic$, 30*(3), 125–126.

Longest, B., Rakich, J., & Darr, K. (2000). *Managing health services organizations and systems* (4th ed.). Baltimore, MD: Health Professions Press.

Mitty, E. (1998). *Handbook for directors of nursing in long-term care*. Albany, NY: Delmar.

National Council of State Boards of Nursing. (n.d.). *About NCSBN*. Retrieved from https://www.ncsbn.org/about.htm

Trautman, D. (2011, April). Healthcare reform 1 year later. *Nursing Management*, 26–31.

CHAPTER 3

Microeconomics in the Hospital Firm: Competition, Regulation, the Profit Motive, and Patient Care

J. Michael Leger, PhD, MBA, RN, and **Mary Anne Schultz**, PhD, MBA, MSN, RN

OBJECTIVES

- Provide a broad view of the economics involved in the hospital environment that includes competition, regulation, and patient care.
- Understand the impact of regulation in the U.S. healthcare system and the costs associated with it.
- Demonstrate the impact of electronic medical records and how this affects the healthcare industry.

ince the introduction of a *prospective payment system (PPS)* for health care 25 years ago, hospital services have become increasingly driven by the market forces of price and quality. Rooted in a tradition of caring, hospitals were once seen as places where people could be healed and have their physical needs met—all through the professionalism and trust of healthcare providers. This was the hospital's *mission.*

Today, hospitals are businesses, big and small, where patient care is but one service and patients are no longer the only constituent. Their caring (and in some cases, curing) processes are now high tech, research-based, and financially driven, and serve a number of stakeholders, such as physicians, investors, patients, and families, and employees, such as nurses, to name a few. Balancing the goals of the players and supporting the many purposes of a hospital require identification of the pressures shaping its operation. Chiefly, these are (1) *competition*, (2) *regulation*, (3) the *profit motive*, and (4) *quality patient care.*

This chapter examines these key forces from the standpoint of theory and practices in both *microeconomics* and cost accounting focused on the hospital firm. Health care once derived its processes almost solely from its mission, but now a hospital's *margin* comes first, because without a (*profit*) margin, the organization, like all businesses, ceases to exist, and hence, there is no mission. This chapter in no way provides a comprehensive survey of these interrelated forces but instead offers an explanatory primer, with examples, for a hospital's economic and business behavior. An overview of the disciplines of both microeconomics and cost accounting is provided to acquaint the reader with what is probably an entirely new way of thinking (and talking) about the institution called a hospital. This way, the profession, through the *nurse leaders*, communicates with key nonprovider hospital decision makers, such as the chief executive officer or chief financial officer, with the same language and thus on a level playing field.

▶ Microeconomics, Cost Accounting, and Nursing

This section addresses the question, "What is microeconomics (and, in turn, cost accounting) and what has it to do with nursing?" *Economics*, the study of how society allocates scarce resources, can be divided into two categories, macroeconomics and microeconomics, which are contrasted in **TABLE 3.1**. *Macroeconomics* (the prefix *macro* meaning large) is the study of the market system on a large scale. Microeconomics is the study of individual consumers in relationship to their markets.

Cost accounting is an element of financial management that generates information about the *costs* of an organization and its components. As such, it is a subset of accounting in general and encompasses the development and provision of a wide range of financial management that is useful to managers in their organizational roles. Keep in mind that the goal in generating this information is to provide a basis for decision making. A quintessential question in our field is this: What should the nurse-to-patient ratio be and on what basis is this decided?

The field of cost accounting, borrowing from *financial accounting* (information generated by firms largely for external purposes—e.g., the Internal Revenue Service), while encompassing *managerial accounting* (information generated by firms for their own internal use), affords us tools to address the tough staffing questions, such as break-even analysis, profitability analysis, make-versus-buy decision making, marginal cost calculations, and cost-quality trade-off analysis. The relationship of the accounting disciplines is depicted in **FIGURE 3.1**. It is the considered opinion of the author that these domains—economics and accounting—were once considered mutually exclusive from the field of nursing. Only as the number of nurses undertaking formal study of these quantitative disciplines, such as in Master of Business

TABLE 3.1 Two Categories of Economics

Macroeconomics:	
Considers:	The aggregate performance of all markets, including the outcomes or performance of all companies or firms in all industries
Gives us:	Indices, or measures (indicators), of a nation's economy, such as stock prices, interest rates, jobless claims, and housing starts
Microeconomics:	
Considers:	The choices made by smaller economic units, such as consumers or individual (hospital) firms
Gives us:	Concepts such as profit, profit maximization, price strategy, and nonprice competition to consider

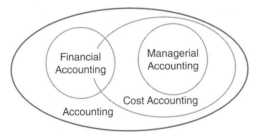

FIGURE 3.1 Relationship of the Accounting Disciplines

Administration (MBA) or Master of Public Health (MPH) programs, increased did our field place itself on equal footing with lay administrators at the top of the hospital hierarchy.

The nurse at the top of the administrative hierarchy, the nurse executive, may have trained with advanced preparation in all three disciplines discussed here: microeconomics, cost accounting, and nursing. The American Organization of Nurse Executives (AONE, 2005) published its view of the core competencies that the nurse executive should have. Among these are analyses of supply and demand data; analysis of financial statements; articulation of business models based on economics, strategic, and business planning; and the development of future business skill sets in leadership team members, all of which are listed under the Business Skills subsection of the AONE's core competencies. This is brought to the attention of the reader to dramatize how important it is for current and future nurse leaders to maintain their own skill set in business and financial matters and to massage this process with key leaders in their organizations, such as *nurse managers*. The deployment of nurse resources at the unit level could quite possibly be the most important decision made in hospital care because it is through the provision of quality nursing care that quality patient outcomes are realized.

Nursing administration, one form of advanced practice (Harris, Huber, Jones, Manojlovich, & Reineck, 2006), is an at-risk specialty, given the numerous reports of dropping enrollment in graduate nursing administration programs (Herrin, Jones, Krepper, Sherman, & Reineck, 2006), a perceived lack of attractiveness of nursing administration as a viable graduate program choice (Rudan, 2002), widespread nurse executive burnout (Rollins, 2008), and the dire situation of the aging nurse faculty workforce (Berlin & Sechrist, 2002). Without this vital specialty, nursing could lose its scientific basis for practice, nurse managers at the unit level might lose recently acquired gains in real autonomy and decision making, and, most of all, research done by nurses on the effectiveness of their measures will continue to be invisible in healthcare quality, health services research, health policy, and healthcare finance initiatives (Lang, 2003). This discussion is an appeal to the reader regarding the uniqueness of the nursing administration specialty, as well as the special challenges afforded the profession if our critical mass of economic and systems thinkers continues to deteriorate.

▶ **Competition**

The *theory of the firm* (the theory of *supply and demand*) explains and predicts price, the quantity of products, and the likelihood of survival of firms in a competitive industry. Before the PPS was introduced into the healthcare market, hospital firms operated on a *cost-plus basis*, billing insurers for the total consumption of resources by an individual patient. After 1983, hospitals were switched to a *diagnosis-related group (DRG)* basis for reimbursement, receiving compensation for what a typical patient within a medical diagnosis and selected other medical conditions would consume. This departure from the cost-plus reimbursement scheme ended the era of price competition in health care, and hospitals began to compete on a nonprice, or quality, basis, which is when patient outcomes magnified in importance.

For centuries, the relationship of the demand for a product or service to its supply has been thought to be largely the result of the intervening variable of price. In the fictional "market for widgets," supply of a product consistently meets the demand for it, given a set of assumptions about the market for *widgets*. This theory (the theory of the firm) explains a lot about the way the world works, pending the strength of these assumptions: large numbers of buyers and sellers, perfect information about the product,

absence of barriers to entry and exit as a business entity in the industry, and homogeneity of the product. Note that a full description of all four assumptions as they pertain to markets for health care is beyond the scope of this text, yet a focus on two of the assumptions—a large number of healthcare buyers and sellers and the existence of good information—is key.

In health care, the four assumptions are less clearly visible than in the fictitious market for widgets for a variety of reasons. Among them are the fact that relatively little is known to the *buyer* of hospital care (the insurance company) about the quality of care purchased from the *seller* (in our case, the hospital), and the demand for hospital care is a *derived* demand. This is to say that it comes from health insurance companies as the intermediary between hospital care providers, such as hospitals, and the individual patient–consumer. When health care entered the competitive arena, decision makers became highly sensitized to the customary business practices of restricting *expenses* and maximizing revenue while producing a service of measurable quality whenever possible.

The change from a system loosely concerned with quality of care, through the professionalism and trust of providers, to a system that prices services strategically while competing on quality has resulted in a cost-conscious era unlike any ever seen before. It is widely recognized that as hospitals compete to provide services, they seek to strike a vital balance between cost reduction and quality of care to adapt successfully to external competitive threats to their survival. In an attempt to successfully adapt, organizations make an effort to (1) optimize profit through pricing strategies, (2) reduce expenses through decisions about personnel and equipment, and (3) achieve reimbursable patient outcomes by satisfying recipients of care through both high tech and caring approaches.

Better care provision (a result of wise resource allocation) may result in better patient outcomes (output), which results in better reimbursement and is alleged to be a benefit of an openly competitive, deregulated hospital market. Hospitals that can demonstrate higher quality of care, or even adequacy of care, will win higher reimbursement, or bids, for reimbursement plans, more patients, and better-qualified care providers. Over time, "good" hospitals will survive because they have established a pattern of good outcomes. The higher the hospital's performance or improvement, the higher the value-based incentive payments.

Additional evidence regarding this theory can be found through such organizations as HealthGrades (see www.healthgrades.com) and *U.S. News and World Report*'s ranking system (see http://health.usnews.com/sections/health/best-hospitals). Both report such measures as risk-adjusted mortality rates, as well as complication rates, such as patient population-specific measures of comparative quality.

In summary, the importance of these hospital ranking systems, or stamps of approval as the public might see them, is this: The information about the quality of the product or service of a hospital is accurate enough to create comparison ratings used by payers as well as by others interested in these data. Hence, the information qualifies as perfect information (not to be taken literally).

What microeconomic theory states regarding the eventual number of hospital firms within an industry under long-run equilibrium (hospitals that are rivals or that compete over the long term) is this: Those hospital firms with better products or services will survive, but those with inferior products and services will not. This is the result of the achievement of quality held by payers and consumers, which, in part, drives the industry's (derived) demand. Unfortunately, relatively little is known about the tenets of competition in health care. More will come to light as variations in the quality of patient outcomes based on reimbursement in hospitals become available in the future. So, the usefulness of this theory for the explanation and prediction of future activities in health care remains challenged. This is not to say that "Supply and demand—it just doesn't work in health care!" is an emotionally charged statement devoid of

reason. It is, instead, appropriate to say that the predictive power of this theory in health care is limited to more than its explanatory power of interpreting the how and why of a hospital firm's behavior. Stated another way, all hospitals seek to maximize patient outcomes/reimbursement and thus maximize performance ratings.

In the world of competitive hospital management, hospitals must innovate with new programs, new patient populations, or quality initiatives to survive and better achieve the continuum of care in the value-based environment. New sources of information on hospital care continually become available in both print and electronic media, so decision makers must be savvy regarding patient outcome comparisons. Just as automobiles are rated for gas consumption and airlines for on-time arrivals, payers and consumers contract for hospital care based on price and quality through *managed care* negotiations.

▶ Regulation and Managed Care

The soaring cost of health care has been one of the most pressing domestic issues for decades. Politicians and pundits speak of how changes in laws could affect this crisis, sometimes provoking a discussion of socialized medicine and cross-country comparison of U.S. versus "other" healthcare expenditures and outcomes. With no clear answer to this type of healthcare ill emerging soon, most would agree that although our healthcare system is among the most market oriented (competitively driven) in the world, it remains *the* most heavily regulated sector of the U.S. economy (Conover, 2004). This author states that the costs of regulation are the benefits we would derive with alternative uses of those resources. After reviewing the literature on 47 different kinds of healthcare regulations, it was estimated that the net burden of health services regulation on society was $169.1 billion annually. For the novice in economic thinking, let's examine what some of the costs of regulation are said to be. In lay terms, it is the sum total of all expenditures by federal or state regulators that oversee, inspect, supervise, monitor, or award privileges to healthcare providers, such as physicians, nurses, and hospitals. In just a quick survey of hospital and nursing regulation costs alone, consider the following:

- The Centers for Medicare and Medicaid Services (CMS) utilization reviews of appropriateness.
- Office of Safety and Health Administration (OSHA) inspection of workplace safety.
- The National Labor Relations Board monitoring of nurse unions.
- National Council of State Boards of Nursing (NCSBN) licensing exam requirements.
- Every state board of nursing, medicine, pharmacy, respiratory therapy, and physical therapy.
- The American Association of Colleges of Nursing (AACN) and the National League for Nursing (NLN) accreditation of nursing schools.
- National Practitioner Data Bank housing information on practitioners.
- Limitations on medical resident or registered nurse (RN) working hours.
- Fraud and abuse protections.

Each one of these organizations or protections has staff, overhead, a place of business to run, and extensive reporting requirements to yet another governmental or quasi-governmental organization. The author makes a convincing case that if health care were deregulated, the cost savings from this could realize gains in health promotion and prevention.

Although in our discussion of rivalry and what hospital firms must do to survive, indeed thrive, a convincing case is made about the benefits of the competitive, or market-driven, environment for hospital care, this is not diametrically opposed to regulatory efforts. This needs to be said because, in essence, a highly competitive market-driven industry is a bit like the polar opposite of one that is highly or completely regulated, as is the case in countries

with a national single-payer health system. In short, the market for hospitals is not what is known as "purely competitive," as is the market for widgets; far from it, in fact. *It holds, instead, a complicated mixture of free-market principles, huge regulatory demands, a demand for sick-care services that is derived and not direct, and the most complicated reimbursement scheme known in modern times in any industry.*

Managed care was originally intended to reduce healthcare costs to the society through the restriction of resource allocation and improve the overall health of individuals. Now, it is a generic term for healthcare payment systems that attempt to control costs and is considered an economic success and a social nightmare. Managed care has, in fact, reduced healthcare costs to society by tying clinical decisions to economic ones that previously were mutually exclusive. In these arrangements, a hospital or group of doctors agrees to provide services in exchange for third-party payment. Managed care networks make available to their members only those providers authorized by the plan. Often, this designation is geographically derived, thereby restricting individuals' choices to go to what they see as the "best" orthopedic or cancer care hospital or doctor if unavailable locally. It is worth mentioning that individuals still have free choice (lots of it)—if they are willing to get out their checkbook!

In managed care, the provider (physician, nurse in advanced practice, or hospital) provides covered services at a discounted rate in exchange for a steady revenue stream. If the novice reading this wonders why providers would "settle for less" by receiving a discounted rate, consider the alternative. Providers would have an uncertain revenue stream that challenges their abilities to cover the basic costs of doing business (reduces *uncertainty*), plus there are few, if any, alternative ways of conducting business, generally speaking. Stated another way, consider what is known as *the first rule of finance*: A dollar today is worth more than a dollar tomorrow, as a result of the time value or opportunity cost of money. That is, any entity that gains revenue in a timely manner not only can retire debt (an asset) but invest; hence, the time value of money is realized. Remember that fee-for-service medicine has all but disappeared, taking with it the old model of the solo-practice physician, and patients who pay out of pocket are rare.

Under a per diem rate agreement, the managed care plan pays the hospital a fixed rate for each day of care, when in fact nurses are in a particularly strategic position to observe that costs per diem to the institution can be (very) variable for one patient stay. Consider the surgical patient who consumes relatively few resources on the morning of admission for a procedure that afternoon. Once the patient enters the operating room, costs to the institution soar steeply and remain high as the patient travels to the postanesthesia recovery room; this can include even more costs if intensive care is involved. For a monthly fee, the hospital must provide the specified services to the third-party payer's enrollees, such as this patient. Under this arrangement, the hospital is ensured money in a relatively timely fashion (based on the average consumption of patients within that DRG and other clinical factors) and the patient–consumer knows he or she will be covered for surgeries that are preapproved.

The overall aim of managed care is to make the patient a better healthcare customer, evaluating whether she or he is getting what she or he is paying for (assuming the individual pays health insurance premiums, which most do). Also, the burden of prevention and wellness increases in importance for the patient, and, presumably, physicians and advanced practice nurses share in this responsibility by virtue of recent changes in medical and nursing education. In this system, the patient has less control over selection of the doctor or hospital and may be responsible for higher deductibles and copayments, as well as penalties for services done outside the network.

From a positive (or factual) point of view, the real cost savings to the healthcare system and society at large are through reduction and *elimination of unnecessary* services, tests, and procedures, as well as time delays through the authorization process where untold numbers of individuals drop off, or attrition out of, the care-seeking process.

▶ Profit Motive and Patient Care

Amid the rhetoric and hysteria regarding hospitals and profit, not enough is said about why a hospital exists. A hospital exists to satisfy the needs of its various stakeholders. Among these are physicians, nurses, and other employees; patients and their families; consumers; researchers; schools of medicine and nursing; and the community at large, to name a few. Although many agree that today's hospitals exist for the provision of sick care, this is not to say there are no other compelling reasons for them to subsist. It is a business entity, and, as such, it responds to many demands from the players, or stakeholders. Among these demands are the volume and morbidity of patients, requests from physicians and nurses in advanced practice for necessary equipment and the efficient flow of patients, concerns from patients and families about inefficient or substandard care, and training opportunities for students of medicine and nursing. The profit motive drives all of these.

In an influential book in its time, *The Profit Motive and Patient Care* (Gray, 1991), the author made the previously unexplored claim that two unique accountability factors exist in health care that do not exist in other organizations: the vulnerability of the consumer (patient) being served and the absence of payers at the point of service. Gray goes on to describe the ways in which the profit motive has come to shape the behavior of all parties, including providers of health care, suppliers of their capital, physicians, employers who provide benefits for their employees, and administrators of health plan benefits. It is this shift in the paradigm of aligning profits with patient care that will shape how providers and purchasers of healthcare service respond to the two great accountability problems.

Gray's explanation of whom the important players (stakeholders) are and how they are motivated to perform has far-reaching implications for the overall philosophical *and* business approaches that healthcare providers, such as nurses, might take. His was among the first credible writings to shake the foundations of why a hospital exists, as well as to articulate the important forces shaping the behavior of the stakeholders.

In this section, it is necessary to debunk some myths still prevailing in certain sections of our society, sometimes even among healthcare providers:

Myth 1: We are a nonprofit entity; we don't have profit.

Myth 2: We are here to provide the highest possible quality of care.

These are among the most important misconceptions forwarded by many stakeholders, among them nurses. Replacing what might be our wishes (myths) with factual statements helps us understand the pervasive economic forces shaping our work and provides resolve for nursing research aims and hypotheses.

Getting the Word Profit Back

The first myth—that of no profit—has hung around for decades. First, it is important to clarify our terminology. Hospitals are now classified as either investor owned (IO), formerly known as "for-profit," or not-for-profit (NFP), formerly known as "nonprofit." All hospitals have profit, *and* each of them chases profit as fast and furiously as the next, period. They may differ on many other factors, chiefly in *how* they approach profit optimization, as well as descriptive characteristics, such as public versus private ownership, urban versus rural, small margin versus large margin, safety net versus nonsafety net, high mortality versus low mortality, and teaching versus non-teaching, to name some. A number of these factors may, in fact, covary with profit status. For example, major teaching hospitals tend to be NFP hospitals, and nearly all IO hospitals

are private, but it is thought that the variable of profit status, and possibly outcomes, is the prime mover of organizational behavior.

Profit, loosely defined as the excess of revenues over expenses, is as necessary to hospitals, irrespective of profit status, as oxygen is to the living system. Almost no hospital could survive without it because it could not remain liquid or solvent. Without it, a hospital eventually goes out of business just like any other entity, leaving services unprovided and employees out of jobs. Profitability, as a construct, is measured by these variables: total margin ratio, operating *profit margin*, nonoperating gain ratio, and return on equity. As you continue reading the next section on the cost inputs for varying levels of quality, keep in mind that costs to the hospital (what is expensed on the hospital's income statement) relative to revenue (money given to the hospital in lieu of care provided) are nearly synonymous with profitability, at least in the short run.

Finally, an accounting note about the differences in IO versus NFP hospitals. In lay terms, the key differences between these two sets of hospitals on the matter of profit goes like this: The dollar line item of profit is found on the income statement of general funds for NFPs versus the profit and loss statement for the corporation; profit is called "profit" in the IO world, versus a "positive fund balance" in the NFP one; and the IO distributes profit (after taxes) at year's end to the shareholders, whereas the NFPs cycle profits back into facility maintenance or expansion after paying no taxes.

Quality of Care: At What Level? At What Cost?

In this chapter's discussion of competition, it was stated that a hospital is *not* in the business of providing the best care money can buy, but that a hospital *is* in the business of providing quality of care at a certain acceptable level where reimbursement is received. It is time to examine why. Measurement of the costs of providing care quality is a function of the cost of providing quality *and* the costs of failing to do so. Lowering quality also has costs to the organization. Besides reimbursement losses, this lowers the quality of care for patients. This can bring about more detrimental effects for patients to deal with, including death, and the organizational reimbursement and reputation suffer; and remember, reputation *is* an asset. So, as lowering quality occurs, this erodes the hospital's competitive position and thus longer-term viability. This cost-quality trade-off explains the behavior of the hospital firm in health care.

In conclusion, what can be said about the profit motive and patient care? Profit, as an incentive, is here to stay. *Profit* is not a dirty word. Furthermore, cost-quality trade-offs drive operational (day-to-day) decisions in all organizations in a competitive industry. Also, cost shifts (costs to the hospital, or expenses) might be borne by the individual, or perhaps the employer, if the individual is discharged prematurely and is too sick to resume employment. Revenues would shift from one governmental organization (such as CMS) to another if they could. And dramatically changing one variable, such as RN staffing, necessitates significant changes in another, such as expenses for other personnel—a topic that will prove essential to our national debate about hospital staffing.

▶ Quality Patient Care

The discussion of profit motive demonstrated how a hospital comes to provide not the best care money can buy but instead an acceptable level of quality. The acceptable level of quality is driven by its cost. Next, to compete on a quality-of-care basis, the hospital must report *measurable* aspects of quality of care—patient outcomes (presumably at an acceptable level)—to various governmental (state health departments and federal agencies) and nongovernmental organizations, such as the Joint Commission. Through processes, such as these, the information about the quality of care in one facility is said to be *perfect information*, a cornerstone of a competitive industry. The information can also be characterized as *symmetric* in

that both the buyer (the insurer) and the seller (the providers) have access to it.

Given the preponderance of information-reporting requirements, it is assumed that hospitals have numerous opportunities for improvement—assuming that these many reporting requirements translate to internal care-improvement processes. Next, through the movement now known as *transparency* (symmetric knowledge), hospitals can bid competitively to purchasers, boasting superior quality outcomes. A third quintessentially important thing this information preponderance gives us is the *incentive* for public programs (e.g., Medicare) and private insurers to reward and reimburse quality of care and efficiency. This incentive program has the overall goal of making hospitals miss reimbursement when they err with never events.

It is essential to note that the *quality and availability of the information* to both buyers and sellers make hospital nonprice competition possible.

Information on Quality and the Risk-Adjustment Process

A time-honored claim that hospitals and other providers have made regarding quality measures in general is that their patient populations contain more *risk* factors than others (e.g., "our patients are sicker"), hence the appearance of "not looking good" to the state or inspection agency. Granted, patient populations from hospital to hospital (or even from doctor to doctor) likely always differ on factors other than the care provided, but, arguably, meaningful points of comparison have been devised by clinical and biostatistical experts within many agencies.

One such agency is California's Office of Statewide Health Planning and Development (OSHPD). California was among the first states to develop a database of risk-adjusted quality measures, and the California Hospital Outcome Project reported to the public for the first time in 1995 and has continuously updated and improved its risk-adjustment processes ever since.

Biostatisticians know that databases this large do, indeed, allow for meaningful points of comparison across hospitals. Generally speaking, risk-adjusted measures of quality of care are in fact useful tools for the comparison of hospitals on the quality of care provided, but imperfectly so. In the California hospital project, for example, the mortality measure was defined as the observed number of deaths from acute myocardial infarction divided by the number of qualifying persons admitted with this primary diagnosis multiplied by the statewide rate. By making the process known to all, agencies such as this assert they have satisfactorily responded to providers' claims about disparate findings based on (unmeasured) risk factors. In fact, on a yearly basis as the press releases come out about new editions of the data, the project offers the opportunity for hospital providers to respond in writing about why their facility "looked worse than expected" in the measures. This way, the project measures are refined yearly, in part on the basis of the responses of participating hospitals. Since inception of this project, the agency has made available other outcome measures, all risk adjusted, that are reflective of common and costly conditions.

Earlier, this chapter expressed the thought that for our profession to be seated at the table of quality initiatives in the context of the hospital business entity, we need expert knowledge of the economic and quality measures being discussed. Furthermore, societal decision makers and gatekeepers, such as the OSHPD and CMS, would benefit from nursing representation to make the hospital measures, now used for reimbursement, meaningful. Fortunately, through the years, as nursing acquired a critical mass of administratively prepared nurses, it has become common for nurse executives from hospitals and/or representatives of our professional societies to be invited to such tables where the decisions are made. Because this was not always the case, it could be considered progress of the profession through acquisition of the same knowledge *and* the same financial language spoken by lay administrators that made this possible. Also look at CMS data.

▶ Healthcare Policy: The Staffing Ratios Debate

The relationship between nurse staffing and patient safety is reasonably well established, especially when patient outcomes, such as medical-surgical mortality rates (Aiken, Smith, & Lake, 1994), acute myocardial infarction mortality rates (Schultz, van Servellen, Litwin, McLaughlin, & Uman, 1997), community-acquired pneumonia mortality rates (Schultz, 2008), failure to rescue (Needleman, Buerhaus, Mattke, Stewart, & Zelevinsky, 2002), and shorter lengths of stay (Lang, Hodge, Olson, Romano, & Kravitz, 2004), to name a few, are considered. How patients fare has long been thought to be due to the result of the number of professional nurse staff available, as well as their preparation, visibility, and experience. Additional organizational variables known to be important include:

- The leadership style of the nurse manager.
- The overall quality of leadership in the institution.
- Whether staffing and other operational decisions are decentralized.
- Physician satisfaction with nursing care.
- The nature of the information system used for patient care.

Research on hospital characteristics and their relationships to patient outcomes has broadened to include additional variables important in the complex relationships of people and technology relative to quality.

Mandated minimum nurse-to-patient staffing ratios were legislated in California in 1999 and implemented January 1, 2004. Also being considered is the importance of having patient classification system data to support the appropriate RN staff requirements. Some of the impetus for the movement toward mandating nurse staffing ratios through governmental and scientific imperatives comes from the challenging conclusions offered by the Institute of Medicine's

(2002) report *To Err Is Human.* This report shook both the scientific and lay communities with its most memorable finding: Between 44,000 and 98,000 deaths occur each year as a result of medical errors. There is hardly a scientific journal that focuses on these types of organizational studies that does not report the influence of nurse staffing, often in the form of RN hours per patient day or RN to all staff hours.

The beginner in politics and policy might ask, "Isn't this a no-brainer? More nurses equals better patient care, right?" Only a fool would disagree. But along the same lines, more police in a neighborhood and fewer pupils per teacher in schools would improve their respective situations, yet these common-sense ideas are difficult to carry out. The following subsections provide the novice nurse–politician some food for thought on the potential implications, or consequences, of such legislation in the context of the (1) operation of a hospital within a community or (2) the market for hospitals as a whole. The implications can be summarized in four parts: hospital operations including closure, feasibility and the nursing shortage, political opportunity costs, and costs to society. The implications—the economic consequences of legislation addressing what staffing *should be* (*normative economics*)—are couched in *positive economics*, or *what is*, factually.

Hospital Operations and Closure

As mentioned previously, the healthcare workforce accounts for at least 50% of a hospital's costs (Kazahaya, 2005). Most of this is nursing personnel costs. Starting with the assumption that some hospitals staff significantly better than the minimum staffing ratios suggest, while some staff significantly lower as a baseline, there is a variance around the regulated minimum ratio (also known as "the floor" ratio). Hospitals staffing well below this floor ratio will experience a rapid rise in *operating expenses* and lost reimbursement, as well as a subsequent drop in operating profit margin. This endangers the hospital's *liquidity* (ability to meet short-term obligations) and

solvency (ability to meet maturing obligations as they become due). Hospitals staffing well above the floor ratio have an incentive to drop nurse staffing levels depending on the cutoff point of where reimbursement is negatively affected, as well as the response to this by their rivals—in other words, it depends on whether neighboring hospitals can afford to remain in business after enactment of this law. Finally, hospitals staffing at about the mandated level may experience no significant change in their financial and, subsequently, business activities, so their staffing may continue as is.

Consider other hospital operations that are disrupted as a consequence of what many nurses thought was a great idea. As reported in *Medical News Report* (2004):

- Elective procedures have been postponed, canceled, or moved to a nearby facility.
- Community hospitals have a more difficult time transferring patients to tertiary care facilities because beds cannot always be staffed.
- Emergency room (ER) wait times have increased.
- ERs have increasingly switched (or requested to switch) to diversion status.
- Night shifts are nearly impossible to staff.
- There is a huge shift to contract (agency or registry) nursing staff, causing a significant rise in expenses, often tens of millions of (unforeseen) dollars in a year.
- The regulations make the hospital increasingly vulnerable to lawsuits, especially on occasions when staffing is less than required.
- When the regulations allow for "licensed" nurses in the equation, RN unions block the effort to fill a void with licensed practical nurse (LPN) hours, thereby inflating union-to-union conflict.

Evidence supporting the view that this mandate was too costly for hospitals to continue operating is seen in the number of hospitals that closed in the years during the implementation phase-in of the California law. Twenty hospitals closed (nine in 2003, eight in 2004, three in 2006; OSHPD, 2006), citing factors on the revenue side of the profitability equation (drop in inpatient revenue and utilization issues). The costs to hospitals of the mandate cannot be underestimated. It is important to note that many forces, both internal and external, cause a business to close and that many of these factors, when they occur simultaneously, push the firm close to the "edge," or more specifically, to the margin. Usually, a hospital firm that closes had both failing business (patient care processes) *and* economic activities (on both revenue and expenditure sides) in the preceding years that ultimately caused its demise. To date, no one empirical effort has isolated the impact of such a law on a hospital's propensity to close due to the complexity of the issues.

Recall from the discussion of profit that when expenses rise in one category, pressure is exerted in the hospital system (or any business) to (1) reduce expenses in another category, (2) make up the expensed activity with an increase in revenue, or (3) both. To formulate a guiding principle on hospital profit-maximizing behavior, Needleman (2008) suggests these questions to consider:

- How much would it cost to increase nurse staffing?
- Would these costs be offset by cost savings from better reimbursement, reduced length of stay (LOS), and fewer complications?
- Would the hospital realize these cost savings, or, because of how the hospital is paid, would these savings be captured by payers?
- Can the hospital attract additional profitable patients on the basis of its nurse staffing?
- Are there cost savings other than those achieved via better patient care that might also be realized if nurse staffing is increased?

So, it should be clear that changing a regulation on the most significant personnel expenditure a hospital budget contains, RN hours, has far-reaching consequences for both hospital business and economic activities. This subsection looks at the core organizational dynamics of a single hospital, which is a very limited aspect of the staffing ratios laws. Even looking at these activities in all hospitals in a state, or in the nation, offers only a partial view of the consequences of mandated ratios as described here. Read on to see how a hospital's behavior cannot be viewed in such a microcosm because of its essential bond to the other subcategories, such as the sporadic nursing shortage.

Feasibility and the Sporadic Nursing Shortage

In the past, hospitals, lawmakers, providers, consumers, and society as a whole were increasingly concerned about the international nursing shortage and its subsequent impact on the quality of care. After implementation of California's safe-staffing law, RN hours per patient day on medical-surgical units rose significantly, perhaps by as much as 21% (Donaldson et al., 2005). Yet the nursing shortage, predicted to be a deficit of 400,000 RNs by 2020 (Buerhaus, Needleman, Mattke, & Stewart, 2002), continued to beg the question of where the nursing hours came from. Over decades, it was a longstanding principle of hospital staffing to "borrow" nurse hours from unit to unit to (1) satisfy short-term patient care demands—for example, a number of new admissions arriving at the same time as intensive care unit transfers—and (2) satisfy regulatory and reporting requirements. Patient care demands may have been met, whereas regulatory and reporting requirements almost certainly were.

Many obstacles hinder compliance with mandated staffing requirements. Consider these real-world examples from *Medical News Report* (2004):

- Hospitals may start a shift in compliance but not end that shift in compliance.
- Hospitals may start and end a shift in compliance, but the middle of the shift is in question.
- Nurse recruitment efforts have been accelerated but often are not associated with the desired result of satisfactory staffing.

- California's law requires nurses to be on standby to cover breaks for bedside nurses, which is a requirement that is practically impossible to meet.
- Penalties exist for noncompliance.
- Nurses increasingly report not taking their breaks, given the lack of coverage while they are to be gone.
- Hospitals could be held *criminally* liable for adverse outcomes in the context of staffing that is less than required by mandate, even in view of evidence of the intent to comply.

These remarks point to regional shortages within one hospital, which carry yet another set of concerns for patient safety. Chiefly, these concerns are costs associated with noncompliance, nurse recruitment (especially as nurses from outside the country are involved), and legal defense. Also, there were no accompanying changes in the revenue side of the hospitals' profit equation. The examples offered in this subsection highlight merely a few of the difficulties hospitals are having with the mandate. Additional issues include workplace safety, nurse injuries, nurse dissatisfaction, turnover, and the propensity to stay in current positions. This subsection emphasizes only some of the more immediate feasibility issues posed by such regulations. And this does not take into account how this will affect reimbursement.

Political Opportunity Costs for Nursing

Highly publicized political wars have taken place, most notably in California and New York, over the staffing ratios debate. Both states had nurse unions that were successful in getting legislation sponsored that evolved into state-wide acute care hospital staffing mandates, but at what political cost? California's 12-year battle (California Nurses Association, n.d.) spanned the reign of two governors, and New York's campaign (Gerardi, 2006) was similarly protracted, both being punctuated by statewide town hall meetings, numerous "call to action" alerts to other professional societies, consumption of resources of nursing associations of all types, and bad press labeling nurses as unyielding and self-serving. In California, such ill will attracted national attention when Governor Arnold Schwarzenegger summarily dismissed both the nurses union's leadership and membership, *as well as* nurses in general by calling nurses "a special interest group" that is just angry because "I kick their butt" (Marinucci, 2004).

These campaigns occurred just as the state of the research was judged *not* to categorically support the thesis of better care provision through more RNs in each case. In fact, the research results are mixed (Burnes Bolton et al., 2007), reporting that although a clear and consistent rise in nurse staffing did exist post-regulation in California, it was not accompanied by a commensurate rise in quality as measured by significantly fewer falls or pressure ulcers. In a study reported by Mark and Harless (2007), a superior distribution of outcomes (mortality and LOS) with a *lower* level of RN staffing was found. In sum, the evidence points to the prevailing conclusion that there is a strong, but not yet totally conclusive, case for an impact of nurse staffing on mortality (Needleman & Buerhaus, 2003) and other adverse outcomes.

If you believe, as some do, that science drives policy and legislation—and that's a leap—you have now identified a gap between just what we recommend on the matter of staffing mandates (the normative economic view) and a recommendation accompanied by a cogent economic rationale (the positive economic position) and plan. Stated another way, consider the words of Keepnews (2007, p. 236):

> Ongoing research on the impact of nurse staffing regulation can yield important information that can guide continued staffing policy efforts. Understanding the impact of such efforts should include evaluating the outcomes of recent legislation in Oregon and Illinois as well as continued examination of staffing ratios

in California. Successful efforts will need to transcend traditional boundaries between researchers, policy analysts, advocates, and organizations.

Costs to Society

Social policy is the domain that aims to improve human welfare and to meet human needs for education, health, housing, and social security. Health is a part of public policy that has to do with social issues. There was a time when *health* was considered the absence of disease. Couple this limited definition of health with the Hippocratic admonition "to do no harm" to identify what the public expects from a hospital: to emerge from the experience with an improved state of health or, at a minimum, to avoid increased morbidity *as a result of* seeking hospital care. Although it is touted as a modern concept, we would do well to remember that the Hippocratic admonition regarding harm emerged centuries ago (Hippocrates, n.d./2004). Previously, it was noted that, at a minimum, quality care is identified as the absence of adversity or the absence of adverse events.

The costs to society of this adversity are understudied or underreported in modern health services research. The costs to society include, but are not limited to, the alternative use of hospital resources in a community (e.g., feeding the poor, housing the homeless), consumption of a tax basis (in the case of NFP hospitals) for the same, the costs of ill health for individuals and employers (such as the opportunity cost of lost time and productivity at work), unreimbursed expenses related to caring for the underinsured or the uninsured, and the alternative use of people and technology resources in other employment. This subsection briefly lists some questions for further study in the context of the costs to society of mandated staffing ratios with respect to the latter two factors—the function and purpose of safety net hospitals and the opportunity realized in the operation of a hospital in a community context.

Safety Net Hospitals

Defined as hospitals disproportionately serving vulnerable, including financially vulnerable, populations, *safety net hospitals* also experienced a sustained significant rise in nurse hours after enactment of safe staffing ratios. It is inaccurate to assume that a higher nurse-to-patient ratio affects the financial structure of hospitals the same way across the board. Safety net hospitals, by definition, are at-risk institutions that have consistently been financially vulnerable organizations when viewed from the revenue side of the profit equation. With large numbers of underinsured or uninsured patients, they have no position from which to compete on price and may not have the resources to compete on the basis of quality. It would stand to reason that although they budget for *bad debt expense*, this line item varies considerably because it is volume dependent and sensitive to changes in the macroeconomic condition. In short, when the region of its location "has a bad year," this institution has an even worse one! It is close to impossible for such a hospital to court more attractive (paying) patients not only because of geography but because of poor internal economic conditions, including liquidity crises.

Having just stated that the competitive position of these hospitals is weak to begin with (they are less able to compete on the basis of price or quality), it stands to reason that they run a high risk of closure, particularly in view of the fact that the patient-to-nurse mandate obliges them to spend more on nurse staffing. With this loss of flexibility to vary the nursing skill mix comes inefficient allocation of scarce resources and an inability to make trade-offs in other hospital services. The subsequent drop in operating profit margin (and perhaps other measures of profitability) could easily cause negative consequences for patients, such as premature discharge, recidivism, and higher complication rates. With the Medicare pay for performance structure, it is easy to see the handwriting on the wall for such environments, with closure looming in the future.

As providers, especially safety net hospital providers, struggle with these enmeshed issues of geographic limitations, a tangible floor in revenue, and dropping profit margins in light of rising bad debt expenses, it is no wonder that the hospital executive has an eye on cash flow relative to debt (cash flow-to-debt ratio) because it is *the* prime predictor of hospital closure. Once again, without a margin there is no mission, despite outcries that health care is a right. Is it? If yes, who pays for it?

A Hospital Firm Within a Community Context

Recall that in the subsections on hospital operations and the nursing shortage, a number of questions were raised relevant to reducing or delaying services (diversion to neighboring ERs), the potential for a hospital to realize other cost savings as RN hours rise (better reimbursement, some *economies of scale*, perhaps, with nursing duties in common with nonlicensed personnel), and the costs to the hospital of recruiting and retaining nurses. The following are some questions posed by the author when considering the impact of such a *government intervention* on small-margin hospitals. Bear in mind that small-margin hospitals include those considered safety net hospitals or those classified as rural.

- Will there be a drop in the employees' *total compensation package*, say, a reduction in health benefits or a rise in premium prices, in an effort to offset the rise in operating expenditures?
- As the line item for RN hours increases, what happens to the expenditures for non-professional nurses and ancillary nursing personnel?
- As these nonprofessional nurse budgets get trimmed, will it be necessary to start outsourcing programs in preparation for layoffs?
- As resources become more constrained, what is the subsequent impact on measurable levels of quality? On reimbursement?

- What is the effect of the change in levels of quality on managed care contract negotiations? In short, will the insurer continue to send covered lives to a facility thought or known to be substandard?
- As measurable levels of quality are affected, what is the impact of this on the hospital's creditworthiness?
- As the hospital's creditworthiness is adversely affected, how compromised is the hospital in borrowing, even in the short term, to meet economic obligations, such as employee wages and other compensatory line items? How will a hospital's payment to its suppliers be affected?
- If the hospital does, in fact, close, what is the impact of this event on the unemployment rate in the surrounding community, especially if the hospital is the largest employer around?
- If the hospital closes, what are the costs to society of airlifting or otherwise transporting the most critical of cases to the appropriate environment of care?

As decision makers in small-margin hospitals wrestle with these tough questions, it remains whether the charge "well, it's a hospital that *should* have closed anyway" is defensible. This discussion does not provide an answer to such normative queries. Instead, the measures (or variables) necessary to construct an individual answer are offered from the logical positivist (factual) economic view.

In concluding this discussion of one of the most challenging healthcare policy questions of modern times, mandated nurse staffing ratios, it is important to remember some guiding principles from positive economics—that is, costs shift, revenues shift, and this will *always* be the case. Costs and revenues shift both within and outside the hospital firm. As in the case of borrowing nurse hours from unit to unit to "look good" or claim compliance with such mandates, what is the subsequent impact on patient care on the unit from which the borrowing occurred? As each hospital chases profit, how long will it continue to play the shell game of shifting ER patients from one safety net hospital to another or allowing premature discharge? This last causes recidivism that results in no reimbursement if patients are readmitted within a month for the same problem. Finally, as far as costs to society are concerned, how is the health of a region or the nation affected by the loss of hospitals that fail seemingly from the economic or quality point of view?

▶ The Business Case: Electronic Health Record Systems in Hospitals

Although information systems, including the electronic health record (EHR), are considered essential to the quality and efficiency of our healthcare system as a whole, the high cost of these systems is prohibitive in successful widespread implementation, especially in hospitals. Vital to daily operations, these systems proclaim to bring many benefits, such as safety, accessibility, retrievability, and convenience. They are a major organizational investment, especially with respect to startup costs (the initial one-time expenses), not to mention the ongoing costs of annual licensing fees, updates, and maintenance to dedicated servers. This section discusses some costs, some benefits, the relationship of these costs and benefits, and the elements of a successful business case for a hospital's EHR system. As done previously, this section offers the reader some measures (variables) to consider when idealizing that healthcare systems, especially hospitals, *ought* to have a computerized record-keeping and decision-support system.

Clinical information systems that computerize the documentation of physicians, nurses, and other care providers, now nearly 20 years old, hold the promise of numerous benefits— for the healthcare system or hospital, for the patient, and for the health of the nation. Among

them are patient safety, accessibility, legibility, process-adherence evidence, data-mining capabilities (Manjoney, 2004), retrievability, convenience, and a reduction in indirect care time. The downside is that privacy issues, costs including upgrades, data transfer inaccuracies, implementation problems, and so on occur. Like the previous section on legislative mandates for professional nurse staffing, the desirability of successful EHR implementation, ongoing maintenance, and subsequent upgrades ensure that the integrity of the system is intact. This could be considered a no-brainer in that more time could be devoted to bedside care and thus generate better patient outcomes, such as fewer medication errors and increased patient satisfaction. However, this is more complex due to ongoing maintenance and subsequent upgrades (including staff time and additional expense) that ensure the integrity of the system.

Costs for the Hospital

The major costs in acquiring an EHR system include the costs of hardware, software, networking, maintenance, installation, and training, as well as opportunity costs (Agrawal, 2002). Direct costs, such as training time, hardware, software, salary, and support fees, are expensed on the hospital's income statement, and big-ticket items, such as the hardware and contracted software, are listed as assets on the balance sheet and depreciated over their useful life. This is a way of spreading out the tremendous cost outlay over time. This is also a way to pair these economic activities with the business or strategic plans the organization might have to determine an asset's future benefits. For example, an EHR system is known to be associated with increasing patient satisfaction and reductions in risk-adjusted mortality or complication rates. It is possible that these improved patient outcomes could be leveraged in a hospital's managed care contract negotiations with insurers. This matching of economic and business activities begins the process of identifying the benefits of the technology relative to its costs.

Indirect costs, those expenses associated with ongoing operational costs, include software maintenance and support fees, salaries for support staff, fees related to space and utilities (Nahm, Vaydia, Ho, Scharf, & Seagull, 2007), and the expenses of safety/security measures. Note that all costs mentioned thus far are borne by the health care-providing institution—in this case, the hospital. The next section, however, discusses that the benefits are shared by more than just this one entity.

Benefits for the Hospital and Patients

Implementation of a system has both tangible and intangible benefits, further complicating a discussion of the dynamics of benefits and costs. Some tangible benefits are concrete measurable gains derived directly from the EHR system, further expanded in the next paragraph. The intangible, or hard-to-quantify, benefits are such things as patient and user satisfaction and safety, increased compliance with federal or state regulations, decreased staff turnover, future leverage derived from the same, and hospital reputation.

Other difficult-to-calculate benefits include reduced resource use (partially from reduced LOS), improved quality through convenient access to information at the point of care, enhanced data capture, enhanced business management, and improved legal compliance with subsequent reduction in claims. In an econometric model making the

business case for electronic medical records (EMR) implementation, Kaiser Permanente justified the costs for an inpatient EMR system through such benefits as increased RN and medical records efficiency; decreased RN overtime; reduced lab expenses, chart review time, and physical therapy wait time along with reduced inappropriate admissions, avoidable days, ER diverts, forms expenses, and medical records supplies; fewer adverse drug events; and redeployment of space (Garrido, Raymond, Jamieson, Liang, & Wiesenthal, 2004). On the revenue side, improved coding accuracy for Medicare risk was mentioned.

Here is where we see a shared-benefit situation. In the case of adverse drug events, the hospital realizes as much as a 2.2-day reduced LOS for those events associated with injury. The patient is spared the inconvenience of the same amount of time, plus the reduced opportunity cost of further morbidity from hospital-acquired conditions and, presumably, a shortened recuperation time with subsequent earlier return to work or productivity. At this point, the patient, the family, and the employer begin to share the benefits that resulted from costs incurred by only the hospital in the business case model. Yet if this is in keeping with a hospital or healthcare organization's mission, the business model is said to be a successful one.

Many different ways of calculating the hospital's return on investment (ROI), the benefits in relation to costs, exist. (See **BOX 3.1**.) Among these are *net present value (NPV)*, payback analysis, and break-even analysis. In each of these, many

---

BOX 3.1 Definitions

Cost-to-benefit analysis compares the cost of program goals that are being considered to the cost of implementing the proposed venture's benefits. If the benefits are greater than the cost, you have a positive cost benefit. A cost-benefit example can be found in Trepanier Early, Ulrich, and Cherry (2012).

Return on investment (ROI) simply calculates the bottom line from your investments in the assets used for the investment—for example, positive ROI of 6% on the investment. Examples of ROI can be found in Pine and Tart (2007).

Break-even analysis identifies the cost and number of units that must be sold at a minimum to recover the fixed costs. This is defined further in Chapters 12 and 16.

other influences must be assessed simultaneously, making the ROI analysis, by definition, very complicated. Among these are inflation, deflation, changes in business and strategic goals, shifts in healthcare management methods, and changes in Medicare reimbursement rates. Well beyond the scope of this text, econometric models identifying the multiple simultaneous influences on a successful analysis of this sort yield a partial solution for justifying the enormous outlay of costs for such information technology projects as EMR. Executive administration would do well to cost-out both sides of the analysis in the short, intermediate, and long terms.

Conventional wisdom leaves little doubt about the ability of information technology to improve clinical outcomes, but equally compelling evidence of the positive financial return of the same has yet to be established. Because the trend in reimbursement mechanisms continues to move toward outcomes achieved, technology may prove to be beneficial. However, equally compelling is pay for performance limiting reimbursements, the downturn in the U.S. economy, and security issues and other unexpected negative side effects of technology. Large purchases may continue not to be good business decisions. This means that there are currently inadequate incentives for hospitals to act on this important aspect of the hospital infrastructure, especially when many of the benefits are difficult to quantify and forecast, not to mention government intervention. This also means that as incentive programs to reward early adoption of technology or other innovations and quality of care are realized, they will act as a catalyst for the implementation of large-scale EMR projects in hospitals everywhere.

Summary

In conclusion, healthcare information systems play a central role in both the quality of care and daily operations (Nahm et al., 2007). They are extraordinarily expensive, even when the potential benefits are considered. Recall some of the lessons learned in this chapter's discussion of profit seeking: Costs shift, revenues shift, and this will *always* be the case. Costs and revenues shift both within and outside the hospital firm, as do costs and benefits, as shown. This is the factual view for any big-ticket item that a hospital might consider (such as substantially increasing professional nurse staffing or EHR implementation). This chapter does not provide an answer to normative queries on whether an EHR system *should be* implemented. Instead, the measures (or variables) necessary to construct an individual answer are offered from the logical positivist (factual) economic view.

As each healthcare organization addresses the issue of widespread implementation of an EMR, it will be increasingly important for decision makers to evaluate the nuances of their own business cases. Given that many factors obscure the construction of a clear business case for EMR, hospitals are forced to consider the *avoidance of an expense* (e.g., future litigation costs, less reimbursement if pay for performance mandates are not met) as parallel with *actual expense reduction* (including less reimbursement, if that has already occurred), especially in the short term. Similarly, they are forced to identify benefits that are realized by the hospital, as well as those gained by the individual patient, his or her employer, or society as a whole. The propensity of a hospital to invest this way will likely be enhanced by the changing CMS rules on nonreimbursement for selected hospital complications. Forcing a hospital to pay for its own mistakes, such as certain hospital-acquired infections, raises the question of what type of electronic system it will take to capture the processes associated with these adverse outcomes for purposes of both quality improvement and revenue sustainability.

This chapter offers background information on the nature of competition and why it is important in the market for hospital care. In the discussion of profit motive and patient care, the reader was asked to join in debunking some myths about why a hospital exists to fulfill its purpose—to satisfy the needs of various stakeholders, such as employees, the community at large, as well as patients and providers, such as physicians and nurses. The regulatory arena was addressed last in the context of the hospital system as a dynamic microcosm of activity affected, sometimes dramatically, by legislative and societal mandates, such as safe staffing laws. All of this reflects the complexity of the system.

Some of this monetary analysis is, in fact, a brand new way of thinking for those who have not studied formally in the fields of economics, accounting, or finance. It is hoped that, through this examination of what it takes for a hospital firm to survive competitive circumstances, future cohorts of nurses can preserve the only sustained hospital foundation—the practice of professional nursing. As stated by Buerhaus et al. (2002), "Nursing matters greatly in the hospitals' ability to provide quality of care and prevent avoidable adverse outcomes" (p. 130). The prevention of avoidable adversity is going to contribute most significantly to the survival of hospital firms through the coming years.

Most of the statements on hospital conditions and the business activities therein are from the domain of positive economics ("what is" or "what exists"), leaving the reader to draw his or her conclusions in the normative economic ("what *should* be") field of endeavor. Nursing's history, of course, has been to embrace the *mission* of caring, often with less investment in the *impact* of ideals, such as safe staffing on the hospital's *margin*. The chapter-opening quote, "No margin, no mission" (quoted in Langley, 1998), focused discussion on the consequences of nursing's advocacy. This is to say that without a sustainable *margin* of profit, a hospital, like all businesses, fails to provide service, employ personnel, pay its suppliers, or fulfill its *mission*.

Discussion Questions

1. Support or refute the statement "Well, supply and demand . . . it just doesn't work in health care!"
2. Discuss how margin and mission are related, or not related, in the hospital environment.
3. Frame some arguments for or against the policy of mandated minimum staffing ratios in the positive versus normative economic dichotomy.
4. Are hospitals competing on the basis of price, quality, or both? Explain.
5. Is hospital care overregulated? Cite some examples to support your argument.
6. What is healthcare regulation and what are some of its costs?
7. Why is the provision of sick care (hospital) services said to be a *derived* demand?
8. Should there be minimum safe staffing ratios—from the standpoint of the patient? Why or why not?
9. Should there be minimum safe staffing ratios—from the standpoint of the hospital? Why or why not?
10. Should there be minimum safe staffing ratios—from the standpoint of the profession? Why or why not?
11. From an economic perspective, describe the cost of regulation in the healthcare environment.
12. What is your definition of profit?

Glossary of Terms

American Nurses Credentialing Center the world's largest and most influential nurse credentialing organization and a subsidiary of the American Nurses Association. American Nurses Credentialing Center is best known for promoting excellence in practice through its Magnet Recognition Program and Pathways to Excellence Program.

Asymmetric Knowledge a state or condition in which buyers and sellers of a product or service have significantly different sets of information.

Bad Debt Expense accounts receivable that will likely remain uncollectible and will be written off. It is a line item for which the hospital budgets.

Buyer one who purchases healthcare services; often the health insurance company.

Competition the efforts of two or more parties to gain the business of a third by offering preferably favorable terms.

Cost the dollar value of inputs used in the production of goods and services (output). Types of costs are variously termed and defined. These include direct, indirect, medical, nonmedical, future, intangibles, fixed, variable, marginal, and opportunity. Not to be confused with *expenses;* it is a broader term.

Cost Accounting an element of financial management that generates information about the costs of an organization and its components. A subset of accounting, in general. Encompasses the development and provision of a wide range of financial information useful to managers in their roles.

Diagnosis-Related Groups (DRGs) Medicare initiated payment to hospitals on this basis beginning in 1984. The prices for the groups are updated yearly by Medicare to reflect changes in reimbursement protocols.

Economics the study of how a society allocates scarce resources and goods.

Economies of Scale also known as "returns to scale," it is the degree to which the cost of providing a good or service falls as quantity (measured by patient days) increases because fixed costs are shared by the larger volume of units.

Expense a more exact concept than *cost*; the exact dollar amount a firm spends on a unit of production. Divided into two major types on a hospital's income statement, there are operating expenses (direct line items for the cost of inputs) and nonoperating expenses (less directly assigned costs—e.g., overhead).

Financial Accounting system that records historical financial information and provides summary reports to individuals outside of the organization of what financial events have occurred and what the financial impact of those events has been.

Firm the company, the hospital.

Government Intervention actions on the part of government that affect economic activity, resource allocation, and especially free choice regarding the purchase of products or services.

Healthcare Economics economics concerned with issues related to scarcity in the allocation of health and healthcare service provision.

Incentive reward to an organization or individual for a behavior. Differs from *motive*, which is a psychological term describing an inner state.

Liquidity ability of a firm to meet its short-term financial obligations—that is, pay bills as they become due.

Macroeconomics a branch of economics concerned with how human behavior affects outcomes in highly aggregated markets, such as the markets for labor or consumer products. In the healthcare context, the behavior of all hospital firms.

Managed Care a system that manages healthcare delivery with the aim of controlling costs. Typically reliant on a physician or nurse in advanced practice, the clinical activity is paired with the economic activity that is thought to reduce frivolous expenses and moral hazard.

Managerial Accounting the process of identifying, analyzing, interpreting, and communicating financial information so that an organization can pursue its goals. Differs from financial accounting in that it is an internal process, whereas financial accounting focuses on reporting financial activity to an outside source.

Margin the point at which one more unit of input no longer yields one more unit of output—instead it yields less.

Microeconomics a branch of economics concerned with the behavior of individuals and a (hospital) firm. The activities of individuals and businesses with regard to the allocation of resources and the production and distribution of goods and services.

Mission a healthcare organization's raison d'être; why it says it exists.

Motive internal psychological state of arousal propelling a person (or organization) to approach a goal.

Net Present Value (NPV) future stream of benefits and costs converted into equivalent values today. Today's value of an investment's future net cash flow minus the initial investment.

Normative Economics judgments about "what ought to be" in economic matters. By definition, they cannot be proved false because they are based on assessments, but they can (and should) be supported by facts or positive economics to be most useful.

Nurse Manager supervisory nurse who has complete operational and financial authority for a unit or units on a 24/7 basis; her or his practice is said to be decentralized.

Operating Expenses line-item entries on the income statement traceable to a hospital's day-to-day business—for example, salaries and bad debt expense. These are different from nonoperating expenses, such as insurance and maintenance of equipment.

Perfect Information a state of complete knowledge about the product of a firm and possibly the actions of other players in it. Not to be taken literally, it is the basis for the purchase of a certain volume of products at a particular price.

Positive Economics study of "what is" in economic relationships.

Profit the excess of revenue over expenses.

Profit Margin the excess of revenue over expenses divided by total revenue. An index of the amount of profit generated by each dollar of revenue.

Prospective Payment System (PPS) introduced by the federal government in 1983, a system by which Medicare reimburses hospitals at a predetermined rate, largely based on discharge medical diagnoses, for its patients. Aimed at influencing hospital behavior through financial incentives that encourage more cost-efficient care, the hospital receives a flat-rate reimbursement for a DRG into which each patient falls based on clinical information, such as age, gender, and comorbidities for a medical diagnosis, irrespective of the actual consumption of services.

Regulation a form of government intervention designed to shape the behavior of an economic entity, whether organizations or individuals. Healthcare providers, such as physicians, nurses, and hospitals are said to be highly regulated, referring to such things as approval by boards of medicine or nursing and licensure by states.

Risk state of uncertainty containing possible adversity or undesired outcomes. If quantifiable, this expectation of loss is said to carry a certain probability.

Seller economic agents who are accountable for the production and sale of healthcare services— for example, the hospital.

Solvency ability of a firm to meet its maturing obligations as they become due.

Symmetric Knowledge knowledge about a hospital's performance (patient outcomes) possessed by both the healthcare buyer and seller.

Total Compensation Package the sum total of an employee's payment for services rendered, including salary and benefits.

Uncertainty lack of certainty, either subjective or objective. It differs from risk in that it cannot be easily quantified.

Widget an abstract unit of production.

References

Agrawal, A. (2002). Return of investment analysis for a computer-based patient record in the outpatient clinical setting. *Journal of the Association for Academic Minority Physicians, 13*(3), 61–65.

Aiken, L., Smith, H., & Lake, E. (1994). Lower Medicare mortality among a set of hospitals known for good nursing care. *Medical Care, 32*, 771–787.

American Organization of Nurse Executives. (2005). *The AONE Nurse Executive Competencies.* Retrieved from www.aone.org/resources/leadership%20tools/PDFs/AONE_NEC.pdf

Berlin, L., & Sechrist, K. (2002). The shortage of doctorally-prepared nurse faculty: A dire situation. *Nursing Outlook, 50*, 50–56.

Buerhaus, P., Needleman, J., Mattke, S., & Stewart, M. (2002). Strengthening hospital nursing. *Health Affairs, 21*, 123–132.

Burnes Bolton, L., Aydin, C., Donaldson, N., Brown, D., Sandhu, M., Fridman, M., et al. (2007). Mandated nurse staffing ratios in California: A comparison of staffing and nursing-sensitive outcomes pre- and postregulation. *Policy, Politics & Nursing Practice, 8*, 238–250.

California Nurses Association. (n.d.). *CNA's 12-year campaign for safe RN staffing ratios.* Retrieved from http://www.nationalnursesunited.org/page/-/files/pdf/ratios/12yr-fight-0104.pdf

Conover, C. (2004, October 4). Health care regulation: A $169 billion hidden tax. *Policy Analysis, 527*. Retrieved from http://www.cato.org/pubs/pas/pa527.pdf

Donaldson, N., Bolton, L., Aydin, C., Brown, D., Elashoff, J., & Sandhu, M. (2005). Impact of California's licensed nurse–patient ratios on unit-level nurse staffing and patient outcomes. *Policy, Politics & Nursing Practice, 6*, 198–210.

Garrido, T., Raymond, B., Jamieson, L., Liang, L., & Wiesenthal, A. (2004). Making the business case for hospital information systems—a Kaiser Permanente investment decision. *Journal of Healthcare Finance, 31*(2), 16–25.

Gerardi, T. (2006). Staffing ratios in New York: A decade of debate. *Policy, Politics & Nursing Practice, 7,* 8–10.

Gray, B. (1991). *The profit motive and patient care: The changing accountability of doctors and hospitals.* Cambridge, MA: Harvard University Press.

Harris, K., Huber, D., Jones, R., Manojlovich, M., & Reineck, C. (2006). Future nursing administration graduate curricula, Part 1. *Journal of Nursing Administration, 36,* 435–440.

Herrin, D., Jones, K., Krepper, R., Sherman, R., & Reineck, C. (2006). Future nursing administration graduate curricula, Part 2: Foundation and Strategies. *Journal of Nursing Administration, 36,* 498–505.

Hippocrates. (n.d./2004). Book 1, Section 2. (F. Adams, Trans.). In *Of the epidemics* (p. 5). Kessinger Publishing.

Institute of Medicine. (2002). *To err is human: Building a safer health system.* Washington, DC: National Academy Press.

Kazahaya, G. (2005). Harnessing technology to redesign labor cost management reports. *Healthcare Financial Management, 59*(4), 94–100.

Keepnews, D. (2007). Evaluating nurse staffing regulation. *Policy, Politics & Nursing Practice, 8,* 236–237.

Lang, N. (2003). Reflections on quality health care. *Nursing Administration Quarterly, 27,* 266–272.

Lang, T., Hodge, M., Olson, V., Romano, P., & Kravitz, R. (2004). Nurse–patient ratios: A systematic review on the effects of nurse staffing on patient, nurse, employee, and hospital outcomes. *Journal of Nursing Administration, 34,* 326–337.

Langley, M. (1998, January 7). Nuns' zeal for profits shapes hospital chain, wins Wall Street fans. *The Wall Street Journal,* pp. A1, A11.

Manjoney, R. (2004). Clinical information systems market— an insider's view. *Journal of Critical Care, 19,* 215–220.

Marinucci, C. (2004, December 8). A tribute for women, Schwarzenegger angers nurses. *San Francisco Chronicle,* p. A1.

Mark, B., & Harless, D. (2007). Nurse staffing, mortality, and length of stay in for-profit and not-for-profit hospitals. *Inquiry, 44,* 167–186.

Medical News Report. (2004, February). *New nurse-to-patient ratios present challenges in California.* Retrieved from

http://www.nursingworld.org/MainMenuCategories /Policy-Advocacy/State/Legislative-Agenda-Reports /State- StaffingPlansRatios

Nahm, E., Vaydia, V., Ho, D., Scharf, B., & Seagull, J. (2007). Outcomes assessment of clinical information system implementation: A practical guide. *Nursing Outlook, 55,* 282–288.

Needleman, J. (2008). Is what's good for the patient good for the hospital? Aligning incentives and the business case for nursing. *Policy, Politics & Nursing Practice, 9,* 80–87.

Needleman, J., & Buerhaus, P. (2003). Nurse staffing and patient safety: Current knowledge and implications for action. *International Journal for Quality in Health Care, 15,* 275–277.

Needleman, J., Buerhaus, P., Mattke, S., Stewart, M., & Zelevinsky, K. (2002). Nurse-staffing levels and the quality of care in hospitals. *New England Journal of Medicine, 346,* 1715–1722.

Office of Statewide Health Planning and Development. (2006). *Hospital closures in California.* Retrieved from www.calhealth.org

Pine, R., & Tart, K. (2007, January–February). Return on investment: Benefits and challenges of a baccalaureate nurse residency program. *Nursing Economic$, 25*(1), 13–19, 39.

Rollins, G. (2008). CNO burnout. *Hospitals & Health Networks, 82*(4), 30–34.

Rudan, V. (2002). Where have all the nursing administration students gone? Issues and solutions. *Journal of Nursing Administration, 32,* 185–188.

Schultz, M. (2008, July). *The association of hospital structural and financial characteristics to mortality from community-acquired pneumonia.* Paper presented at the Congress on Nursing Research of Sigma Theta Tau International, Singapore.

Schultz, M., van Servellen, G., Litwin, M., McLaughlin, E., & Uman, G. (1997). Can hospital structural and financial characteristics explain the variations in hospital mortality caused by acute myocardial infarction? *Applied Nursing Research, 12,* 210–214.

Trepanier, S., Early, S., Ulrich, B., & Cherry, B. (2012, July–August). New graduate nurse residency program: A cost-benefit analysis based on turnover and contract labor usage. *Nursing Economic$, 30*(4), 207–214.

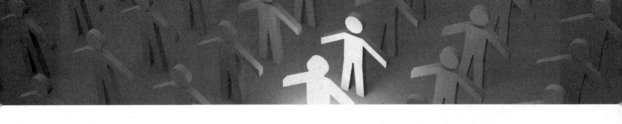

CHAPTER 4

Providing Patient Value While Achieving Quality, Safety, and Cost-Effectiveness

J. Michael Leger, PhD, MBA, RN, **Sandy K. Diffenderfer**, PhD, MSN, RN, CPHQ, **Janne Dunham-Taylor**, PhD, RN, **Karen W. Snyder**, MSN, RN, and **Dru Malcolm**, DNP, MSN, RN, NEA-BC, CPHRM

OBJECTIVES

- Articulate the goal of quality patient care.
- Explain the four most important hospital strategies to be implemented to prepare for value-based payments.
- Describe administrative practices that support performance improvement efforts.
- Analyze the nurse leader's role in patient safety.
- Propose ways that nurse leaders can promote evidence-based practice.
- Synthesize how nurse leaders can promote patient value while achieving quality, safety, and cost-effectiveness.

▶ Introduction

The most important priority in all healthcare settings is to determine what the patient wants and values; to provide safe, loving, quality care; and to constantly improve care delivery and continuity across the continuum in a cost-effective way. This is true for staff and physicians at the point of care and for administrators in all decisions and actions.

This is a demanding goal! Thankfully, at times it is achieved. When this goal is met, the patient and caregivers recognize that it was worth the effort. As healthcare payments are transformed from volume-based to value-based reimbursement over the next decade (American Hospital Association 2011 Committee on Performance Improvement [AHA], 2011), this goal *must* be met.

There are four significant challenges and related goals confronting contemporary health care that are the focus of this chapter (**BOX 4.1**):

1. **To habitually determine what our patient/client/resident wants and values.** Healthcare workers often miss the goal related to this challenge. Many individuals in health care do not know how to discover what the patient wants and values. Often, workers are focused only on the current care setting rather than continuity across the continuum. Determining what the patient wants and values needs to be assessed by staff at the point of care. In addition, everyone in the organization from board members and the chief executive officer (CEO) to the nurse aide and housekeeper should make regular rounds to speak and interact with patients to determine whether their needs are being met. Often, healthcare workers are not good listeners; active listening must begin with those in administrative roles because executive leaders set the tone for the organization.

   Thus far, healthcare leaders have not clearly identified how to determine what the patient wants and values, and the current quantitative outcome measures do not capture whether this goal has been accomplished. Instead, healthcare measures focus on patient satisfaction scores, complications, financial ratios, and/or staffing or turnover metrics—none of which captures whether the patient got what was wanted or valued. The core principle of patient care quality is to determine what the patient wants and values and to make the patient the leader of his or her care. These are misunderstood principles.

2. **To provide the very best quality care, once we know what the patient wants and values.** Care that is provided must take into account what the patient wants and values while collectively using the nurses' professional judgment along with evidence-based care. What we believe is quality care may be at odds with what the patient wants and values. Nevertheless, healthcare providers must be cognizant of their patient

---

BOX 4.1 Four Significant Challenges in Health Care

1. To habitually determine what our patient/client/resident wants and values
2. To provide the very best quality care, once we know what the patient wants and values
3. To keep our patient/client/resident safe
4. To accomplish the first three challenges in a cost-effective way

advocacy and teaching responsibilities because the patient may not be aware of quality and safety standards.

3. **To keep our patient/client/resident safe.** To accomplish this, everyone in health care must constantly consider ways to improve safety. Healthcare organizations and systems are complex. As the complexity of healthcare delivery increased, bureaucracies were formed. The complexity has resulted in increased healthcare errors. Our goal is to simplify our organizational environment by carefully examining what we do to determine whether these activities reflect the organization's mission and values. This means that everyone is a leader, especially the staff nurse and nurse aide, who make 90% of their work decisions at the point of patient care. These leaders continuously make small incremental changes as they interact with each patient and determine the need for change. Thus, it is important that administrators recognize, value, and support leaders at the point of care, and for administrators to be a part of the patient care team.

   When problems are identified, the issues are recognized as critical opportunities to simplify the patient environment and make it safer. Interdisciplinary shared governance and the accompanying complex communication are essential to hear the "voice of the customer" (National Institute of Standards and Technology, 2013, p. 13) and keep patients safe. Failure to identify these problems and issues result in an increase in errors that result in poorer patient outcomes and reimbursement.

4. **To accomplish the first three challenges in a cost-effective way.** Cost-effectiveness is listed fourth because it should never be given a higher priority than the previous three

goals. As stated in other discussions, "If we do what is right for the patients, financial well-being will follow." The bottom line is never the first priority. To accomplish this goal, financial information needs to be transparent across the organization because staff at the point of care must understand the costs to complete delivery of care in the most cost-effective way. Everyone in the organization needs to make decisions based on the organization's mission and values—what is best for patients—with the bottom line always being second.

To present the information in this chapter in a more meaningful manner, it is being subdivided into three (3) sections:

Part 1: Problems We Must Address

Part 2: What Does the Patient Want?

Part 3: The Impact of Quality

PART 1: PROBLEMS WE MUST ADDRESS

▶ We Have a L-O-N-G Way to Go to Fix Our Healthcare System

We are facing major healthcare problems in the United States. According to the World Health Organization (WHO, 2013), in 2011 the United States spent more per capita ($8,607.88) on health care than any other country but "with third world outcomes" (p. 244). In addition, the Commonwealth Fund (2013) reported that the 2011 *National Scorecard on U.S. Health System Performance,* which assessed health and health care in the United States based on quality, access, efficiency, and equity, assigned the United States a score of 52 out of a possible score of 100.

This is far short of what is attainable considering the U.S. per capita expenditure on health care.

Care is often fragmented and depersonalized. Unintentional harm to patients is common. At times, the patient's condition becomes worse rather than better—or the patient dies when he or she comes in contact with healthcare workers. Patients' needs and values are often not considered in the plan of care. This is compounded by the sheer number of the U.S. population that is uninsured. It is a primary goal of the Patient Protection and Affordable Care Act (PPACA; U.S. Government Printing Office, 2010), otherwise known as the Affordable Care Act (ACA), to provide many of these individuals with health insurance; nevertheless, some individuals, for example, migrant workers, will remain uninsured. How ACA will be impacted by the results of the 2016 Presidential and Congressional elections remains to be seen.

Preparing for the future state of health care requires leadership, planning, and change management. In the seminal work *Hospitals and Care Systems of the Future* (AHA, 2011), an outline of 10 must-do strategies was recommended that hospitals must implement in preparation for the future value-based market dynamic, termed the "second curve" (p. 3). An organizational culture of performance improvement (PI), accountability, and quality is critical to implementation of these strategies (AHA, 2011). The entrenched hierarchal, patriarchal culture that continues to thrive in the U.S. healthcare system will need to change in organizations that intend to remain viable. Nevertheless, organizational culture develops over time and is resistant to change. What is needed are transformational change agent leaders who understand the complex nature of the healthcare system.

Complexity change agents refute the traditional assumptions of organization change that envision organizations as machines (Crowell, 2011). The complexity view of the leader/change agent recognizes that change starts with those closest to the work of the organization, efficiency does not come from control, and prediction is not possible (Crowell, 2011). Leaders who will be successful in navigating the turbulent coming years in healthcare recognize that improvements are emergent, not hierarchical. Successful leaders/change agents may arise at any level of the organization or even outside the organization; nevertheless, they recognize how and when to influence the system toward self-organization. Although incremental improvements are positive and need to continue, the entire healthcare system must change to meet the challenges of the upcoming healthcare reality.

Of the 10 strategies set forth by the American Hospital Association (AHA) (2011), four are identified as major priorities. The underpinnings for all four of these strategies are concomitant with quality and value: (1) seamless patient care across the continuum, (2) use of evidence-based practice to improve quality and safety, (3) improved efficiency, and (4) development of integrated information systems.

The first priority addresses the need for seamless patient care across the continuum (AHA, 2011). Whereas all members of the healthcare team are involved in implementation of this priority, it is recognized that nurses play a key role in patient continuity of care, including patient education and communication. As the focus of healthcare transitions to value across the continuum of care, the role of nurses, nurse practitioners, and case managers will come to the forefront. This priority is also linked to priority 2, second-curve metrics, "Utilizing evidenced-based [*sic*] practice to improve quality and patient safety" (p. 4) because the expectation is measurement and management of care transitions (AHA, 2011).

The second priority set forth by the AHA (2011) proclaims the use of evidence-based practice to improve quality and safety. In addition to measurement and management of care transitions, second-curve metrics related to this priority include the following:

- Management of utilization variation
- Preventable admissions, readmission, nonemergent/nonurgent emergency department (ED) visits, and mortality
- Reliable patient care processes
- Active patient engagement in design and improvement (AHA, 2011, p. 4)

Most contemporary nurse leaders have experienced the challenge of linear measurement models. Nevertheless, successful nurse leaders recognize the potential for integration of complexity principles into such measurement models and are positioned to lead change related to current measurement assumptions to create models that reflect the complex nature of healthcare delivery (Porter-O'Grady & Malloch, 2011). Because leaders are duty bound to ensure regulatory compliance—especially considering value-based purchasing mandates—measurement models must include industry standards and measures that reflect the mission, values, and context of the organization, as well as what the patient wants and values.

The third priority identified by the AHA (2011) is improved efficiency. It is well known that unnecessary operational inefficiency is a significant source of healthcare costs. Fortunately, healthcare workers have some control over this dynamic (de Koning, Verver, van den Heuvel, Bisgaard, & Does, 2006). This priority is a familiar one; nevertheless, robust PI work must continue using methods, such as Lean Thinking and Six Sigma, to increase productivity and improve financial management. These methods can be combined to provide a framework for systematic improvements in health care (de Koning et al., 2006). It is important here to point out that there is tension among professionals in regard to the best approach to improving quality, specifically whether an incremental approach or a systems approach is most effective. It is our opinion that both approaches are needed to survive in the ever-changing healthcare environment.

The final top priority for hospitals in preparation for the value-based market is the development of integrated information systems (AHA, 2011). Technological advances contribute significantly to the increasing cost of care. However, it is evident that data must be readily available for analysis and improvement work. Regardless of what happens financially, health care will change!

Patient Safety Issues

The priority for quality improvement work is always to provide a safe environment. The focus is to design quality and safety into our processes. The focus on safety is evident because publications about patient safety are published daily. For example, the Leapfrog Group (2013) published recommended "leaps" that organizations should take that promote quality. The recommendations include: (1) implementing computerized physician order entry (CPOE), (2) having an electronic health record (EHR) (also called electronic medical record [EMR]), (3) implementing intensive care unit staffing with physicians experienced in critical care medicine, and (4) attaining a high Leapfrog Safe Practices score. The safe practices score measures the organization's progress in meeting and implementing the safe practices endorsed by the National Quality Forum that are aimed at reducing the risk of harm in certain processes, systems, or environments of care (Leapfrog Group, 2013). It is estimated that if all hospitals implemented the first three leaps, "over 57,000 lives could be saved, more than 3 million medications errors could be avoided, and up to $12.0 billion could be saved" (para. 3) annually. Again, focusing on prevention of human pain and suffering is the priority.

In a groundbreaking report, the Institute of Medicine (IOM, 1999) estimated that as many as 98,000 hospital deaths per year were the result of avoidable medical errors. The landmark study noted that hospital medical errors were the eighth leading cause of death in the United States. These statistics did not take into account errors that may have occurred in the vast array of other healthcare settings. This report startled the healthcare community and consumers to action, yet authors noted in a 2005 follow-up report that progress toward improved patient safety was slow (Leape & Berwick, 2005). In 2007, the IOM published findings from a workshop, *Creating a Business Case for Quality Improvement Research* acknowledging a "reluctance to invest in quality improvement" (p. 1) throughout the country. Resources are limited and tend to be spent on "highly visible technology-driven programs" (IOM, 2007, p. 1). Although technology can improve systems, it is not the single answer to a safer healthcare system.

The Eighth Annual HealthGrades Patient Safety in American Hospitals Study (Reed & May, 2011) reported that from 2007 through 2009:

- There were 708,642 identified patient safety events. This is daunting considering that only 13 potential patient safety indicators were evaluated in the study, and thus this number represents only a small portion of total patient safety events.
- Based on the total hospitalized Medicare patients, 1.6% experienced one or more patient safety events.
- Patient safety events cost Medicare nearly $7.3 billion and resulted in 79,670 potentially preventable deaths.
- One in 10 surgical patients died following serious but treatable complications.
- A total of 52,127 Medicare patients developed a nosocomial (hospital acquired) bloodstream infection; of these patients 8,114 died. Nosocomial acquired bloodstream infections cost the federal government approximately $1.2 billion.
- If all hospitals performed at the level of top-ranked facilities, approximately 174,358 patient safety events and 20,688 deaths could have been avoided, saving the federal government $1.8 billion.

These authors noted that preventable medical errors are so prevalent and expensive that selected indicators will be part of a hospital's performance score for the value-based incentive plan. The Hospital Value-Based Purchasing Program, which was established by the PPACA of 2010 (U.S. Government Printing Office, 2010), represented the first time that U.S. hospitals were paid for inpatient service based on quality rather than quantity. Beginning in fiscal year 2013, Medicare made incentive payments to hospitals based on how well they performed on clinical measures,

as well as measures based on patients' experiences or based on improvement of the measures compared to their baseline (Centers for Medicare and Medicaid Services [CMS] 2011). Although the definitions of several of the indicators in the study were changed from the previous report, it is clear that patient safety events remain a problem in U.S. hospitals (Reed & May, 2011). The *most important issue* is human pain, suffering, and loss and death related to these preventable events. The healthcare system must be fixed.

Being proactive, preventing patient safety events is important. However, when mistakes occur, administrators must react from the complexity, "no blame" perspective rather than from the patriarchal Industrial Age view. The traditional approach to patient safety violations was to identify what an individual practitioner did wrong. Serious errors resulted in occurrences being "reported to the board for disciplinary investigation because of an error or breach in the standards of safe practice" (Woods & Doan-Johnson, 2002, p. 45). Many facilities have adopted "no-blame" policies rather than focusing on blame and punishment.

There are two issues here. First, assigning blame encourages individuals to hide or not report errors. Second, even when one individual made the error, upon critical examination, usually there are underlying process problems. Most often, there are multiple factors that caused the error. Administrators must consider the most important issue about errors—what can be done to prevent the error from occurring again?

A more effective solution is to report the error and undertake a root cause analysis to determine what process changes—or patterns or trends—occurred that provide clues for needed changes. Medical errors usually involve more than one individual and require a systems approach to find solutions. Usually, an organizational systems process went wrong or a better process needs to be implemented. Administrators must establish systems to prevent reoccurrence. A systems approach is best.

Establishing a just or blame-free culture is critical if organizations are to focus on process and system improvements rather than assigning blame. Without the occasion for open discussion, many opportunities for improvement are hidden or go unreported because team members are fearful of losing their jobs or getting into trouble. To this end, the problem will reoccur.

Creating a just culture begins with executive leaders and must be reinforced each time an incident occurs. Administrators must be informed. Once informed, it is important that administrators role model expected behaviors, speak publicly about safety, set expectations, establish policy, and personally participate in significant event root cause analyses.

Another important source for patient safety opportunities is the organization's incident reports or variance reports. Healthcare risk managers have used these tools for years; nevertheless, the information provided in these reports needs to be used more effectively. Incident or variance reports are traditionally used to alert risk managers of potential litigation. The risk manager's role has historically been to identify, manage, and reduce risk to support the delivery of safe health care while reducing organizational legal risks. Most risk management activities occur after an incident; thus, these functions are not the best way to achieve safe care. Nevertheless, administrators need to pay particular attention to these resources because these reports provide valuable information regarding organizational issues that need to be resolved to ensure patient safety.

An emerging role in health care is the patient safety officer. This position promotes safety through education; examination of issues to determine better, safer organizational processes; discovering the root cause; creating system changes to prevent future incidents of the same kind; and involvement in implementing programs designed to foster safety. The patient safety officer works closely with risk management personnel to discover the root cause of patient safety events and create system changes to facilitate a safer environment.

Medication Errors

The IOM released a report in 2006 on prevention of medication errors. The research discovered a frightening statistic: "a hospital patient can expect on average to be subjected to more than one medication error each day" (p. 1). Errors occurred in every step of the medication process, but more occurred during prescribing and administration. Experts estimate that error rates are actually higher than the numbers reported. One of the studies cited in the report documented an additional cost of $8,750 per hospital stay for each adverse drug event. IOM (2004a) reported in an earlier study that "two hospitals over a 6-month period found that nurses were responsible for intercepting 86 percent of all medication errors made by physicians, pharmacists, and others involved in providing medications for patients before the error reached the patient" (p. 3). The IOM (2006) asserts that most of the errors and the additional costs were preventable.

The risks of adverse drug events are higher for nursing home patients. Garcia (2006) predicted that nearly "two thirds of nursing facility residents will experience an adverse drug event over a 4-year period of time, with one in seven of these residents requiring hospitalization" (p. 306). Simonson and Feinberg (2005), in extensive work reviewing the medication issues in elderly adults, identified that *one-half* of adverse drug events in nursing home facilities are preventable.

Caution is advised related to computerized provider order entry (CPOE). Although EHRs, which include CPOE and clinical decision support (CDS), have improved some aspects of patient safety (Agency for Healthcare Research and Quality [AHRQ], n.d.), Wetterneck et al. (2011) reported an increase in duplicate medication order errors following implementation of EHRs with CPOE and CDS. These researchers identified improved communication, teamwork, and CPOE usability and functionality as approaches to reducing such errors. This is important because EHRs are expensive and technology is often viewed as a fail-safe way to prevent medication errors. Medication administration is a complicated process; most errors are system errors rather than user errors. Healthcare leaders need to monitor and analyze medication errors carefully because identified problems may warrant the time and expense of a PI team.

Healthcare-Associated (Nosocomial) Infections

Healthcare-associated (nosocomial) infections continue to be an issue in organizations across the country. *Healthcare-associated infections* that occurred in U.S. hospitals were estimated at 1.7 million and were associated with approximately 99,000 deaths (Klevens et al., 2007). Scott (2009) estimates the range of overall annual direct medical costs of hospital-associated infections as between $28.4 billion and $33.8 billion. Scott estimated the range for the cost benefits of prevention as $5.7 billion to $6.8 billion (low) to $25.0 billion to $31.5 billion (high). Reed and May (2011) reported that hospital-acquired bloodstream infections among hospitalized Medicare patients for the period of 2007 to 2009 were serious and costly: hospitalized Medicare patients acquired 52,127 bloodstream infections, 8,114 patients died, and the cost to the federal government was an estimated $1.22 billion. Again, the *most important issue* is human pain, suffering, and loss and death, related to these preventable events. *Methicillin-resistant Staphylococcus aureus, or* MRSA, has reached endemic levels in hospitals and long-term care facilities, and rates continue to rise. The increasing numbers of patients with healthcare-associated infections provide evidence that *healthcare workers are not following the most basic preventive measure: good hand hygiene.* The healthcare system must be fixed.

Nevertheless, complexity theory provides an underpinning for approaching such dearth. Crowell (2011) describes complexity science as "nonlinear, dynamic, often uncertain, and very much relationship-based" (p. 3). The focus needs to be bottom-up rather than top-down management. Lindberg and Clancy (2010) propose that

within organizations some individuals or groups have different "deviant" practices that produce better "positive" (p. 152) outcomes. *Positive deviance* holds that staff members at the point of care are best equipped to solve the problem. The job is to discover positive deviant practices, and then through widespread engagement spread these best practices throughout the organization and system. Positive deviance is a potentially dramatic breakthrough related to the culture of change for hospitals. An increasing number of hospitals are using this philosophy to solve the problem of MRSA (AHC Media, 2008).

Falls

Falls among older adults (age 65 and older) continue to be a safety issue. Falls are the leading cause of death among older adults, with mortality rates from falls increasing over the past ten years. In 2009, 20,400 people 65 and older died from injuries from unintentional falls. In 2010, 2.3 million people 65 and older were treated in EDs for nonfatal injuries from falls and more than 662,000 of these patients were hospitalized (Centers for Disease Control and Prevention [CDC], 2012). In the report of their study, Stevens, Corso, Finkelstein, and Miller (2006) estimated the direct costs of falls was $19.2 billion per year, while the CDC (2012) estimated that the direct medical costs of falls in 2010 alone was $30.0 billion. These figures do include subsequent long-term care costs or loss of quality of life.

The Institute for Healthcare Improvement (IHI, 2013) reported that patient falls are the most prevalent adverse events in hospitals. Of upmost concern is that ". . . injuries from falls are often associated with morbidity and mortality" (IHI, 2013, para 1). Research suggests an increasing risk of falls with lower nurse staffing levels (Whitman, Kim, Davidson, Wolf, & Wang, 2002).

Missed Care

Missed care is distressing to nurses, but most important, these omissions can result in patient morbidity and mortality. The omission of simple yet missed vital care tasks, such as turning, ambulating, feeding, mouth care, and toileting, can lead to patient complications—for example, decubitus ulcers and pneumonia. Although the patient is always the priority, pay-for-performance/value-based purchasing emphasizes the significant reimbursement ramifications of these two complications alone. It is important to acknowledge that nurses must be accountable for the patient care they provide.

Nurses cannot abandon efforts to improve quality and safety; however, leaders can use complexity theory to adapt to the natural aspects of life within the healthcare system. Missed care may be related to poor professional nurses' delegation skills or failure to properly supervise assigned care. When opportunities to improve are identified, real-time corrections must be made. Or, if the issue is more complex, follow-through is needed to determine next steps, improve and sustain the gains, and never give in to complacency where people say "that's just the way it is." Regardless of the method used to improve quality, the complex nature of health care mandates a culture change in which all health care workers make safety the priority focus every day and in all settings.

Interruptions

Interruptions in the work environment are frequently occurring safety issues. When the work of nurses is interrupted, errors occur and efficiency is decreased (Biron, Lavoie-Tremblay, & Loiselle, 2009; Trbovich, Prakash, & Stewart, 2010). An example of process improvement that decreased the frequency of interruptions during medication administration involved the use of red aprons (Relihan, O'Brien, O'Hara, & Silke, 2010) worn by the medication nurse which identified that the nurse was not to be disturbed (AHRQ, 2008; Relihan et al., 2010). This improvement example demonstrated Lean thinking related to unevenness of flow (Cookson, Read, Mukherjee, & Cooke, 2011).

These are a few of the safety issues facing today's healthcare system. Administrators must find ways to create a culture of safety that does not tolerate continuation of these problems. Ethical principles and standards of care mandate a focus on patient safety.

Workforce Management Issues

We examine what happens when registered nurses (RN) or nursing budgets are cut. Studies have shown that the dissatisfaction rate of nurses is four times greater for hospital nurses than all other U.S. workers (Aiken, Clarke, Sloane, Sochalski, & Silber, 2002). Dissatisfaction is often related to high patient-to-nurse ratios. A poll of RNs by the American Nurses Association (ANA, 2008) revealed that close to half of the respondents are considering leaving their job because of inadequate staffing. Data from respondents were reported as follows:

- 73% of nurses asked do not believe the staffing on their unit or shift is sufficient.
- 59.8% of those asked said they knew of someone who left direct care nursing because of concerns about safe staffing.
- Of the 51.9% of respondents who are considering leaving their current position, 46% cite inadequate staffing as the reason.
- 51.7% of respondents said they thought the quality of nursing care on their unit has declined in the last year.
- 48.2% would not feel confident having someone close to them receiving care in the facility where they work (para. 2).

Research supports the gravity of inadequate staffing. Aiken et al. (2002) reported that nurse staffing ratios are linked to quality of care and patient outcomes. Adding one additional patient to the nurse assignment increases the likelihood of patient death by 7% within 30 days of hospital admission. On a positive note, ANA (2013b) cited that "*each additional patient care RN employed (at 7.8 hours per patient day) will generate over $60,000 annually in reduced medical costs and improved national productivity*" (para. 5). Evidence supports that improving the work environment for nurses can lead to improved job satisfaction and increased patient satisfaction and safety (Dunton, Gajewski, Klaus, & Pierson, 2007; Vanhey, Aiken, Sloane, Clarke, & Vargas, 2004). Likewise, Boev (2012) found preliminary support for the relationship between nurses' and patients' satisfaction in adult critical care.

Researchers analyzed data from the National Database of Nursing Quality Indicators (NDNQI) regarding the nursing environment in relation to patient outcomes. These researchers concluded that multiple factors, including nurse staffing, percentage of RN staff, and RN years of experience, affect patient safety and nurse-sensitive outcomes. For example, the incidence of hospital-acquired pressure ulcers decreased with a more experienced staff, along with having a higher percentage of RNs caring for the patient (Dunton et al., 2007).

The IOM (2004b) supported the following impact that leaner nurse staffing levels have on patient outcomes in their report Keeping Patients Safe: Transforming the Work Environment of Nurses (IOM, 2004b). The report contends that not only has nurse staffing levels been associated with an increased length of stay, higher nosocomial infection rates, and increased pressure ulcer rates, but there is evidence that indicates patient mortality increases when there is less nursing time provided to patients. In summary, nurses are "indispensable to our safety" (p. 3).

Based on these data, the ANA (n.d.) called for support of the Registered Nurse Safe Staffing Act that would create reliable nurse staffing levels. The ANA (n.d.) proclaimed that managing the patient-to-RN ratio improves job satisfaction and patient outcomes. Nurses' dissatisfaction with inadequate staffing is often supported by the research and is linked to less than satisfactory patient outcomes. This is only the beginning of the problem. In *Keeping Patients Safe: Transforming the Work Environment of Nurses*, the IOM (2004b) noted the following (**BOX 4.2**):

- **Loss of trust in hospital administration is widespread among nursing staff.** . . . This loss of trust stems in part from a perception that initiatives in patient care and nursing work redesign have emphasized efficiency over patient safety. . . . Poor communication practices have also led to mistrust.
- **Clinical nursing leadership has been reduced at multiple levels, and the voice of nurses in patient care has diminished.** Hospital reengineering initiatives often have resulted in the loss of a separate department of nursing. . . . At the same time, nursing staff have perceived a decline in chief nurse executives with power and authority equal to that of other top hospital officials, as well as [a decline] in directors of nursing who are highly visible and accessible to staff. . . . These changes—along with losses of chief nursing officers without replacement; decreases in the numbers of nurse managers; and increased responsibilities

---

BOX 4.2 IOM Notes Negative Quality/Patient Safety Effects of Work Redesign

- Loss of trust in hospital administration
- Work redesign emphasized efficiency over patient safety
- Loss of a separate department of nursing
- Decline in nurse executives with the power and authority equal to the rest of the executive team
- Decrease in the number of nurse managers
- Remaining nurse managers have responsibility for more than one unit

Data from Institute of Medicine. (2004b). *Keeping patients safe: Transforming the work environment of nurses.* Washington, DC: The National Academies Press.

for remaining nurse managers for more than one patient care unit, as well as for supervising personnel other than nursing staff . . . —have had the cumulative effect of reducing direct management support available to patient care staff. This situation hampers nurses' ability to fix problems in their work environments that threaten patient safety (p. 4).

Evidence has shown that understaffing, negative cultures, burdening nurse managers with more than 50 full-time equivalents (FTEs), 12-hour shifts, the lack of interdisciplinary shared governance, allowing physician or other staff disruptive or abusive behaviors, and moral distress issues are linked to poor patient outcomes; decreased patient, nurse, and physician satisfaction; higher staff turnover; and decreased reimbursement.

Complexity Issues

All of the preceding problems are complexity issues; everything is interconnected. With a sentinel event as an example, the event causes disorder. A root cause analysis restores order, *but hopefully with some small incremental change or changes in the way the work is done.*

Consider the following example of a sentinel event. During the time that the sentinel event occurred, staffing was inadequate, turnover was high because of a negative unit culture, and the nurse manager's leadership skills were inadequate. All these issues created complexity and contributed to the error. There was no single cause and "fixing" only one of the problems will not prevent the event from reoccurring. Such quick fixes increase complexity, which is counterproductive to PI work because more complexity creates more errors. This is the reason that all stakeholders are involved in the review and resolution of sentinel events, because what is needed is to determine ways to fix the causes and simplify processes. Sharing the lessons from root cause analyses with all staff demonstrates transparency. Secrets have a way of eventually becoming public knowledge.

Cultural Issues

Another factor related to what patients want and value is culture. Increasingly, the U.S. population is becoming more racially and culturally diverse. The following is the U.S. population breakdown by race, according to the 2010 U.S. census (U.S. Census Bureau, 2011):

- 72% white (223.6 million) (includes 16% Hispanic, [50.5 million])
- 13% black or African American (38.9 million)
- 5% Asian (14.7 million)
- 2.9% American Indian and Alaska Native (2.9 million)
- 0.2% Native Hawaiian or other Pacific Islander (0.5 million)
- 6% other races (19.1 million)

The U.S. Hispanic population almost doubled in the last decade (43% growth), yet the U.S. Asian population grew faster than any other major race for the same time period (U.S. Census Bureau, 2011). It is common to see Spanish television stations or to buy a product with instructions written in several languages. Obviously, the U.S. population is ethnically diverse.

This diversity constitutes a new perspective toward not only culturally diverse patients, but also toward culturally diverse staff. We are often unaware of specific cultural beliefs, values, and traditions, and so we may inadvertently tread on those beliefs and practices as we deliver health care. Just as there is a need for improvement related to patient-centered care, quality, and safety, there is room for improvement related to culturally competent care.

As Healthcare professionals, it is important to recognize the wonderful differences that exist between cultures and to support the cultural beliefs and norms of others. It is important to educate all staff regarding cultural differences, to value these differences, and to encourage everyone to respect and give radical loving care to each person based on that person's cultural beliefs.

Healthcare workers are ethnocentric in giving care to clients when they do not provide care based on what patients want and value.

It is imperative that we take the time to learn about patients' cultural or ethnic differences. Care based on cultural differences affects nutrition, family functioning, lifestyle differences, spiritual or religious differences, biological variations, the way one relates to both health and disease, communication issues, differences in locus of control, differences in views about independence versus collectivism, and socioeconomic realities.

Additional cultural differences exist between physicians, nurses, and nonclinical administrators. In medical school, physicians often learn that they are autonomous and independent (although this is changing with group practices). This can lead to autocratic, domineering, and paternalistic behaviors because often teamwork and collaboration are not stressed nor valued. Also, nurses may determine that they are in a lower position in the hierarchy of importance because administrators tend to provide more support to physicians (who have the power to admit; thus, they affect revenue). These differences can be overcome. It is important that each member of the healthcare team is valued and respected and that everyone upholds the same organizational values to provide quality care for patients. When administrators do not support organizational values and give too much autonomy to physicians, disruptive physician behaviors may continue, creating a less effective or even hostile work environment. Patient care, as well as reimbursements, can be compromised when this occurs.

Disparities Issues

Significant healthcare access issues continue. The fifth *National Healthcare Disparities Report* (AHRQ, 2008) described disparities related to the quality of and access to health care. Although some progress has been made, the report highlights gaps that did not improve (**BOX 4.3**). A primary problem has been to decrease the identified gaps related to lack of insurance.

Those without insurance often do not get needed medical care. Miller, Vigdor, and Manning (2004) claimed that lack of insurance creates hidden costs for society. These authors based this claim on data from the IOM report that estimated the cost in terms of foregone health, shorter lives, and demands on the healthcare infrastructure to be $65 billion to $130 billion a year. Using this hidden cost to provide insurance coverage would be more effective.

Currently, the healthcare "safety net" provides care for the uninsured or underinsured. The largest provider in this safety net is hospital EDs. Community clinics, public health departments, and hospital-based clinics, created to provide this care, cannot accommodate the demand. Hospital ED visits classified as nonurgent continue to increase. Key reasons for this include

---

BOX 4.3 Disparities Among Races

- Blacks had a rate of new AIDS cases 10 times higher than whites.
- Asian adults aged 65 and over were 50% more likely than whites to lack immunization against pneumonia.
- Native Americans and Alaska Natives were twice as likely to lack prenatal care in the first trimester as whites.
- Hispanics had a rate of new AIDS cases over 3.5 times higher than that of non-Hispanic whites.
- Poor children were over 28% more likely than high-income children to experience poor communication with their healthcare providers.

Reproduced from Agency for Healthcare Research and Quality. (2008). *National healthcare disparities report: 2007.* AHRQ Pub. No. 08-0041. Rockville, MD: U.S. Department of Health and Human Services.

difficulty obtaining timely appointments with a primary care provider, the lack of affordable transportation, and the lack of insurance. Much of this is not reimbursed; thus, hospitals incur more and more of the expense of providing this care.

Regulatory Response: Restricting or Eliminating Reimbursement

As healthcare expenses rise, federal and state governments are faced with deficits. At the same time, there is a growing elderly group who is eligible for Medicare. The CMS, which represents more than 50% of the health insurance in this country, responded by reimbursing for quality care and withholding reimbursement when quality issues were identified (pay for performance or value-based purchasing).

Hospitals

Acute care facilities must demonstrate compliance with the guidelines for care of certain conditions to receive the highest possible reimbursement. In this case, the CMS (the payer) specified certain patient care paths, based on evidence-based practice, to obtain reimbursement. If the patient care path is not followed as specified, the healthcare organization does not receive reimbursement for the care. For example, if antibiotics are not given within 2 hours of a pneumonia diagnosis (the care path specification), the payer will not reimburse the hospital. This emphasizes the importance of clinician timeliness in treating the patient, or everyone loses, including the patient.

In 2008, additional indicators were put in place restricting or eliminating reimbursement for certain hospital-acquired conditions that were not present on admission (CMS, 2012d). These hospital-acquired conditions were expanded to 11 categories for fiscal year 2013 (CMS, 2012c). (See **BOX 4.4**.) These conditions have been termed *never events*.

The CMS (2013g) quality initiatives encompass the gamut of the healthcare system, from

---

BOX 4.4 2013 CMS Hospital-Acquired Conditions

Foreign Object Retained After Surgery
Air Embolism
Blood Incompatibility
Stage III and IV Pressure Ulcers
Falls and Trauma

- Fractures
- Dislocations
- Intracranial Injuries
- Crushing Injuries
- Burn
- Other Injuries

Manifestations of Poor Glycemic Control

- Diabetic Ketoacidosis
- Nonketotic Hyperosmolar Coma
- Hypoglycemic Coma
- Secondary Diabetes with Ketoacidosis
- Secondary Diabetes with Hyperosmolarity

Catheter-Associated Urinary Tract Infection (UTI)
Vascular Catheter-Associated Infection
Surgical Site Infection, Mediastinitis, Following Coronary Artery Bypass Graft (CABG)
Surgical Site Infection Following Bariatric Surgery for Obesity

- Laparoscopic Gastric Bypass
- Gastroenterostomy
- Laparoscopic Gastric Restrictive Surgery

Surgical Site Infection Following Certain Orthopedic Procedures

- Spine
- Neck
- Shoulder
- Elbow

Surgical Site Infection Following Cardiac Implantable Electronic Device (CIED)
Deep Vein Thrombosis/Pulmonary Embolism Following Certain Orthopedic Procedures

- Total Knee Replacement
- Hip Replacement

Iatrogenic Pneumothorax with Venous Catheterization

Reproduced from Centers for Medicare and Medicaid Services. (2012c). Hospital-acquired conditions (present on admission indicator). Retrieved from http://www.cms.gov/Medicare/Medicare-Fee-for-Service -Payment/HospitalAcqCond/Hospital-Acquired_Conditions.html providers to hospital care, and include quality measures information that CMS recommends that consumers use when faced with healthcare decisions. The CMS quality initiatives span several years and thus only an overview is provided here.

The Hospital Inpatient Quality Reporting Program was originally mandated by the Medicare Prescription Drug, Improvement, and Modernization Act (MMA) of 2003 (CMS, 2003). The MMA authorized CMS to pay hospitals a higher annual update on their payment rates based on reporting of identified quality measures. The initial MMA rate was a 0.4% reduction for hospitals that did not successfully report. In 2005, the Deficit Reduction Act increased the reduction to 2.0 percentage points (CMS, 2013b).

The Hospital Outpatient Quality Reporting Program was mandated by the Tax Relief and Health Care Act of 2006 (CMS, 2006). This program required hospitals to submit outpatient quality measures data. The data included process, structure, outcome, and efficiency measures. Outpatient care encompassed ED services, observation, outpatient surgical services, laboratory tests, and radiology (CMS, 2013a).

An example of a quality initiative is the Hospital Value-Based Purchasing Program (CMS, 2013c), effective fiscal year 2013, which provides value-based incentive payments based on the hospital's performance on quality measures (pay for performance) or based on the hospital's improvement on quality measures from the baseline period. *The higher the hospital's performance or improvement, the higher the value-based incentive payment.* If a hospital does not meet these guidelines, reimbursement will be decreased by a percentage for the following year. Thus, hospitals not only lose on a never event, but are penalized further for reimbursement the next year.

Home Health

There are three types of home health quality measures: (1) process, (2) outcomes, and (3) potentially avoidable events (CMS, 2012b).

Details related to home health measures are extensive and can be found at www.cms.gov /Medicare/Quality-Initiatives-Patient-Assessment -Instruments/HomeHealthQualityInits/HHQI QualityMeasures.html.

Long-Term Care

The CMS nursing home measures are also extensive. There are five short-stay quality measures and 13 long-stay nursing home quality measures (CMS, 2013c). Details related to nursing home quality measures are vast and can be found at www .cms.gov/Medicare/Quality-Initiatives-Patient -Assessment-Instruments/NursingHomeQualityInits /NHQIQualityMeasures.html.

Postacute Care

Finally, additional CMS quality initiatives are in place for postacute care (CMS, 2012e) and for end-stage renal disease (ESRD) (CMS, 2012a). The ESRD Quality Initiative, which became effective in 2012, was the first pay for performance (also known as value-based purchasing) quality initiative implemented as mandated by the Medicare Improvements for Patients and Providers Act (MIPPA) of 2008 (U.S. Government Printing Office, 2008). Its goal was to enhance the quality of care provided to ESRD patients as they battle this devastating disease (CMS, 2012a). Additional information regarding the CMS quality initiatives can be found at www .cms.gov/Medicare/Quality-Initiatives-Patient -Assessment-Instruments/QualityInitiativesGenInfo /index.html?redirect=/qualityinitiativesgeninfo/.

Quality Reporting System Mandate

In an effort to align payment incentives across the healthcare system, CMS (2013f) implemented payment incentives and adjustments to promote reporting of quality information by identified providers. The quality reporting system is mandated by federal legislation. Beginning in 2015, the program also applies to eligible providers who do not satisfactorily report quality measures data (CMS, 2013d). Details related to the Physician Quality Reporting System can be found at www.cms.gov/Medicare/Quality -Initiatives-Patient-Assessment-Instruments /PQRS/index.html.

Medicaid programs are funded at both state and federal levels; thus, these restrictions on reimbursement are being linked to Medicaid payments as well. Next, the AHA developed guiding principles for nonpayment for all insurance companies for certain serious adverse events (that are preventable, may indicate a hospital system error, or where there are published guidelines for prevention of these errors if the hospital deems the event was preventable) from the National Quality Forum's list of 28 serious reportable events (Tennessee Hospitals & Health Systems, 2008) (see **BOX 4.5**).

Patient safety was of such concern to the public that The Joint Commission (TJC) implemented National Patient Safety Goals in 2003 (TJC, 2013b). Accredited facilities must demonstrate compliance with the intent of these goals to maintain their accreditation status. Details regarding the 2013 National Patient Safety Goals (TJC, 2013c) can be found at www .jointcommission.org/standards_information /npsgs.aspx.

▶ Our Reality Is Changing—Ready or Not!

As you read this chapter, begin to think of the many ways nurses can change how healthcare services are provided—ways that are much more effective and that involve the patient in care decisions. This leads us to something that we need to make top priority as we give care: *finding out what the patient wants and values.*

There are opportunities all around us. Patients have access to more information about

---

BOX 4.5 The American Hospital Association Guidelines for Reimbursement Restriction

The American Hospital Association recommends that hospitals not seek payment from patients or their insurance companies for the following serious preventable adverse events if the hospital deems the event was preventable:

- Surgery on a wrong body part
- Surgery on the wrong patient
- Wrong surgical procedure
- Unintended retention of a foreign object
- Patient death or serious disability associated with an air embolism that occurs while being treated in a healthcare facility
- Patient death or serious disability associated with a medication error
- Patient death or serious disability associated with a hemolytic reaction due to administration of ABO/HLA incompatible blood or blood products
- Artificial insemination with the wrong donor sperm or wrong egg
- Infant discharged to the wrong person
- Death or serious disability (kernicterus) associated with failure to identify and treat hyperbilirubinemia in neonates
- Patient death or serious disability associated with a burn incurred from any source while being cared for in a healthcare facility

Data from Tennessee Hospitals & Health Systems. (2008). *THA develops nonpayment policy on serious adverse events.* Nashville, TN: Tennessee Hospital Association.

their care, yet they need our help in translating the meaning of various options available to them when they experience disease. At the same time, they are turning to healthier lifestyles so they can live longer, healthier lives. Nurses have an advantage in this environment because, although we learn about disease and how it is treated, we also learn about prevention and health. In healthcare organizations, nurses are with patients far more than are physicians. Patients value our interpersonal skills because we are more likely to listen and to help. Thus, for us, moving into this new age is not as difficult as it is for physicians who are mainly focused on disease and which medications to prescribe to deal with disease.

Nurses also have a lot to offer to bottom-line healthcare administrators who do not necessarily understand the care side of health care. We can help them in this shift because we are closer to the patient and can bring that perspective to the table. The important place for survival is at the point of care. As administrators, we need to encourage and empower staff at the point of care to make 90% of the decisions about that care. Staff need to become leaders, helping the patients become leaders in their own care decisions. We administrators are here to facilitate staff being able to do this. We need to be sure that staffing is adequate, and more staff may be needed during peak times. We need to protect staff so that they can do their work. We need to support interdisciplinary shared governance at the bedside with everyone in the organization doing regular rounds.

One purpose of this book is to help nurse leaders express what is needed, using statistics, so that linear administrators are more likely to listen. This helps make it possible for patients to get what they value while they are with us. Linear administrators understand, and need, numbers. If we format what we believe is needed in a way that shows numbers and dollars, our suggestions are more likely to be supported within an organization. Along with this, we need to involve staff in budgets, sharing financial information. Transparency throughout the organization is the end goal.

PART 2: WHAT DOES THE PATIENT WANT?

▸ Our First Priority: Discovering What the Patient Wants and Values

Value from the patient's perspective is the most important concern. Sometimes patients believe that the healthcare provider does not listen, and does not care to listen to what the patient actually wants or needs. The old paternalistic medical model—we will just tell you what is best for you—is outdated, is resented, and no longer applies to most patients. Patients often feel depersonalized, experience long waits, and, worse yet, receive substandard care especially if they are in a lower socioeconomic group or if they are a racial or ethnic minority.

Porter-O'Grady and Malloch (2011) discuss the change in the patient–provider relationship:

- Patients now determine the parameters of the patient–provider relationship, setting the stage for a different kind of interaction than has historically occurred.
- Patients need to develop partnerships with providers to sort through the available choices and pick the best. They need providers to act as educators who are willing to assist them in making healthcare decisions.
- Patients need help from providers both in verifying the accuracy of the data they have independently garnered from a host of sources and in interpreting the data.
- Patients are interested in options, not an order to undergo a particular treatment. They want to be able to consider a range of options within the context of their own personal values and priorities and choose the one option that best fits these.

■ Providers now need to be concerned with what patients know and can do with regard to controlling their own health decisions in a "user-driven" world. More of the responsibility for health care will be placed on patients and their loved ones. Providers must now transfer skills to others and surrender ownership of care to others (p. 17).

It is important for the nurse leader to constantly think, *"What does the patient want and value?"* along with *"safety, safety, safety," "quality, quality, quality,"* and *"cost-effectiveness, cost-effectiveness, cost-effectiveness."* The nurse leader can facilitate what is valuable to patients. The expectation is that staff at the point of care do the same thing. This is a change for most of us, who are accustomed to providing care with no consideration of the *patient's* perspective.

Administrators are not alone in needing to change their perspective. All staff, board members, physicians, and the executive team must change their perspectives. Everyone has to talk with each patient and listen to what he or she has to say. *The most important place is at the point of care, and administrators must support those who are at this point of care.* Paying attention to what the patient values as *first priority,* with safety and quality second, enables us to make better decisions, be more effective, and save money and risk to the patient. This perspective has a positive impact on the financial bottom line as well. Thus, everyone wins!

Values depend on the circumstances and whose point of view is being considered. Patient perceptions, and what the patient wants, are more important than what we believe the patient *should* want when determining quality indicators. Once we have determined what evidence-based care might be necessary for a specific patient (after we have determined what the patient wants), there is still more to do. We need to then offer the patient choices in remedies and therapies that fall under that evidence-based care rubric, while ensuring that the patient is fully informed. Currently, healthcare team members fail in healthcare delivery because we often consider what we want instead of consulting the patient and finding out the patient's wishes.

Value has another implication. We all must understand the importance of including our *patients as leaders in the decision-making process of their care, otherwise known as patient-centered care.* The patient has to be involved in deciding which services will be provided. This pivotal point will change health care as we know it.

The Consumer-Driven Health Care Institute (2013) promotes policy that empowers individuals to make decisions about their health care, advocating the following:

■ Consumers will work with their physicians and healthcare providers to create a better healthcare outcome for themselves and their families.

■ Healthcare usage is more cost efficient with empowered and knowledgeable consumers who use information tools.

■ Price and quality transparency about healthcare professionals is a key method for effective consumer healthcare choices (para. 2).

Transparency means that we share all pertinent information. Consider that if we did not share, the Internet nevertheless provides voluminous information, and CMS provides information to the general public, including facility quality ratings. We cannot stop the tide—information is accessible to the public. Some of the information is helpful and excellent; some is erroneous and misleading. Nurses can assist patients to appropriately evaluate this information to make the best decisions.

Another trap for nurses is to lament that improvements cannot be made because of inadequate resources. Active listening does require a lower patient-to-nurse ratio so that the nurse can take the time to determine what patients value and desire. In addition, traditionally there have been cyclical nursing shortages. But bemoaning shortages and financial constraints **does not improve patient care**. The excuse of inadequate resources needs to be discarded, and instead nurses must determine how to make a positive difference. However, that being said, it is important that administrators make sure that staffing *is* adequate for current patient needs. And all of us, including staff, need to be creative and make sure we are using the resources we have in the most advantageous way possible. This is important because, if nurses do not find a way to do things better, someone else will.

Nurses need to be innovative and encourage all staff and physicians to be innovative. When contemplating current practice, nurses must evaluate what needs to be changed. For example, are limited visiting hours really necessary? Why most procedures are scheduled Monday through Friday? It is interesting that consumer groups advocate *not* having procedures scheduled on Friday because staff are often limited on weekends and are thus less equipped to deal with patient complications. If a patient has an acute episode on Friday evening, why does the patient have to wait until Monday for most services? We must question everything we do!

Not much has been discussed about quality and safety in this section because the issues that were reviewed are important if nurses are to deliver patient-centered quality services. It is important to emphasize listening to the patient, providing sufficient information for decision making, and supporting the patient in treatment decisions—all within a safe, cost-effective environment.

The Healing Relationship

The IOM (2001) advocates, "Care is based on continuous healing relationships" (p. 3). At times in this chapter, we mention "loving" care. Love is necessary for healing. By *love*, we mean a caring relationship. Jean Watson (2004) examined the relationship between caring and curing in her book *Postmodern Nursing and Beyond*. The author examines both the technical side of nursing and the holistic side, which is traditionally associated with caring. Over the years, a lot of emphasis has been put on the caring component of nursing practice.

Chapman (2004) made the connection between loving and healing and stressed the importance of listening to the patient. This means that as we listen to each patient, we read between the lines

using our intuition. The physical diagnosis may not be the most important issue for the patient. Instead, nurses must determine what the patient wants and values and focus the patient's care on what is important to the patient.

Chapman (2004) encourages us to see that what the patient needs goes beyond the physical needs to the emotions. Significant life changes are often thrust upon a patient. The patient may be in pain, and pain can be a lonely experience. The term "radical loving care" (Chapman, 2004) stresses the importance of making a significant connection with each patient. It is a trinity that is very beneficial to have present in a healthcare organization: the Golden Thread (the loving thread that connects us), the Sacred Encounter (each time we interact with a patient), and the Servant's Heart (we serve others).

Patient and Family Advisory Councils

One way to find out what patients want and value is to conduct focus groups with patients and families. Focus groups or patient advisory councils can be very beneficial in determining what patients and families value and want related to health care. Many organizations find that focus groups augment other forms of feedback, such as results from patient satisfaction surveys. Consumers Advancing Patient Safety (2012) has a step-by-step guide with examples on how to partner with patient groups to enhance value and safety (Leonhardt, Bonin, & Pagel, 2007). Additional information regarding Consumers Advancing Patient Safety can be found at www.patientsafety.org.

In addition, it is important to include the patient and family in interdisciplinary rounds and shift reports *at the patient's bedside*. In some organizations, interdisciplinary rounds and shift reports are completed just outside the patient's room. This is disrespectful to the patient, who is the leader of his or her plan of care, and these conversations may also pose confidentiality issues. Often, the healthcare workers focus on their needs rather than the needs and values of the patient. Of course, the patient's acuity and state of rest may preclude report at the bedside.

Replace Patient Compliance with What the Patient Wants and Values

Recall that the patient is the leader in his or her care. Value is based on what the patient wants and needs; thus, the phrase *patient compliance* should be eliminated from our healthcare vocabulary. The term originates from the patriarchal medical system. *Patient compliance* assumes that healthcare workers know better than the patient what the patient wants and values. This term has negative connotations, and thus many healthcare workers use the term *adherence* instead of *compliance*.

The ethical principle of autonomy applies here. Special pause is needed related to this issue because the *ANA Code of Ethics with Interpretive Statements* (2001) upholds the patient's right to self-determination, or autonomy. Patients have the moral and legal right to make knowledgeable, informed healthcare decisions, with the support of family and significant others, by:

- Receiving accurate, complete, and understandable information in a manner that facilitates informed judgment;
- Being provided available treatment options, including no treatment, and the risks & benefits of those options; and,
- Feeling supported by healthcare providers in the patient's decision to accept, refuse, or terminate treatment, including the choice of no treatment (Provision 1.1.4).

The patient has a right to choose, and what is termed "noncompliant" may be due to what the patient wants and values, or it may result from a lack of knowledge. Thus, it is the healthcare worker's responsibility to educate the patient related to current evidence-based care. Then, the patient is equipped to make decisions based on what is valued and needed.

To further understand "patient noncompliance," consider the side effects that can occur with medications. When the physician or nurse practitioner prescribes a medication—for example, a steroid—and the patient decides that the harmful side effects outweigh the benefits and does not take the medication, perhaps being "noncompliant" is smart and safe.

Health literacy has come to light as a problem that influences patient adherence to recommended treatment. The U.S. Department of Health and Human Services (n.d.) defined *health literacy* as the "degree to which individuals have the capacity to obtain, process, and understand basic health information and services needed to make appropriate health decisions" (para. 1). This includes the individual's basic reading levels. Poor health literacy is associated with poor health outcomes. The IOM (2004a) reported that 90 million people in the United States "have difficulty understanding and acting upon health information" (p. 1). An inability to understand medical language and printed instructions affects the individual's ability to follow recommended treatments. Clear communication in plain language is imperative. It is important to determine that the patient understands the provided education.

Another pervasive "noncompliance" issue is the cost of healthcare services. Again, using a medication example, consider a scenario in the local pharmacy. An elderly woman waits in line for her prescriptions, and the pharmacist tells her that her medications total $568. She says, "I am on a fixed income. I don't have that much money." The pharmacist says, "Well, your doctor insists on not using generic medications, so there is nothing I can do to bring the cost down." They finally agree for her to pay for a week's worth of medications and to wait for her next Social Security check. If this woman uses her Social Security check to pay for medications, how will she pay for other necessities, such as rent and food? Her physician considers the generic medications less effective. However, did the physician take into account *value* as defined by the patient (what she needs)? Would it have been better for the pharmacist to call the physician to discuss the possibility of using generic drugs to save costs for the client? And even if generic drugs were used, can this woman afford to buy the medications and still have money for rent and food? Were *all* of these drugs necessary? Why do the drugs cost so much?

Larger societal issues add to the problem of patient "noncompliance." Consider the difficulties that many patients encounter in seeing their physician when they experience problems. They are charged for an office visit. If they need to be transferred to a specialist, in a health maintenance organization system they may or may not be able to get beyond the gatekeeper to obtain the care they need. The public deals with "compliance" issues by surfing the Internet and reading literature related to their health condition or illness—sometimes becoming better informed than healthcare providers—and by turning to alternative medicine. Perhaps the most important adherence issue is that nurses and other healthcare providers forget that patients have the right to make choices.

It is important to discuss treatments, including medications, with patients. Nurses need to do a better job of patient (and family) education. Healthcare workers must encourage the patient (and family) to ask questions and to understand how to best deal with health problems. Nurses need to have time to do this activity to teach patients in ways that patients understand. When the patient compliance patriarchal system is gone, it will be replaced with what the patient wants and values.

PART 3: THE IMPACT OF QUALITY

▶ The Quality Dimension

Consider quality with the recollection that what the patient wants and values comes *first*. In addition to listening to the patient and involving the patient in decision making about treatments and care from the patient's value perspective, quality (including safety) is paramount. When nurses are effective in the quality arena, our decisions and actions provide care that is needed in the safest, most effective way. What exactly is quality?

This chapter describes a fundamentally different perspective in defining quality and what quality is really all about. Quality has many definitions and can mean different things to different people.

Definitions of quality have been inadequate. In fact, most definitions do not consider the patient's perspective but rather rely heavily on the perspective of the healthcare professional or that of the payer or regulator. Nurses have forgotten the most important person in the equation—our *patient*, our *client*, our *resident*. Most often healthcare professionals do not consult the patient to find out what the patient wants, needs, or values. Perhaps this is best captured in the definition of quality in the book *Through the Patients' Eyes* (Gerteis, Edgman-Levitan, Daley, & Delbanco, 1993). The authors promote the concept that quality has two dimensions: technical excellence and the subjective experience.

Technical excellence is defined as 'the skill and competence of professionals and the ability of diagnostic or therapeutic equipment, procedures, and systems to accomplish what they are meant to accomplish." The subjective experience is what the patient experiences most directly in their interactions with healthcare professionals. It is through these encounters that patients base "their perception of illness or well-being" thereby forming their subjective experience upon which they closely identify as healthcare quality (p. xi).

For this new century, the IOM (2001) recommends that healthcare workers commit to six aims for improvement that will change the perspective of care to one that focuses on what the patient wants and values. These aims are built around the core need for health care to be:

- *Safe*: avoiding injuries to patients from the care that is intended to help them.
- *Effective*: providing services based on scientific knowledge to all who could benefit, and refraining from providing services to those not likely to benefit.
- *Patient-centered*: providing care that is respectful of and responsive to individual patient preferences, needs, and values, and ensuring that patient values guide all clinical decisions.
- *Timely*: reducing waits and sometimes harmful delays for both those who receive and those who give care.

- *Efficient*: avoiding waste, including waste of equipment, supplies, ideas, and energy.
- *Equitable*: providing care that does not vary in quality because of personal characteristics, such as gender, ethnicity, geographic location, and socioeconomic status (pp. 2–3).

Patient-centered means listening to each patient. The patient might value something entirely different from the care that is provided. It is important to understand what the patient values. Often, patients value different things at different times. For example, when a patient is in critical condition, the patient may want a highly skilled, prompt, technologically advanced, yet kind caregiver, whereas a nonacute patient may prefer a rapid turnaround with a kind, personable caregiver. Nevertheless, it is more than that. The answer to the value question depends on how the patient defines quality of life.

Performance Improvement

It must be determined whether the total organization is achieving quality. Of course, all workers can improve. All organizations need PI work to examine quality and safety issues, as well as to identify opportunities to improve processes and outcomes. It is a proactive process, meaning that everyone identifies problems and contributes to improvement efforts. Performance improvement has been implemented with varying success in many healthcare organizations and businesses.

Performance improvement is referenced by several terms—for example, continuous improvement, continuous quality improvement, total quality measurement, and quality management, to name a few. Several methods are used to improve performance; however, many healthcare organizations use some form of "plan, do, study, act," or PDSA, to address quality improvement. The IHI (2012) outlined a model that includes questions the organization must answer followed by the PDSA cycle to test the change to determine whether improvement was made (**BOX 4.6**). This is an efficient practice model that results in increased patient satisfaction and quality.

BOX 4.6 Model for Improvement

The Model for Improvement, developed by Associates in Process Improvement, includes three fundamental questions and Plan-Do-Study-Act (PDSA) cycles to conduct small-scale tests of change.
Questions to answer:

- *What are we trying to accomplish?* Set aims and time-specific measurable goals.
- *How will we know that a change is an improvement?* Establish measures, compare with a baseline measure for evaluating results.
- *What changes can we make that will result in improvement?* Brainstorm ideas and test them one at a time in a pilot setting. The idea is to fine-tune the process before fully implementing it across the organization. Prioritize which change should be tried first.

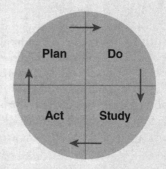

Plan the test of change. Activities, actions, task, or process step.
Do implement the change.
Study the change results. Is the result or outcome better? Was the defined goal met?
Act to keep the change or go back to planning. Is fine-tuning needed or is it necessary to start from scratch? Revisit the fundamental questions.

Modified from the Institute for Healthcare Improvement (IHI). The Model for Improvement, as seen on IHI's website (www .IHI.org), was developed by Associates in Process Improvement [Langley, Nolan, Nolan, Norman, Provost. The Improvement Guide. San Francisco: Jossey-Bass Publishers; 2009].

Six Sigma (Smith, 2003) is a popular approach to performance that was previously used in businesses other than health care. It provides a systematic approach to improve patient outcomes, and acts as a PI tool that incorporates data analysis to identify and reduce variation, thereby reducing patient safety events (**BOX 4.7**). By reducing variability and promoting standardization, the potential for errors is greatly decreased, resulting in increased patient safety and better outcomes. Standardization is an important concept.

Although it is helpful to have standardization in processes, this approach does not take into account individual patient differences and can increase complexity. When complexity increases, more errors occur. Some advocate making small incremental changes at the bedside, rather than standardization. Each patient's expectations are different because patients want and value different things. Thus, nurses need to listen to patients about what they want and value.

Although *Lean* and *Six Sigma* are separate entities, there is a current effort in health care to combine these two methods into a single approach to perform quality improvement (Glasgow, Scott-Caziewell, & Kaboli, 2010). Using both approaches provides processes focused on measuring and eliminating errors (Six Sigma) while ensuring efficient work flow and value-added time (Lean) (Glasgow et al., 2010). Combining these two approaches also balances the regulatory need to maintain process performance (Six Sigma) while supporting rapid continuous improvement (Lean), and thus also easing the tension between the need for incremental changes and system changes.

An important part of the role of an administrator is to pay attention to, and promote, ways the healthcare team can reframe their work to better achieve each patient's goals. This is complicated because it is a new concept for many individuals in health care. Paying attention to value, along with quality and safety, puts us in an interesting dilemma. Value, quality, and safety are somewhat elusive because they can never be totally achieved. Yet nurses need to constantly improve patient care processes. It is important to dedicate time and effort to striving to achieve value, quality, and safety. When nurses believe that they have done their best, they have satisfying work experiences. When excellent, safe care is delivered, and the patient values the service, everyone on the healthcare team feels good about his or her work, and, most important, the patient benefits by experiencing the best possible care.

Input and participation by staff are essential to the success of PI teams. Front-line staff are most familiar with the problems and opportunities and can be instrumental in identifying and implementing change or in orchestrating sabotage when they are not consulted. Involvement in PI programs is often mandated in annual employee evaluations and reflected in bonuses for incentive plans.

Former patients are particularly valuable members of PI teams. Improvement efforts

---

BOX 4.7 Critical Elements of Six Sigma

- Genuine focus on the customer.
- Data and fact-driven management: the numbers speak.
- Processes are where the action is; processes are the key vehicle to success.
- Proactive management: acting in advance of a problem rather than reacting.
- Boundaryless collaboration: break down barriers between departments, organize work teams across the organization.
- Drive for perfection but tolerate failure.

Data from Smith, B. (2003). *Lean and Six Sigma—a one-two punch*. Quality Progress, 37–41.

are meant to improve patient care, and input from these stakeholders may reveal what was important to them during their encounters with the healthcare system. It is also helpful if project members include patients' family or significant others because these individuals experienced the difficulties inherent in a healthcare crisis or in encounters with the healthcare system. Input from all stakeholders related to the project is invaluable. They have the best ideas about what needs to be done, or changed, to achieve value.

Performance improvement efforts must involve all stakeholders to critically evaluate current practice, processes, potential environmental hazards, and other unsafe situations before incidents occur. Again, the goal is to be proactive rather than reactive. The PI plan should be integrated with the organization's operations and financial plan, as well as education and strategic plans to provide enhanced safety for patients. It is imperative that administrators focus on safety when considering budget requests. Nurses need to be assertive and consistently tout the importance of these expenditures.

This means that all healthcare workers must look around with "new eyes" to see potential issues that, if recognized, could be prevented. Consider the following list:

- Drug packaging looks the same for different drugs or drug names are similar. Bar coding is critical.
- Errors involve a breakdown in communication. High-risk communications include times of transition, such as shift change, patient transfer to another area, or transfer to another facility. Adopting a standard communication method is helpful. **BOX 4.8** provides an example of an effective communication method that resulted in 96% to 100% retention of information.
- When staffing is inadequate, more safety issues occur. It may be better to employ more staff, close beds, merge units, or use other planned strategies so that everyone knows what to do when this occurs.

BOX 4.8   SBAR Communication

S situation (the current issue)
B background (brief, related to the point)
A assessment (what you found/think)
R recommendation/request (what you want next)

Data from Haig, K., Sutton, S., & Whittington, J. (2006). SBAR: A shared mental model for improving communication between clinicians. *Journal on Quality and Patient Safety, 32*(3), 167–175.

- It is important for every RN routinely to make rounds and talk with the patients. These activities provide opportunities to discover what the patient wants and values.
- It is equally important for nursing assistants to make regular rounds and make sure patients are routinely turned and given important care.
- Poor teamwork and ineffective leadership bring on a multitude of safety issues.
- Sometimes an RN does not assume leadership of a team—for example, in the case of a new graduate RN. This brings to light the importance of mentors and preceptors.
- Woods and Doan-Johnson (2002) analyzed 21 disciplinary case files from nine boards of nursing to develop a taxonomy of nursing practice errors (**BOX 4.9**). In an effort to raise awareness, it is important to share this information with staff. These errors must be addressed through staff education and PI efforts.
- Lack of critical thinking can cause errors. Staff members need to be educated to go beyond "task orientation" to understand systems thinking before they select actions.
- Interdisciplinary miscommunication is a serious safety issue. Markey and Brown (2002) noted that a team of RNs, physical therapists, occupational therapists, patient care assistants, and physicians, when working together on teams, discovered that each discipline had a different vocabulary for the same activities.

BOX 4.9 Categories of Nursing Errors

- Lack of attentiveness
  Attentiveness refers to the nurse's ability to find out and remember assessment data on each patient "paying attention to the patient's clinical condition and response to therapy, as well as potential hazards or errors in treatment" (p. 46).

- Lack of agency/fiduciary concern
  Lack of agency/fiduciary concern gets back to what the patient values. Here, the nurse needs to be an advocate for the patient, by questioning physician orders, calling physicians, and paying attention to patient/family requests.

- Inappropriate judgment
  The nurse's judgment and clinical expertise is important if the nurse is to intervene on the patient's behalf.

- Medication errors
  A medication error is any preventable event that may cause or lead to inappropriate medication use or patient harm while the medication is in the control of the healthcare professional, patient, or consumer. Such events may be related to professional practice, healthcare products, procedures, and systems, including prescribing; order communication; product labeling, packaging, and nomenclature; compounding; dispensing; distribution; administration; education; monitoring; and use (p. 47). Many medication errors are never reported.

- Lack of intervention on the patient's behalf
  Often, symptoms that the nurse does not recognize or respond to in a timely manner result in a complication or death that could have possibly been prevented.

- Lack of prevention
  Teach all employees to identify any potential problems and rectify them as soon as the problems are noticed. Infection control, immobility hazards, and a safe environment are areas of concern.

- Missed or mistaken physician or healthcare provider orders
  Use of a provider order entry and a computerized documentation system could more effectively prevent this occurrence.

- Documentation errors (p. 46)
  Additional documentation errors are problematic in two areas:
  1. *Charting procedures or medications before they were completed.* Such a documentation error can cause a patient to miss a dose of medication or a treatment and can confuse, misrepresent, or mask a patient's true condition.
  2. *Lack of charting of observations of the patient* causes serious harm when a nurse fails to chart signs of patient deterioration, pain, or agitation or particular signs of complications related to the illness or therapies (p. 48).

Data from Woods, A., & Doan-Johnson, S. (2002, October). Executive summary: Toward a taxonomy of nursing practice errors. *Nursing Management,* 45–48.

These authors found that each department had its own activity and mobility vocabulary and because staff members' duties for mobilizing patients were not defined, specific guidelines were most helpful in carrying out the activities specified by nurses, patient care assistants, physicians, physical therapists, or occupational therapists. These guidelines were also shared with patients and families, which accomplished better consistency when working with patients. For example, the patient care assistants understood specifically what to have the patient do, as well as what the aide should do for the patient. These guidelines provided a set of scripted behaviors that achieved a more consistent approach.

Evidence-Based Practice

When contemplating quality patient care, consider whether the most appropriate, up-to-date care is provided. Research has shown that both physicians and nurses plan care and treatment based on what they learned in school, even if that was 20 years ago. In addition, the nurse may not know what is best for a certain individual with a particular need. Nurses must have access to the latest research related to the problem, and/or treatment of the problem, and must use that information and professional judgment to determine the most appropriate approach. Evidence-based practice is a synthesis of research and clinical expertise that has demonstrated to be successful related to particular conditions. This is a challenge because there is so much information available. Knowing where to find the best information, how to evaluate the information to determine what is the best or most appropriate research, and how to apply it to practice is complicated.

The Internet and technology systems are powerful resources. For example, a lot of research on patient outcomes is available. When a physician or nurse practitioner writes a medication order, he or she may not know which of several drugs might be most effective. Evidence-based decision-support systems can quickly determine the best available research for specific topics. These systems also provide evidence-based plans of care and therapy recommendations.

Evidence-based practice is important, but only 15% of the nursing workforce consistently implements practice based on evidence (Shirey, 2006). One problem is that nurses and providers do not realize how easily information can be accessed, or they do not take the time to look up current research results. Many lack the skills to translate research knowledge into practice. Obtaining the information is only the first step. Administrators can encourage evidence-based practice by removing barriers to access, by providing technology (such as a computer or handheld device), and by establishing the expectation that practice must be based on current evidence. Sometimes evidence is available in the EMR system. Additionally, administrators and leaders must use evidence to guide our leadership and management practices.

Clinical Pathways and Protocols

When delivering care, evidence-based practice can be achieved by using clinical pathways, order sets, or clinical protocols as long as the pathways or protocols are kept current. An effective clinical pathway is the result of interdisciplinary teamwork; the team includes the physician, nurse, social worker, dietitian, and patient and may include other members, such as a chaplain or nurse aide or significant family members. Approved protocols can automatically be implemented without an additional order. A caution related to clinical pathways is that all caregivers must continue to take into account patient idiosyncrasies or differences (and what the patient wants and values) that might change the pathway.

Changing Administrative Practices

Variation in the success of PI programs is often related to administrative leaders who do not support the work. Thus, problem processes proliferate that may negatively affect the success of the organization. Often, PI endeavors are not perceived as important. Nurse leaders need to complete an organizational assessment and learn how to identify and make systems changes effectively. Note that the most effective changes are small, incremental, and at the point of care. Little by little, better quality is achieved. This is better than adding to the complexity with quick fixes, which create more issues to be dealt with later. As complexity increases, errors increase. Nurses need to know how to find information related to their administrative work to remain up-to-date in administrative practices and must encourage staff and physicians to use these resources.

The IOM (2001) provides the best signpost, to date, for us to use as our ultimate goal. It advocates the redesign of our healthcare delivery systems based on 10 fundamental rules. *Redesign* has been so mismanaged in health care that the word has negative connotations. The difference here is that *redesign,* as described by the IOM, uses the administrative practices discussed in this text. It is *not* a bottom-line approach to downsize. The 10 rules of redesign are as follows:

1. **Care is based on continuous healing relationships.** Patients should receive care whenever they need it and in many forms, not just in face-to-face visits. This implies that the healthcare system must be responsive at all times, and access to care should be provided over the Internet, by telephone, and by other means, in addition to in-person visits.

2. **Care is customized according to patient needs and values.** The system should be designed to meet the most common types of needs, but should have the capability to respond to individual patient choices and preferences.

3. **The patient is the source of control.** Patients should be given the necessary information and opportunity to exercise the degree of control they choose over healthcare decisions that affect them. The system should be able to accommodate differences in patient preferences and encourage shared decision making.

4. **Knowledge is shared and information flows freely.** Patients should have unfettered access to their own medical information and to clinical knowledge. Clinicians and patients should communicate effectively and share information.

5. **Decision making is evidence-based.** Patients should receive care based on the best available scientific knowledge. Care should not vary illogically from clinician to clinician or from place to place.

6. **Safety is a system property.** Patients should be safe from injury caused by the care system. Reducing risk and ensuring safety require greater attention to systems that help prevent and mitigate errors.

7. **Transparency is necessary.** The system should make available to patients and their families information that enables them to make informed decisions when selecting a health plan, hospital, or clinical practice, or when choosing among alternative treatments. This should include information describing the system's performance on safety, evidence-based practice, and patient satisfaction.

8. **Needs are anticipated.** The system should anticipate patient needs rather than simply react to events.

9. **Waste is continuously decreased.** The system should not waste resources or patient time.

10. **Cooperation among clinicians is a priority.** Clinicians and institutions should actively collaborate and communicate to ensure an appropriate exchange of information and coordination of care (pp. 8–9).

Provider Accountability in the Cost–Quality Dilemma

The linear healthcare administrator, heavily committed to the bottom line, may question, "Where is the money coming from for all this?" Reframing is in order. Finding the value of a healthcare service requires healthcare leaders and care providers to ask the following questions:

- What is the actual service provided?
- How do organizational processes support this service?
- What are the interactions between these processes?
- What impact does the service have on the patients and the community? (Porter-O'Grady & Malloch, 2011, pp. 300–301)

Striving for value will make a difference. The nurse leader is situated between senior leaders and staff, and thus is in a pivotal position to influence change. The nurse leader is a teacher for staff and a role model for all healthcare workers. Focusing on what the patient values and wants is a wise choice, as opposed to focusing on those things that do not make a difference for patients. Often, this is a new concept for patients and families as well. A proportion of patients will not accept the new role, some because of culture, others because of health literacy, lack of knowledge, or a host of additional reasons (Longtin et al., 2010).

This brings the nurse back to the foundational document, the ANA *Code of Ethics with Interpretive Statements*, which demands that nurses provide the patient with the needed knowledge. Patients have the moral and legal right "to be given accurate, complete, and understandable information in a manner that facilitates informed judgment" (ANA, 2001). Habitually seeking what the patient wants and values is *not optional*; rather it is our mandate. The issue is a serious one.

A "bottom-line" administrator, simply on the basis of salary alone, may deem that RNs are more expensive to employ. To save money, the administrator may demand the staffing mix be changed by decreasing the number of RNs and adding licensed practical nurses (LPNs) or nursing assistants. This demand is not supported by evidence. Melberg (1997) examined budgets and staffing at five hospitals, documenting that a hospital budget with a 96% RN staff mix is *less expensive* than another hospital budget with a 64% RN mix. In fact, the hospital with the highest costs had the *lowest* RN skill mix (64%). Melberg (1997) noted:

> A high RN mix does not correlate with higher nursing costs per patient day in acute or critical care. Diluting the RN mix does not always reduce staffing costs. Although hospital A has a 96 percent RN-skill mix, the highest in the system, total nursing salary per patient day falls exactly in the middle. The highest costs occurred at hospital C where, in fact, the 64 percent RN mix is the lowest in the system (p. 48).

Likewise, a study by Lindrooth, Bazzoli, Needleman, and Hasnain-Wynia (2006) corroborates that it is more cost-effective to provide a higher RN ratio. Thus, cost may be *higher* with a higher ratio of non-RN staff.

This is only the beginning of the cost issue because RNs save costs in other areas in addition to salaries. Consider patient outcomes and the cost of patient safety events. Recall earlier in this chapter that the IOM (2004a) documented that each patient safety event added an additional $8,750 to each hospital stay. Also recall research that notes higher RN ratios are linked to better patient outcomes. When lower RN staffing leads to death or injury, it is a *very high cost*. Thus, determining the appropriate nursing skill mix requires analysis of the care environment, population served, patient acuity, patient turnover, the type and manner in which care is delivered, culture, budget, staff competencies, and evidence-based findings. There are no easy answers. What works best in one setting (for example, in a step-down unit) may not be best in another (for example, a skilled unit). Thus, the nursing skill mix is determined by the current circumstances and changes to meet new situations as they occur.

Administrators must critically analyze issues of adequate staffing and the RN staffing mix. Research supports the fact that increased RN staffing affects patient safety. This provides the impetus for administrators to focus on RN recruitment and retention efforts. Recall from earlier in this chapter that the ANA (2013b) cited, *"each additional patient care RN employed (at 7.8 hours per patient day) will generate over $60,000 annually in reduced medical costs and improved national productivity"* (para. 5).

What Does It Mean to Be in the Information Age?

Performance improvement in the Information Age means that nurses must use technology effectively. In the past, many computer systems were not integrated. The transition to a fully integrated computerized system moves the organization to a more viable state that enables improved access and use of information. Integration allows use of CDS at the point of care, which is crucial to implement evidence-based practice. This presents a major financial undertaking because computer systems are expensive. Costs extend beyond the walls of the organization, which brings about additional challenges. Physicians and other providers need to be able to access the system from multiple locations, not just when they are in the facility. For true point-of-care access, computers must be mobile or at every point of care.

Online Clinical Documentation Systems

The Leapfrog Group (2013) identified the importance of CPOE and is especially pertinent in large healthcare systems. Online documentation provides integration of documentation from all disciplines. All disciplines chart together, and thus there is immediate access to relevant information, as well as better continuity of care. In addition, preformatted charting presents an easy, time-saving format for the clinician to follow. Patient safety is enhanced through decision support. Built-in clinical alerts identify abnormal results, allergies, stop dates on medicines, incompatible medicines, times to administer medications, and provide a variety

of other safeguards that promote patient safety and quality.

Online systems also provide immediate and virtual access to laboratory and radiology results in both the healthcare facility and the physician's office. In addition, physicians can interact with the CPOE system from their office location. Prescriptions and discharge instructions can be generated. From a safety standpoint, the liability related to legibility problems is decreased.

In these systems, documentation is thorough and better reflects patient status, resulting in enhanced safety and increased reimbursement as a result of accurate coding for billing. The systems can also link cost and quality data.

An alert to clinicians using computers in the patient's presence is that patients may erroneously think that providers are using the computer in a way unrelated to patient care. Thus, it is important for providers to explain computer work to clarify their actions for patients.

Bar Coding

A closed-loop system comprising a scanner to bar-code the medication, the clinician administering the medication, and the patient's armband has proven very successful in reducing medication errors, when appropriately used, related to the five rights of medication administration: right patient, right route, right dose, right time, and right medication. Medication-dispensing systems are available in many facilities to assist with medication administration. Some facilities have implemented robotics to assist with medication identification in the pharmacy, as well as with delivery from the pharmacy. These strategies also decrease the possibility of error. Although costs are significant, the savings realized from diverted errors, increased patient satisfaction, and promotion of quality more than makes up for the expense.

Portable Electronic Devices

Portable electronic devices are used to promote efficiency and decrease transcription errors.

Access is available from remote locations, for example, during the admission process to retrieve demographic and insurance information. In addition, clinicians can retrieve information about medications, diagnoses, and other health data immediately as needed.

▶ Recognition of Value and Quality

A number of programs in healthcare focus on value and quality. Some have gained national awareness.

The Leapfrog Group

Organizations have implemented voluntary programs that measure and report safety data and outcomes. An example is the Leapfrog Group, which supports pay for performance, whose primary focus is to improve and implement best practices. The Leapfrog Group is a consortium of major companies and other large private and public healthcare purchasers. . . . Members and their employees spend tens of billions of dollars on health care annually. Leapfrog members have agreed to base their purchase of health care on principles that encourage quality improvement among providers and consumer involvement (Leapfrog Group, 2013, para. 3).

Magnet Recognition Program

Earning the esteemed designation of a Magnet facility has become a renowned indicator of quality. This is an expensive process in terms of both money and resources for the facility. Magnet recognition is a voluntary process encompassing strenuous evaluation of nursing excellence and innovation in nursing practice (American Nurses Credentialing Center [ANCC], 2013). The Magnet Recognition Program has three goals:

■ Promote quality in a setting that supports professional practice

■ Identify excellence in the delivery of nursing services to patients/residents
■ Disseminate best practice in nursing services (ANCC, 2013, para. 7)

The National Database of Nursing Quality Indicators

The NDNQI was developed by the ANA 2013a) to collect and report nurse-sensitive outcomes data in an effort to show how nursing care promotes quality and patient safety. Participation is voluntary, and thus data may not provide an accurate picture of nursing care across the nation. Nevertheless, the NDNQI data provide nurse administrators a tool to compare outcomes, staffing, and other nurse-sensitive measures. Some of the data include incidents of hospital-acquired pressure ulcers, fall rates, and restraint use in relation to nursing hours per patient day and skill mix.

▶ Performance Measurement

In an effort to contain costs, performance measurement became popular in the early 1990s when companies purchasing health plans needed to examine cost and quality data to determine which plan was best for the dollars spent. At first, these efforts were called report cards and only summary performance data were included. Later, report cards were used internally by healthcare organizations to improve services. (Details can be found at www.healthgrades.com/.)

The idea behind performance measurement is that patient outcomes could be used to determine the effectiveness of organizational performance. Although this measurement is an improvement on past practices, there are several problems with this measurement: (1) future performance cannot be determined from historical data; (2) no one asked the patient what the patient wanted or valued; (3) organizations are inundated with data, leaving little time to analyze or use the data effectively; and (4) sometimes the data were used punitively when outcomes were poor, which only impeded future improvements.

As report card data became available, TJC (2013a) expanded performance measurement to include two sets of measures: core or standardized measures and noncore measures. In 2003, TJC joined forces with CMS to align efforts and required organizations to report on certain measures depending on the populations served (TJC, 2013a). Measures are identified for hospitals, long-term care facilities, and home care. The results are available to the public at www.qualitycheck.org (TJC, 2013d).

Benchmarking

Many healthcare organizations benchmark quality measures. Often, when *benchmarking*, the organization sets a goal, for example, to be in the top 25th quartile. However, benchmarking can be fraught with problems. Rudy, Lucke, Whitman, and Davidson (2001) reported that while benchmarking is a common approach to

establishing quality, the value of the benchmarks weigh heavily on the origination of the data: Is it from the literature, from hospital-specific sources, or from an integrated hospital system? **TABLE 4.1** provides a summary of some of the pros and cons with the three primary sources of benchmarking data.

There is an additional problem with benchmarking. Comparisons do not take into account what has value from the patient's perspective. For example, when benchmarking the wait time for an ED visit, a wait time of 1 hour might compare favorably with other ED wait times. Nevertheless, consider this statement from the patient's perspective: The patient does not enjoy experiencing an hour wait in the ED to be seen by the provider. From the patient value perspective, it is better to eliminate the wait time and have the patient seen by the provider immediately. Some EDs already use 30 minutes as the benchmark; even a 30-minute wait is not as valuable to the patient as no wait time.

Patient Satisfaction

Patient satisfaction is one early performance measure that focuses on what the patient

TABLE 4.1	Pros and Cons with Three Primary Sources of Benchmarking Data	
Types of Benchmarking	**Pros**	**Cons**
Literature	Broad range of access to benchmarking data and metrics	Relevant to populations or clinical practice? What is the standard error of the benchmark?
Internal	Ease of access	Invalid assessment of performance when compared to other institutions
System	Avoids pitfalls of Literature and Internal sources	Requires coordinated database resources and sophisticated statistical analyses

values. Patient satisfaction instruments are a beginning measurement of value, although they take place *after* the healthcare experience. Hospitals have used patient satisfaction measurements for some time because measuring patient satisfaction has been an important core outcome measure for Joint Commission accreditation.

Examples of companies that provide patient satisfaction instruments and services to healthcare organizations include Gallup® (2013) and Press Ganey Associates* (2013). Generally, hospitals pay these companies to collect and tabulate the data. This is considered more effective because patients are more likely to be forthright with an outside vendor, as opposed to those providing their care. There are other advantages to using an outside vendor: The organization's results are ranked among similar organizations, thus providing benchmarking opportunities.

To adequately assess patient satisfaction, both the patient's and the provider's expectations must be clearly identified. In the past, patients were seen as customers in need of health care; now they are viewed as informed consumers looking for quality care. Health care has become a competitive business. Many facilities are using contract agencies to market their services and measure their success, and they have implemented service excellence initiatives to improve patient satisfaction. Some even have scripted behaviors and protocols to standardize dialogue in difficult situations. This is an example of standardization previously discussed.

It is important to remember that nurses deal with people. What has value to one individual may not have value to another. For example, one individual may welcome talking about emotions with a healthcare provider, whereas another individual may find this invasive. One individual may respond to pain by being stoic, whereas another who experiences even mild pain may scream and yell.

Staff evaluations may be directly linked to satisfaction results. Results from patient satisfaction surveys can be very useful and can be used to do the following:

- Improve and measure the quality of care
- Manage complaints
- Implement strategic planning and marketing decisions
- Evaluate and/or provide bonuses to departments or individual (physician and nonphysician) staff
- Enhance public relations
- Meet accreditation standards
- Monitor for risk management
- Link survey results to clinical data
- Use survey results for contract payer negotiations
- Compare the results for benchmarking
- Link the results to financial data

Performance Measurement and Patient Value

It is questionable as to whether these measures reflect what patients want and value. The CMS Quality Initiatives (CMS, 2013e) and the Joint Commission's National Patient Safety Goals (TJC, 2013c) are patient-centered, but, again, it is uncertain whether these measure the patient's perception of value. Outside vendors measure patient satisfaction, but, again, do the operational definitions capture the patient's perception of value?

Empirical data have dominated the healthcare system. What is needed in addition to quantifiable data is capture of the complexity of healthcare work including qualitative data— for example, "patient–provider relationships, effectiveness of the procedure, patient satisfaction, and health behaviors practiced is not considered in the reimbursement categories" (Porter-O'Grady & Malloch, 2011, p. 85). This links to the patient and family advisory focus groups discussed earlier in this chapter. The data received from these groups provide rich information for PI work.

Administrators must maintain the focus on what patients want and value. If leaders lose sight of this goal, statistics are useless. The organization may be profitable and have stellar patient outcomes, but if patients are not getting what they need, want, and value, they have a choice as to whether or not to return to the facility. As organizations collect data from focus groups, or even as they organize the groups, they must consider the data in terms of populations served because voluminous qualitative data can become overwhelming. The emphasis must move from individuals to populations. As nurses examine patient populations, their focus should move beyond identified diseases or problems. For example, parents of young children have concerns that are different from those of older adults who are experiencing chronic diseases and who are on fixed incomes. Focus group participants may need to be organized to better identify these populations.

Balanced Scorecard: Best Approach to Performance Measurement

Balanced scorecards (BSC) are the best way to conduct improvement work (IHI, 2012). Metrics captured in the organization's BSC are tied directly to the strategic plan. A primary utility of the BSC is the tie between strategic management and performance management. Measurement of key financial, quality, market, and operational indicators provides management with an understanding of performance in relation to established strategic goals and graphically displays a snapshot of the institution's overall health (Health Care Advisory Board, 1999). Plotting the data for these measures using a run chart (and then a control chart when sufficient data points are collected) is a simple and effective way to determine whether changes are leading to improvement or whether the gains are sustained (IHI, 2012). Run charts and control charts are graphs of data over time and are important tools for assessing effectiveness

of change (IHI, 2011b). Benefits of run charts include the following:

- They help improvement teams formulate aims by depicting how well (or poorly) a process is performing.
- They help in determining when changes are truly improvements by displaying a pattern of data you can observe as you make changes.
- They give direction as you work on improvement and offer information about the value of particular changes (IHI, 2011b, para. 2).

It is vital that administrators and managers understand the type data collected and the correct type of chart to be used. This information is beyond the scope of this chapter.

Utilization Review

Another measurement related to the care provided is *utilization review*.

Utilization management has a quality dimension in that the primary purpose is to ensure appropriate use of available services and resources. Many organizations integrate utilization management into the case management role, creating a more complete system of quality management. Historically, healthcare organizations established a person or department to complete utilization review through the relay of clinical information to payers so that the payers could determine whether they would pay for additional care for patients. In the managed care climate, providers cannot provide the care and then submit the bill; rather, they must get preapproval for the care. The payers determine whether the care is allowable. Once the payers determine that the care meets their criteria, the patient is certified for payment.

▶ Employee Issues

When discussing value and quality, it is important to remember employees. When administrators value employees, employees value patients. Thus, this section describes value and quality related to employees.

OSHA Standards for Employee Safety

The first issue is employee safety. There are many possible hazards in the healthcare industry. The Occupational Safety and Health Administration (OSHA) provides nationally mandated standards for the workplace (U.S. Department of Labor, n.d.). Detailed information is available at the U.S. Department of Labor OSHA website (www.osha .gov). Administrators and other leaders must be regularly oriented to OSHA standards. In addition, OSHA has record-keeping requirements that mandate that organizational leaders keep records updated to document compliance with OSHA standards. In larger healthcare systems, both quality and infection control personnel are often concerned with workplace compliance with OSHA standards. In smaller systems, OSHA compliance often becomes an additional responsibility of staff who already have many other roles and responsibilities. Regardless, the nurse leader must be aware of the current standards, ensure that employees are oriented to these standards, and ensure that the patient-care environment is in compliance with the standards.

Promoting a Healthy Workplace

Achieving a healthy workplace includes examining the environment. This can be quite complicated. For example, a sharps injury from a needle used by a patient is a major hazard.

> Of the nearly 14 injury cases per 100 long-term-care employees, a significant number are related to patient lifting or repositioning tasks. OSHA recommends "that manual lifting of residents be minimized in all cases and eliminated when feasible." . . . Possible solutions . . . include using mechanical lifts and ceiling-mounted lift systems. . . . For patients with the ability to assist, or who are able to bear weight completely, equipment, such as sit-to-stand devices, ambulation-assist devices, transfer boards, and lift cushions or chairs, can minimize assistance needed in transferring. [This includes height-adjustable beds with electric controls rather than cranks and showering and bathing assistive devices.] (Weber, 2008, p. 30)

The general public, patients, employees, and administrators frequent healthcare facilities. The volume of people who have access to healthcare facilities presents a number of ways that employees and others could be put at risk (infectious diseases, violence, and so forth). Administrators are responsible for maintaining a safe environment for staff as well as patients.

Disaster Planning and Preparedness

Disaster planning and preparedness has assumed new significance. With the many weather-related events, facilities must be prepared to deal with these issues, even when the facility has been decimated. In addition, the issue of bioterrorism must be addressed for the safety of patients and employees. Procedures to address the identified emergency are dictated by the Federal Emergency Management Administration (FEMA, n.d.), but facility-related issues, such as lack of available nurses and methods to contain or quarantine, are facility specific and should be addressed in policy. Sadly, these issues must be considered at budget time to designate appropriate funds for protective apparel, vaccinations, preparation and training for staff, and public education.

Chaos Theory

Another scientific field of thought is chaos theory. In this theory, the world all around us seems chaotic, but even when it seems that total chaos surrounds us, we must rise above it and look down to find the order and perfection.

Sometimes when unexpected events happen or setbacks or difficult situations occur, it is comforting to know that these experiences accomplish good things for us. Nurses can learn from such situations and become better persons and providers of care. In addition, these experiences can lead to something different or new that we would probably never have tried if the difficulties had not occurred.

When considering planning for change, chaos theory tells us that we cannot possibly plan, or map out, all of the details of the change because of chaotic occurrences. As these occurrences happen, they necessitate adjustments in the plan. This is why all staff need to be involved in understanding the plan and need to be empowered to accomplish it—because the final product, or components of the final product, will ultimately be different from what was planned. Really, there is no final product. Chaos continues to change what was implemented. No one can stop change; rather, it continually moves on into uncharted territory.

Many administrative leaders do not understand the concept of constant change. Instead, they try to cling to the Industrial Age idea that everything is rational and can be planned out in minute detail. It is as if they think they can just order others to follow through on their plan, and then they become frustrated when people do not follow through. This is not the new reality. Continuing to believe this opens us up to unnecessary frustration, and employees will be frustrated as well.

Instead, all of us must be open to the reality around us, see the changes that are occurring, and help interpret the chaos for one another. Although everyone has their own views of reality, chaotic reality happens, and changes will occur and leave us behind, obsolete and unfulfilled.

A good leader is one who can read the signposts suggesting that a change is imminent and can discern the direction of the change and the elements indicating its fabric. The good leader synthesizes rather than analyzes and views the change thematically and/or relationally, drawing out of it what kind of action or strategy should be applied—the response, that is, that best positions for the organization to thrive in the coming circumstances.

For a leader to act as a strategist today means not detailing the organization's future actions, but analyzing the relationship of the system to its external environment, determining the ability of the system to respond and adapt in a sustainable way, and translating that relationship and ability into language that has meaning for those who must do the work of the organization. Translating the signposts into understandable and inspiring language is more critical than almost any other strategic task. It is vital that a change have implications for those who are doing the work. Another way of saying this is that it must have meaning to them within the framework of their work activities so that they can commit to it, which they must do if they and the organization are to adapt to the change successfully. The leader's job is to describe the change in a way that allows the workers to understand its value and how it will affect their own efforts.

(Porter-O'Grady & Malloch, 2011, pp. 23–24)

See **BOX 4.10**.

BOX 4.10 Interdependence

In nature, everything is interdependent. There is an ebb and flow between all the elements of life. Leaders must see their role from this perspective. Most of the work of leadership will be managing the interactions and connections between people and processes. Leaders must remain aware of these truths:

- Action in one place has an effect in other places.
- Fluctuation of mutuality means authority moves between people.
- Interacting properties in systems make outcomes mobile and fluid.
- Relationship building is the primary work of leadership.
- Trusting feeling is as important as valuing thinking.
- Acknowledging in others what is unique in their contribution is vital.
- Supporting, stretching, challenging, pushing, and helping are part of being present to the process, to the players, and to the outcome.

Reproduced from Porter-O'Grady, T., & Malloch, K. (2003). Quantum leadership: A textbook of new leadership. Sudbury, MA: Jones and Bartlett, p. 22.

Summary

Chapter 4 is concerned with how to best support patients being the leader in their care. To do this, we need to find out and provide only what patients value within a safe environment. In healthcare settings, we have not always stressed the importance of listening to our patient to find out what s/he wants and needs. Also, we must give our patient information so that s/he can make the best decisions on needed care.

The old patriarchal system where we made decisions for the patient, and many times did not tell our patients what would happen, is outdated. Along with this, we, as nurses, need to get out of the "task" box and become leaders to make sure that patients are receiving only what they really want. So, this new perspective is so important and, as leaders, we need to support patient decisions.

Chapter 4 also includes information on both quality and patient safety. Nurses understand more about quality and patient safety than our patients do. This is another aspect of leadership that is needed at the point of care. However, we are still harming too many patients in our healthcare systems. Many patient safety issues are caused by a series of events or organizational processes that are broken. It is time to fix these problems and leave blame behind.

As we provide care patients value in a safe environment, chances are we healthcare providers have a knowledge deficit – it is not possible to keep up with all the current treatments, drugs, and research results that could improve our practice and benefit our patients. Now that we are in the Information Age, this research evidence is not a big secret anymore. Yet, despite the readily-accessible research data, we tend to go on doing what we were taught in school, even though evidence-based practices have been identified that should change our practices. Thus, in the end, we must ask ourselves *what does each patient value*? Is this what we are providing? And, as previously noted, this is first priority, not the bottom line.

Discussion Questions

1. Describe strategies used by the nurse administrator that provide patients with what they want and value.
2. What administrative practices support PI efforts?

3. Provide examples of the 10 IOM (2001) rules for redesign applied to your healthcare setting.
4. State five ways that administrators promote patient safety.
5. Why is it important to provide evidence-based care? Discuss some of the challenges nurse administrators face in creating an environment in which bedside nurses use evidence-based care.
6. Discuss the use of run charts and control charts to improve quality.
7. Discuss how Lean thinking and Six Sigma can be used together to improve healthcare quality.
8. What are ways to promote employee safety?
9. Describe how complexity theory applies to your practice.
10. Explain reasons that chaos theory offers hope for the future of health care.

Glossary of Terms

Balanced Scorecard (BSC) a tool used to measure key financial, quality, market, and operational indicators which provides management with an understanding of performance in relation to established strategic goals and graphically displays a snapshot of the institution's overall health.

Benchmarking comparison of quality measures with quality measures from a different source (for example, a similar unit or organization or from the literature).

Bioterrorism term first used in 1991; terrorism which involves biological weapons.

Bureaucracy organizations with specializations, adherence to rules, and a hierarchy of authority.

Chaos Theory recognizes that human and organizational systems are self-organizing; there is constant tension between stability and chaos.

Complexity Science scientific ideas derived from quantum physics, chaos theory, and systems theory which recognize that human and organizational systems are self-organizing; acknowledges that everything is related at some level.

Complexity Theory recognizes that behavior is nonlinear and that order is found in seemingly random complexity.

Ethnocentric the belief that one's own faction is superior.

Health Literacy the ability of individuals to obtain, process, and understand health information and services in order to make appropriate health decisions.

Healthcare Disparity health care that is markedly less in regard to access and availability of facilities or services.

Healthcare-Associated Infections infections associated with the delivery of health care; caregiver-to-patient, environment-to-patient, or patient-to-patient.

Institute of Medicine an independent, nonprofit, nongovernmental organization that provides advice to decision makers and the public.

Kaizen Blitz collaborative work held over 3–5 days in which staff evaluate, develop, and redesign identified processes, followed by monitoring to measure whether the gains are sustained.

Lean uses standard solutions to common problems with a focus on the customer; processes assure efficient work flow and value-added activities; the primary analytic tool is value-stream mapping.

Malcolm Baldrige National Quality Award the highest level of national recognition for performance excellence in the United States.

Meaningful Use in order to receive incentive payments from CMS, providers must demonstrate that they are "meaningfully using" EHRs through compliance with objectives; organizations must "meaningful use" certified computerized health record (CHR) technology to improve patient care.

Missed Care the omission of vital care tasks, such as turning, ambulating, feeding, mouth care, and toileting, which can lead to patient complications—for example, decubitus ulcers and pneumonia.

National Database of Nursing Quality Indicators (NDNQI) consists of nurse-sensitive indicators; the only database of indicators at the nursing unit level.

National Patient Safety Goals actions that organizations accredited by TJC are required to take in order to prevent medical errors.

National Quality Forum a nonprofit, public service organization committed to the transformation of health care to a safe, equitable, and high-value system.

Non-Value-Added Time excessive amounts of nursing time being spent on support activities.

Outcome Measures the effects of healthcare practices and interventions.

Patient Care Quality the determination of what the patient wants and values; to make the patient the leader of his/her care.

Patient-Centered Care care that is focused on the patient's experience of illness and health care and on systems needed to meet the individual patient's needs.

Patient Safety Officer position that promotes safety through education; examines issues to determine better, safer organizational processes; discover the root cause; create system changes to prevent future incidents of the same kind; and then involvement in implementing programs designed to foster safety.

Positive Deviance proposes that within organizations some individuals or groups have different "deviant" practices that produce better "positive" outcomes; holds that staff at the point of care are best equipped to solve the problem.

Quality definitions have been inadequate; most importantly, to determine what the patient wants and values; consists of two dimensions, technical excellence and the subjective experience measured by the patient.

Rapid Improvement Events (RIEs) collaborative work held over 3–5 days in which staff evaluate, develop, and redesign identified processes followed by monitoring to measure whether the gains are sustained.

Risk Management role which has historically been to identify, manage, and reduce risk in order to support the delivery of safe health care while reducing organizational legal risks.

Root Cause Analysis a tool used to identify process variation by asking "Why?" related to each finding in order to drill down to discover why a portion of the process occurred or did not occur.

Sentinel Event an unexpected occurrence including death or serious physical or psychological injury (or the risk thereof).

Six Sigma a popular approach to PI focus is on measuring and eliminating errors; used to reduce patient safety events through reduction of process variation; tools incorporate data analysis to identify and reduce variation; provides a systematic approach in order to improve patient outcomes.

The Joint Commission (TJC) an independent, not-for-profit organization that accredits more than 20,000 healthcare organizations in the United States; TJC accreditation symbolizes an organization's commitment to meeting identified performance standards.

Transparency the availability (free flow) of information that allows informed decisions.

Value-Based Reimbursement reimbursement based on quality rather than quantity; incentive payments based on performance measures or improvement of performance from the baseline.

Value-Stream Mapping the primary analytical tool in Lean activities which can be used effectively to identify interruptions in order to make improvements in work flow; this tool is an extended process flowchart that focuses on speed, continuity of flow, and work in progress in order to identify non-value-added steps and bottlenecks.

Voice of the Customer the process for capturing patient- and other customer-related information which is intended to be proactive and continuously innovative so that it captures customers' stated, unstated, and anticipated requirements, expectations, and desires.

Volume-Based Reimbursement reimbursement based on quantity rather than quality.

References

Agency for Healthcare Research and Quality. (n.d.). *Patient safety and quality: Duplicate medication order errors increase after computerized provider order entry is implemented.* Retrieved from http://www.ahrq.gov /legacy/research/jan12/0112RA12.htm

Agency for Healthcare Research and Quality. (2008). *National healthcare disparities report: 2007.* AHRQ Pub. No. 08-0041. Rockville, MD: U.S. Department of Health and Human Services.

AHC Media. (2008). Change the culture, protect the patient using "positive deviance" to prevent MRSA. *Hospital Infection Control, 35*(9), 97–101.

Aiken, L., Clarke, S., Sloane, D., Sochalski, J., & Silber, J. (2002). Hospital nurse staffing and patient mortality, nurse burnout, and job dissatisfaction. *Journal of the American Medical Association*, *288*(16), 1987–1993.

American Hospital Association 2011 Committee on Performance Improvement. (2011, September). *Hospitals and care systems of the future*. Chicago, IL: Author.

American Nurses Association. (2008). *Nurse staffing impacts quality of patient care*. Retrieved from http://www.nursingworld.org/FunctionalMenuCategories/Media Resources/PressReleases/2008PR/NurseStaffing ImpactsQualityofPatientCare.aspx

American Nurses Association. (2013a). *NDNQI: National Database of Nursing Quality Indicators*. Retrieved from http://www.pressganey.com/solutions/clinical-quality /nursing-quality

American Nurses Credentialing Center. (2013). *Program overview*. Retrieved from http://www.nursecredentialing .org/Magnet/ProgramOverview

Biron, A., Lavoie-Tremblay, M., & Loiselle, C. (2009). Characteristics of work interruptions during medication administration. *Journal of Nursing Scholarship*, *41*(4), 330–336.

Boev, C. (2012). The relationship between nurses' perception of work environment and patient satisfaction in adult critical care. *Journal of Nursing Scholarship*, *44*(4), 368–375.

Centers for Disease Control and Prevention. (2012). *Falls among older adults: An overview*. Retrieved from http://www.cdc.gov/HomeandRecreationalSafety/Falls /adultfalls.html

Centers for Medicare and Medicaid Services. (2003). *Medicare Prescription Drug, Improvement, and Modernization Act (MMA) of 2003*. Retrieved from http://www.cms.gov /Medicare/Demonstration-Projects/DemoProjects EvalRpts/downloads/MMA649_Legislation.pdf

Centers for Medicare and Medicaid Services. (2006). *Tax Relief and Health Care Act of 2006*. Retrieved from https://www.cms.gov/Regulations-and-Guidance /Legislation/LegislativeUpdate/index.html

Centers for Medicare and Medicaid Services. (2011, April). *Fact Sheets: Details for: CMS issues final rule for first year of hospital value-based purchasing program*. Retrieved from http://www.cms.gov/apps/media/press/factsheet. asp?Counter=3947

Centers for Medicare and Medicaid Services. (2012a). *End-stage renal disease (ESRD) quality initiative*. Retrieved from http://www.cms.gov/Medicare/End-Stage-Renal-Disease /ESRDQualityImproveInit/index.html

Centers for Medicare and Medicaid Services. (2012b). *Home health quality initiative: Quality measures*. Retrieved from http://www.cms.gov/Medicare/Quality-Initiatives-Patient -Assessment-Instruments/HomeHealthQualityInits /HHQIQualityMeasures.html

Centers for Medicare and Medicaid Services. (2012c). *Hospital-acquired conditions*. Retrieved from http://www .cms.gov/Medicare/Medicare-Fee-for-Service-Payment /HospitalAcqCond/Hospital-Acquired_Conditions.html

Centers for Medicare and Medicaid Services. (2012d). *Hospital-acquired conditions (present on admission indicator)*. Retrieved from http://www.cms.hhs.gov /HospitalAcqCond/01_Overview.asp#TopOfPage

Centers for Medicare and Medicaid Services. (2012e). *Post acute care reform plan*. Retrieved from http://www .cms.gov/Medicare/Medicare-Fee-for-Service-Payment /SNFPPS/post_acute_care_reform_plan.html

Centers for Medicare and Medicaid Services. (2013a). *Hospital inpatient quality reporting program*. Retrieved from http://www.cms.gov/Medicare/Quality-Initiatives -Patient-Assessment-Instruments/HospitalQualityInits /HospitalRHQDAPU.html

Centers for Medicare and Medicaid Services. (2013b). *Hospital outpatient quality reporting program*. Retrieved from http://www.cms.gov/Medicare/Quality-Initiatives -Patient-Assessment-Instruments/HospitalQualityInits /HospitalOutpatientQualityReportingProgram.html

Centers for Medicare and Medicaid Services. (2013c). *Hospital quality initiative*. Retrieved from http://www.cms.gov /Medicare/Quality-Initiatives-Patient-Assessment -Instruments/HospitalQualityInits/index.html

Centers for Medicare and Medicaid Service. (2013d). *Physician quality reporting system*. Retrieved form http://www .cms.gov/Medicare/Quality-Initiatives-Patient-Assessment -Instruments/PQRS/index.html

Centers for Medicare and Medicaid Services. (2013e). *Quality initiatives—general information*. Retrieved from http:// www.cms.gov/Medicare/Quality-Initiatives-Patient -Assessment-Instruments/QualityInitiativesGenInfo /index.html?redirect=/QualityInitiativesGenInfo/

Chapman, E. (2004). *Radical loving care: Building the healing hospital in America*. Nashville, TN: Baptist Healing Hospital Trust.

Commonwealth Fund. (2013). *Why not the best? Results from the National Scorecard of U.S. Health Systems Performance, 2011*. Retrieved from http://www.commonwealthfund .org/Publications/Fund-Reports/2011/Oct/Why-Not -the-Best-2011.aspx?page=all

Consumer-Driven Health Care Institute. (2013). *Our mission*. Retrieved from http://www.cdhci.org/index.php

Consumers Advancing Patient Safety. (2012). *How to develop a community-based patient advisory council*. Retrieved from https://www.ahrq.gov/research/findings/final -reports/advisorycouncil/adcouncil1.html

Crowell, D. M. (2011). *Complexity leadership: Nursing's role in health care delivery*. Philadelphia, PA: F. A. Davis.

de Koning, H., Verver, J. P. S., van den Heuvel, J., Bisgaard, S., & Does, R. J. M. M. (2006, March–April). Lean Six Sigma in healthcare. *Journal for Healthcare Quality*, *28*(2), 4–11.

Dunton, N., Gajewski, B., Klaus, S., & Pierson, B. (2007). The relationship of nursing workforce characteristics to patient outcomes. *Online Journal of Issues in Nursing.* Retrieved from http://www.nursingworld.org/Main MenuCategories/ANAMarketplace/ANAPeriodicals /OJIN/TableofContents/Volume122007/No3Sept07 /NursingWorkforceCharacteristics.aspx

Eden Alternative. (2009). *About us: The Eden Alternative.* Retrieved from http://www.edenalt.org/about-the-eden-alternative/

Federal Emergency Management Agency. (n.d.). *Home page.* Retrieved from http://www.fema.gov/

Gallup. (2013). *Home page.* Retrieved from http://www .gallup.com/home.aspx

Garcia, R. (2006). Five ways you can reduce inappropriate prescribing in the elderly: A systematic review. *Journal of Family Practice, 55*, 305–312.

Gerteis, M., Edgman-Levitan, S., Daley, J., & Delbanco, T. (1993). *Through the patients' eyes: Understanding and promoting patient-centered care.* San Francisco, CA: Jossey-Bass.

Glasgow, J. M., Scott-Caziewell, J. R., & Kaboli, P. J. (2010, December). Guiding inpatient quality improvement: A systematic review of Lean and Six Sigma. *Joint Commission Journal on Quality and Patient Safety, 36*(12), 533–540.

Haig, K., Sutton, S., & Whittington, J. (2006). SBAR: A shared mental model for improving communication between clinicians. *Journal on Quality and Patient Safety, 32*(3), 167–175.

Health Care Advisory Board. (1999). *Balanced scorecards.* Retrieved from http://www.advisory.com

Institute for Healthcare Improvement. (2011a). *Run chart tool.* Retrieved from http://www.ihi.org/knowledge /Pages/Tools/RunChart.aspx

Institute for Healthcare Improvement. (2011b). *Strategies for leadership: Hospital executives and their role in patient safety.* Retrieved from http://www.ihi.org/knowledge /Pages/Tools/StrategiesforLeadershipHospitalExecutive sandTheirRoleinPatientSafety.aspx

Institute for Healthcare Improvement. (2012). *Measures.* Retrieved from http://www.ihi.org/knowledge/Pages /Measures/default.aspx

Institute for Healthcare Improvement. (2013). *Falls prevention.* Retrieved from http://www.ihi.org/explore /falls/Pages/default.aspx

Institute of Medicine. (1999). *To err is human: Building a safer health system.* Washington, DC: National Academies Press.

Institute of Medicine. (2001). *Crossing the quality chasm: A new health system for the 21st century.* Washington, DC: National Academies Press.

Institute of Medicine. (2004a). *Health literacy: A prescription to end confusion.* Washington, DC: National Academies Press.

Institute of Medicine. (2004b). *Keeping patients safe: Transforming the work environment of nurses.* Washington, DC: National Academies Press.

Institute of Medicine. (2006). *Preventing medication errors.* Washington, DC: National Academies Press.

Institute of Medicine. (2007). *Creating a business case for quality improvement research: Expert views, workshop summary.* Washington, DC: National Academies Press.

The Joint Commission. (2013a). *Core measures sets.* Retrieved from http://www.jointcommission.org /core_measure_sets.aspx

The Joint Commission. (2013b). *National patient safety goals.* Retrieved from http://www.jointcommission .org/standards_information/npsgs.aspx

The Joint Commission. (2013c). *2013 national patient safety goals.* Retrieved from http://www.jointcommission.org /standards_information/npsgs.aspx

The Joint Commission. (2013d). *Quality check.* Retrieved from http://www.qualitycheck.org/consumer/search QCR.aspx

Klevens, R. M., Edwards, J. R., Richards, C. L., Horan, T. C., Gaynes, R. P., Pollock, D. A., & Cardo, D. M. (2007, March–April). Estimating health care-associated infections and deaths in U.S. hospitals, 2002. *Public Health Reports, 122*, 160–166.

Leape, L. L., & Berwick, D. M. (2005). Five years after *To err is human*: What have we learned? *Journal of the American Medical Association, 293*(19), 2384–2390. doi:10.1001/jama.293.19.2384

Leapfrog Group. (2013). *The Leapfrog Group fact sheet.* Retrieved from http://www.leapfroggroup.org/about_us /leapfrog-factsheet

Leonhardt, K., Bonin, D., & Pagel, P. (2007). *How to develop a community-based patient advisory council. Aurora Health Care and CAPS Toolkit.* Retrieved from http:// patientsafety.org/page/109387/;jsessionid=7vhlrvtobuim2

Lindberg, C., & Clancy, T. R. (2010). Positive Deviance: An elegant solution to a complex problem. *Journal of Nursing Administration, 40*(4), 150–153.

Lindrooth, R., Bazzoli, G., Needleman, J., & Hasnain-Wynia, R. (2006). *The effect of changes in hospital reimbursement on nurse staffing decisions at safety net and nonsafety net hospitals.* Retrieved from http://www.pubmedcentral.nih. gov/articlerender.fcgi?tool=pubmed&pubmedid=16704508

Longtin, Y., Sax, H., Leape, L.L., Sheridan, S. E., Donaldson, L., & Pittet, D. (2010). Patient participation: Current knowledge and applicability to patient safety. *Mayo Clinic Proceedings, 85*(1), 53–62. doi:10.4065/mcp.2009.0248

Markey, D., & Brown, R. (2002). An interdisciplinary approach to addressing patient activity and mobility in medical-surgical patient. *Journal of Nursing Care Quality, 16*(4), 1–12.

Melberg, S. (1997). Effects of changing skill mix. *Nursing Management, 28*(11), 47–48.

Miller, W., Vigdor, E., & Manning, G. (2004, January–June). Covering the uninsured: What is it worth? *Health Affairs,* W4157–W4167.

National Institute of Standards and Technology. (2013). *Healthcare criteria for performance excellence.* Gaithersburg, MD: Author.

Planetree. (n. d.). *About us.* Retrieved from http://planetree .org/?page_id=510

Porter-O'Grady, T., & Malloch, K. (2003). *Quantum leadership: A textbook of new leadership.* Sudbury, MA: Jones and Bartlett.

Porter-O'Grady, T., & Malloch, K. (2011). *Quantum leadership: Advancing innovation, transforming health care* (3rd ed.). Burlington, MA: Jones & Bartlett Learning.

Press Ganey Associates. (2013). *Home page.* Retrieved from http://www.pressganey.com/index.aspx

Reed, K., & May. R. (2011). HealthGrades patient safety in American hospitals study. *HealthGrades.* Retrieved from http://patientsafetymovement.org/wp-content /uploads/2016/02/Resources_Reports_Patient_Safety _in_American_Hospitals_Study.pdf

Relihan, E., O'Brien, V., O'Hara S., & Silke, B. (2010, October). The impact of a set of interventions to reduce interruptions and distractions to nurses during medication administration. *Quality & Safety in Health Care, 19*(5), 52–57.

Rudy, E., Lucke, J., Whitman, G., & Davidson, L. (2001). Benchmarking patient outcomes. *Journal of Nursing Scholarship, 33*(2), 185–189.

Scott, R. D. (2009). *The direct medical costs of healthcare-associated infections in U. S. hospitals and the benefits of prevention.* Retrieved from http://www.cdc.gov/HAI /pdfs/hai/Scott_CostPaper.pdf

Shermont, H., Mahoney, J., Krepcio, D., Baccari, S., Powers, D., & Yusah, A. (2008). Meeting of the minds: Ten-minute "huddles" offer nurses an opportunity to assess unit workflow and optimize patient care. *Nursing Management, 39*(8), 38–44.

Shirey, M. (2006). Evidence-based practice: Impact on nursing administration. *Nursing Administration Quarterly, 30*(3), 252–265.

Simonson, W., & Feinberg, J. (2005). Medication-related problems in the elderly: Defining the issues and identifying solutions. *Drugs and Aging, 22*(7), 559–569.

Smith, B. (2003, April). Lean and Six Sigma—a one-two punch. *Quality Progress,* 37–41.

Stevens, J., Corso, P., Finkelstein, E., & Miller, T. (2006). *The costs of fatal and non-fatal falls among older adults.* Retrieved from http://injuryprevention.bmj.com /content/12/5/290.full

Tennessee Hospitals & Health Systems. (2008). *THA develops nonpayment policy on serious adverse events.* Nashville, TN: Tennessee Hospital Association.

Trbovich, P., Prakash, V., & Stewart, J. (2010). Interruptions during the delivery of high-risk medications, *Journal of Nursing Administration, 40*(5), 211–218.

U.S. Census Bureau. (2011). *Overview of race and Hispanic origin: 2010.* Retrieved from http://www.census.gov /prod/cen2010/briefs/c2010br-02.pdf

U.S. Department of Health and Human Services. (n.d.). *Quick guide to health literacy: Fact sheet.* Retrieved from http://www.health.gov/communication/literacy /quickguide/factsbasic.htm

U.S. Department of Labor. (n.d.). *Occupational Health and Safety Administration.* Retrieved from http://www. osha.gov/

U.S. Government Printing Office. (2008). *Medicare improvements for Patients and Providers Act of 2008.* Retrieved from http://www.gpo.gov/fdsys/pkg/PLAW-110publ275 /pdf/PLAW-110publ275.pdf

U.S. Government Printing Office. (2010). *Patient Protection and Affordable Care Act of 2010.* Retrieved from http:// www.gpo.gov/fdsys/pkg/PLAW-111publ148/pdf/PLAW -111publ148.pdf

Vanhey, D., Aiken, L., Sloane, D., Clarke, S., & Vargas, D. (2004). Nurse burnout and patient satisfaction. *Medical Care, 42*(2 Suppl.), II57–II66.

Watson, J. (2004). *Postmodern nursing and beyond.* New York, NY: Elsevier.

Weber, S. (2008, July). Ergonomics standards: An overview. *Nursing Management,* 28–31.

Wetterneck, T. B., Walker, J. M., Blosky, M. A., Cartmill, R. S., Hoonakker, P., Johnson, M. A., . . ., Carayon, P. (2011). Factors contributing to an increase in duplicate medication order errors after CPOE implementation. *Journal of the American Medical Informatics Association, 18,* 774–782.

Whitman, G., Kim, Y., Davidson, L., Wolf, G., & Wang, S. (2002). The impact of staffing on patient outcomes across specialty units. *Journal of Nursing Administration, 32*(12), 633–639.

Woods, A., & Doan-Johnson, S. (2002, October). Executive summary: Toward a taxonomy of nursing practice errors. *Nursing Management,* 45–48.

World Health Organization. (2013). *Health financing: Health expenditure per capita by country (latest year).* Retrieved from http://apps.who.int/gho/data/node.main.78?lang=en

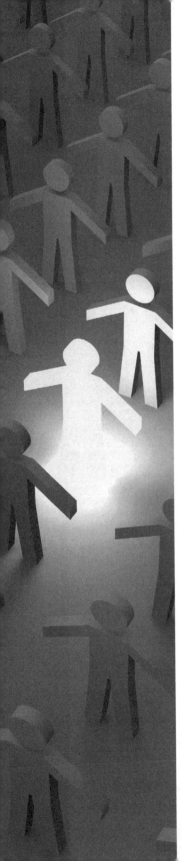

PART II
Budget Principles

CHAPTER 5

Budgeting

Paul Brown, MSN, RN, **Gary Eubank** MSN, RN, and **J. Michael Leger**, PhD, MBA, RN

OBJECTIVES

- Understand a high-level overview of the budgeting process.
- Describe how variable costs and fixed costs impact an organization's budget.
- Discuss the impact of productive and non-productive hours.
- Demonstrate the steps in budget preparation for a nursing department.

▶ An Introduction to Budgeting

Budgets are an organization's formalized financial plans, and planning is an important activity in budgeting. The budget represents the organization's goals that focus on operations improvement through defining specific, quantifiable financial performance measures. Budget planning involves making predictions for next year's volume, revenue, and expenses that are routinely based on (1) prior years' historical, or actual, performance and (2) projected estimates for growth. Budget planning is also a way to introduce and reinforce budget control by setting financial performance targets that require reporting and efficient management throughout the organization's fiscal year. Unfortunately, until recently most nursing leaders have had low influence on the budgets in the departments under their purview with the exception of monitoring expenses and explaining variances.

For most nurse leaders, budget information and activities are involved with spending, whereas having revenue information is not as common. In recent years, nurse leaders have become more accountable for all aspects of their budget management, as well as the influence they play in the budget planning processes. This is one reason why it is important for the nurse leader to understand the vital link between the amounts of money received from all payer sources (e.g., Medicare, Medicaid, insurance, and private pay) and the critical role of balancing that revenue with incurred expenses at the unit level (e.g., equipment, supplies, staffing).

Another budget responsibility of the nurse leader is to be an advocate for patients, ensuring that the patient receives the best and safest services possible. As the level of management closest to the services at the point of care, a nurse leader with a sound knowledge of relevant budget information influences patient care. All nurse leaders are most effective when they are able to make sound decisions and defend those decisions by having the skills and the vocabulary to (1)

determine what financial information is available, (2) acquire that information, (3) interpret its impact on patient care, and (4) communicate that to others within the organization. The budget management terms and techniques discussed in this chapter provide the nurse leader with a high-level overview of the budgeting process.

▶ Budgeting Principles and Terminology

Understanding the budgeting process requires first an understanding of the terminology commonly used. Stepping into the world of finances can be intimidating for a nurse leader, but a familiarity with basic finance and budgeting language makes this transition more seamless. While this chapter does not intend to prepare the nurse leader to fully comprehend the many intricacies of financial budgeting, or to become fully proficient at the budgeting process that occurs in every healthcare organization, it will provide an appreciation of the process and the important role of the nurse leader.

Capital Budgeting Versus Operational Budgeting

While there are many types of budgets that comprise an organization's annual budget, the two primary types of budgets the nurse leader will most often work with include an operating budget and a capital budget. Operating budgets cover the day-to-day costs of a unit, including such things as wages for regular and per diem staff, supplies, equipment, repair and maintenance, travel and education, and dues and subscriptions. Like all budgets, operating budgets represent the "best guess" for costs over a coming period. Historical data are most often the starting point for developing future budgets.

The capital budget, on the other hand, covers the purchase of long-term investments that are often referred to as capital assets. These assets, or investments, include such purchases as land, buildings, and, most appropriate to the nurse leader, equipment (e.g., IV pumps, patient beds, point of care equipment). The capital budget is developed separately from the operating budget and is often funded through separate funding sources, or accounts. Nurse leaders are most involved in capital budgeting when they request expensive, long-lived equipment for their units (this equipment may last 2 years, but it varies by organization). In most organizations, a financial rationale must be provided to support the capital spending request. This process is called *capital budgeting*. The rationale for purchasing capital assets may include replacing older or nonworking items, buying a newer and better piece of equipment that improves productivity or patient safety, or meeting the needs of a new line of service to generate new revenue. The threshold dollar limit for an item to be considered for the capital budget varies by organization; however, the only requirement for an asset to be deemed a capital asset is that it must provide useful service that extends beyond the year in which it is put into service.

Cost Concepts

Expenses are the cost of doing business that decreases the equity of an organization. Thus, controlling the outflow of money from an organization requires a watchful eye to minimize excessive spending that negatively impacts the inflow of revenue. Because cost control is a major function in the role of the nurse leader, having basic knowledge of cost concepts and their behavior is key to successfully maneuvering through cost management. Fundamental to cost control is an understanding of the relationship of fixed and variable costs.

Fixed Costs

Fixed costs are those that stay the same regardless of the level of activity. The first example of fixed costs is those costs that would exist even if the organization were shutdown: rent, insurance, taxes, depreciation, a minimal level of utilities,

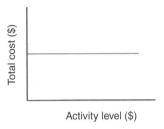

FIGURE 5.1 Fixed Costs: Cost for a Nurse Manager

etc. From a nursing perspective, fixed costs include those minimum costs that are always paid regardless of the volume of activity. Regardless of patient activity—whether measured by patient visits, patient acuity, or patient minutes, hours, or days—certain costs are always present. Examples include minimum staffing requirements, the salary and benefits of the nurse leader, rent, telephone service, and other cost center supplies that do not fluctuate with volume. Some consider these costs to be *direct costs*, or the costs of resources that are necessary in order to provide direct care to patients. **FIGURE 5.1** depicts the nurse manager's salary as a fixed cost. Also to consider are what some would identify as the *indirect* (resource costs that are not directly related to providing patient care), or shared, *costs* related to patient care, such as administration, quality improvement/assurance, risk management, and infection control.

Variable Costs

Variable costs are those that change, or fluctuate, depending on the level of activity or volume. In the healthcare environment, volume is a complex concept because volume not only includes the census numbers but also patient acuity, patient minutes/hours/days, and patient visits. Variable costs occur in addition to fixed costs to yield the organization's total costs:

TOTAL COSTS = FIXED COSTS + VARIABLE COSTS

Staffing, beyond the minimum staffing requirements, is a variable cost based on the

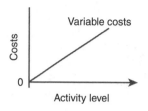

FIGURE 5.2 Variable Costs: Cost for Supplies as Unit Volume Increases

variable patient census and acuity. Other typical variable costs are medical and surgical supplies, linen, and food costs. Variable costs vary in direct proportion to fluctuations in activity levels, as depicted in **FIGURE 5.2**.

TABLE 5.1 illustrates variable and fixed costs for a nursing department's budget.

Revenue Concepts

Revenue is the amount of money that is earned by an organization and is most easily explained as the charges billed to patients when services are provided for which the organization expects to be paid. There are two types of revenues: actual (paid at the time services are rendered) and

expected (payment that is expected sometime after the services are rendered). The largest portion of healthcare reimbursement is based upon expected revenue.

Gross revenue is the sum of all charges for the care provided to the patient for all services provided during an episode of care.

NET REVENUE = GROSS REVENUE – DEDUCTIONS FROM REVENUE

However, healthcare organizations can no longer expect, in most situations, to be reimbursed for full charges. Net revenue is calculated by deducting projected reductions in payment, such as fixed payments (e.g., diagnosis-related group (DRG) payments from Medicare), contractual allowance (e.g., a negotiated amount contracted by insurance companies), and charity care (e.g., patients with no healthcare benefits who cannot afford to pay for charges) from the gross revenue (expected amount of payment). **TABLE 5.2** illustrates the calculation of projected net revenue based on a contractual allowance with an insurance payer source.

There are three primary revenue sources for health care in the United States: Medicare,

TABLE 5.1 Variable and Fixed Costs for a Nursing Department's Budget			
Account	**Total**	**Fixed**	**Variable**
Salary: nurse manager	$100,000	$100,000	
Office supplies	$15,000		$15,000
Telephone	$24,000	$24,000	
Travel expense	$10,000		$10,000
Medical supplies	$58,000		$58,000
Rent	$85,000	$85,000	
Total costs	$292,000	$209,000	$83,000

TABLE 5.2 Illustration of Net Revenue Calculation

Type of Procedure	Payer Source	DRG Reimbursement	Contractual Allowance	Projected Net Revenue
DRG 209 – Major Joint Procedure Lower Extremity	Insurance Company A	$10,034	10% below DRG	$9,030.60

DRG, diagnosis-related group.

Medicaid, and other programs/self-pay. (For more information on the history of Medicare and Medicaid in the United States, see Chapter 1 or visit www.cms.gov.)

Medicare

Currently, there are some 44 million beneficiaries—some 15% of the U.S. population—who are enrolled in the Medicare program, with enrollment expected to rise to 79 million by 2030 (*http://assets.aarp.org/rgcenter/health/fs149_medicare.pdf*). Total spending from Medicare grew to $626.2 billion in 2015.

Medicaid

While the Medicaid program is state specific, the program is both a federal and state matching entitlement program. Now, more than 70 million people in the United States receive their healthcare benefits through this program, with total spending reaching $545.1 billion in 2015 (*http://www.usnews.com/news/articles/2015/02/24/medicaid-enrollment-surges-across-the-us*).

Other Programs/Self-Pay

Commercial payers make up the largest revenue stream for U.S. health care, although each individual market might see different payer mixes (or, sources for reimbursement of healthcare services identified by payer type). In 2015, Centers for Medicare and Medicaid Services (CMS) reported that more than $1.072 trillion of healthcare revenue, or more than 33% of the national healthcare

dollars spent, comes from private healthcare spending. Out-of-pocket spending, sometimes categorized as "Self Pay" constitutes $338 billion of total healthcare spending in 2015.

Break-Even Analysis

To stay in operation, the *minimum* long-term goal of any organization must be to at least *break even*. When one breaks even, the costs of operations exactly equal the revenues. There is no profit and no loss. More revenues result in a profit, and fewer revenues (or more costs) result in a loss. When an entity operates below the break-even point, it must borrow or pull from savings from earlier periods when profits were made. Clearly, these are short-term solutions, and when they are exhausted, the entity will be forced to close.

Breakeven can be shown graphically and calculated mathematically. Both the visual and mathematical approaches are based on the definitions of costs. Remember that there are two kinds of costs: fixed costs and variable costs. **FIGURE 5.3** provides a graphical representation of

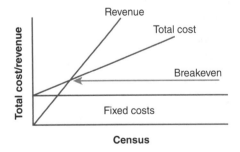

FIGURE 5.3 Graphical Breakeven

breakeven. Notice that the *variable* costs begin to rise from the base of fixed costs—costs that continue even when activity drops to zero. The revenue line begins at zero—*no activity, no billing.* Thereafter, it climbs at a steady rate toward the upper right corner of the graph. The slope of the revenue line (the rate at which it climbs) is dependent on the rate of billing—the bigger the bills, the steeper the climb. Our revenue slope would be based on the total revenue as it related to the average census or patient day. That is a crude measure, and many other measures could be used. Nevertheless, at best, the break-even chart is a tool that will give you a rough idea of the activity level needed to remain solvent.

Remember, the more detailed your cost analysis, the better this tool will work for you. A break-even analysis for a procedure will be more accurate than a break-even analysis for a unit or department. Similarly, a break-even analysis for a unit or department will be more accurate than a break-even analysis for an entire healthcare institution. Unfortunately, at some point, the break-even point for the organization as a whole becomes the issue in question.

Mathematically, breakeven is calculated using the formula that follows. It indicates that one breaks even when the revenues equal the expenses. Because both revenues and variable costs are a function of activity level—in this case, patient days—*we must know both the average cost and the average revenues as we add patients to the census.* Given that, breakeven occurs when revenues per patient day equal fixed costs plus variable costs per patient day. The question we want to answer is this: *How many patients do we need in house, on average, to break even?* What is the break-even census?

> *Breakeven occurs when Revenues*
> */Patient day × Census*
> *= Fixed costs + Variable costs*
> */Patient day × Census*

Assume the following data:

Revenues per patient day	$ 2,000
Variable cost per patient day	$ 110
Fixed costs per year	$ 1,000,000

> *Revenues per Patient day × Census*
> *= Fixed costs + Variable costs per*
> *Patient day × Census*
> *$2,000 × Census = $1,000,000*
> *+ $110 × Census (2,000 − 110)*
> *× Census = $1,000,000*
> *Census = $1,000,000 / 1,890*
> *Census = 529 per year*

You can verify your answer:

> *Revenues/Patient day × Census*
> *= Fixed costs + Variable costs/*
> *Patient day × Census*
> *$2,000 × 529 = $1,000,000 + $110 × 529*
> *$1,058,190 = $1,000,000 + $58,190*

Your answer may not be exact. First, these are estimated numbers. You cannot be certain that your fixed costs will be $1,000,000, or that your average daily patient revenue will be $2,000, or that your average daily variable cost will be $110. What the break-even analysis has given you is a rough estimate. If, as you move into the year, you find your estimates of revenues or costs are badly off target, or you find your average census is only 475, you can go back to the drawing board and change the underlying realities.

Similarly, *if your variable revenues do not exceed your variable costs, you can never break even.* If, in this example, the revenues per patient day had been $2,000 but the variable costs per patient day had been $2,001, no amount of activity will result in a break-even situation. You will lose $1 per patient day, and the harder you work, the deeper in a hole you will find yourself. This understanding of the fact that variable revenues must exceed variable costs leads to an alternative way to think about the break-even calculation. This is not a change in either the concept or the calculation. It is simply an approach that avoids the manipulation of an algebraic equation and is easier for some people to remember.

Start with your fixed costs. They exist *whether or not* there are patients in the beds. To cover your fixed costs, you must make more revenues on the patients than you have costs caused by the patients. This "extra" revenue can then be used to cover your fixed costs.

Next, think about the revenues and the variable costs. These elements change with activity. In essence, if there were no patient in the bed, neither the revenue nor the variable cost exists. So, a patient, in a bed, creates both a variable revenue and a variable cost. The term for the difference between these two is *contribution margin*. Contribution margin is the amount available to *contribute* toward covering fixed costs. When you have just enough contribution margin to cover fixed costs, you arrive at breakeven:

$$\text{Breakeven} = \frac{\text{Fixed costs}}{\text{Revenues / patient day} - \text{variable costs / patient day}}$$

$$\text{Breakeven} = \frac{\$1,000,000}{\$2,000 - \$110}$$

$$\text{Breakeven} = \frac{\$1,000,000}{1,890}$$
$$= 529 \text{ patients per year}$$

If one approach to calculating break-even works, so will the other. Perhaps the most important concept of breakeven is the understanding that some costs and most revenues are a function of activity. Some costs, however (perhaps most costs in a typical small healthcare institution), are fixed and continue even after the shutdown point. When you consider actions that will improve profitability or reduce a loss situation, you must clearly identify which elements of cost and revenue you can best affect to improve profitability.

▶ Budgeting Implications for Nurse Leaders

The process of budgeting, both in annual preparation and in ongoing monitoring, consumes a large portion of the nurse leader's time. The two primary components of a budget are costs and revenues. It is a clear expectation that variable costs are well budgeted, closely monitored, and any variances are quickly adjusted to positively impact an organization's overall financial health status. And while revenue and fixed costs are often considered less vital to the role of the nurse leader, as healthcare organizations realign to provide a more patient-centric healthcare model, nurse leaders will be required to have a better understanding of the patient's payer source and the impact this has on the revenue side of the budget.

Budget responsibilities usually include an evaluation of the adequacy of the budget and, at times, the development of a new budget. Budget evaluation is an important activity because a cost center budget may not have been thoroughly evaluated for some time. What has been appropriate for the past 10 years is not necessarily what is needed presently. This chapter is designed to help the nurse leader determine whether the overall budget—in particular, the staffing budget—is appropriate and adequate to meet present patient needs.

▶ An Introduction to Nursing-Specific Budgeting Principles

At its most fundamental level, budgeting comes down to a predetermined amount of funding that is allocated for a particular "cost center." A nursing department, for example, represents a cost center for the organization. The funding allocated each year for the nursing department is the department's budget. The nurse leader is expected to staff the department with an appropriate skill mix of nursing staff, while staying within the allocated budget.

Depending on the clinic setting, a variety of nursing staff may be required to meet patient care needs. In health care, these positions are calculated as full-time equivalents (FTEs). An

TABLE 5.3   FTE Hours

FTEs	Hours Per Week*	Hours Per Year*
0.1	4	208
0.2	8	416
0.3	12	624
0.4	16	832
0.5	20	1,040
0.6	24	1,248
0.7	28	1,456
0.8	32	1,664
0.9	36	1,872
1.0	40	2,080

*Based on an 8-hour day (this would need to be changed for a 12-hour day.)
FTE, full-time equivalents.

FTE is a unit of measurement that represents one person who works a full-time position. In other words, an FTE is essentially a calculation of a person working 2,080 hours per year. This number is derived from the premise of an employee working 8 hours per day, 5 days per week, 52 weeks per year ($8 \times 5 \times 52 = 2080$).

1 FTE = 40 hours per week × 52 weeks per year = 2,080 hours per year

However, more than one person can fill one FTE. For example, multiple part-time employees who work less than full time can combine to equate to one FTE. To calculate hours worked, let's consider that an employee works 32 hours per week. What is that employee's FTE status?

32 hours/week worked/40 hours (1 FTE) = 0.8 FTE

See **TABLE 5.3** for a table of FTE hours.

Units of Service

Units of service is used by healthcare organizations to measure specific services a patient uses within a specific time frame (i.e., patient minutes, hours, days, visits, births, treatments, operations, or other patient encounters). Patient days, for example, are the number of inpatients present on any given day at midnight. One patient day is given for each day the patient is present on an inpatient unit.

Nursing Workload

Using the same various units of services causes a problem in that all patients do not require the same amount of nursing care. For instance, one treatment could take a half hour, whereas another could take 2 hours. Or one patient requires intensive care, whereas another needs only the stepdown unit. Or a home care nurse could drive 30 miles to make a visit, whereas other visits require only a 5-mile drive. Therefore, further unit-of-service specification is needed to accurately reflect nursing workload, or the volume of work performed by nurse caregivers.

Developing a Nursing Department Budget and Staffing Plan

In order to develop a budget and staffing model, we must first gather data that stand to influence staffing workloads. This section provides an overview of the development of a staffing model and the projected financial impact. In the next chapter, we will dissect each of these key areas to develop staffing models and budgets for specific clinical settings.

Establish Volume

Our first step will be establishing expected patient volume. Depending on the setting, this information can be collected from various sources, including average patient days, the percentage of direct admits from emergency room (ER) visits, or the number of outpatient visits. It is important to recognize that various factors can influence volume and to be cognizant of these potential influencers. Examples of potential factors include medical staff admission trends, increases or decreases in the number of medical staff, market share (are new hospitals being built or existing hospitals closing in the area? are new free-standing emergency departments being introduced into the market?), patient satisfaction, and the percentage of visits from the ER that are converted to inpatients.

Determine Nurse–Patient Ratio

Once volume is established, the nurse leader can begin the calculations to determine the appropriate

nursing workload. In this instance, the workload is defined as the nurse–patient ratio. This ratio is necessary in order to determine how to optimally provide the minimum standard of care. Hospital policy, accreditation standards, community standards, and clinical outcomes will drive this ratio. It is also important to note that specific clinical settings will have different nurse-to-patient ratios (Med/Surg versus intensive care unit [ICU], for example).

Establish Skill Mix Necessary to Meet Patient Needs

The percentage of staff comprised of each job class is referred to as a *skill mix*. In addition to organization policy, which can direct specific skill mixes of nursing staff, community standards and trends should be observed and incorporated into skill mix calculations if your organization wants to stay competitive with local healthcare organizations. For example, healthcare organizations in many areas are moving toward Registered Nurse (RN)-only patient care models. If your organization does employ RNs exclusively for licensed nursing care, you may want to consider whether there exists a defined need for non-RN licensed staff and unlicensed assistive personnel (UAP), and if the budget will allow for such positions.

While larger metropolitan hospitals are moving toward this RN-only patient care model, smaller community hospitals in rural areas depend on Licensed Practical/Vocational Nurses, as well as UAP to make up a portion of their nursing workforce. In these cases, the nurse leader will need to carefully consider the skill mix of RNs and these other roles. A review of staffing models of healthcare organizations in similar markets will give insight into community standards.

▶ Non-Productive Time

Personal Time Off

Once volume, nurse–patient ratio, and skill mix are established, the nurse leader will need to factor the annual personal time off (PTO) per employee.

Annual PTO is generally the combination of vacation, holiday, and sick leave afforded to an employee each year. Organizational Human Resource policies often govern the percentage of total work hours to be factored for PTO.

Overtime

The nurse leader will need to project the percentage of total work hours that will be accrued and paid as overtime. Historical information and future forecasts, including increases in average daily census and staff vacancies, are important determining factors.

Education and Orientation

With PTO and overtime established, the nurse leader determines the amount of time each job class will require for education and orientation. The Joint Commission, if applicable, and an organization's policies govern the frequency of required staff meetings and education requirements. The nurse leader must identify the number of hours by job class for each role necessary to achieve required educational offerings. These hours include the time necessary to accomplish required annual competencies or educational programs offered to promote excellence and innovation in clinical practice.

The nurse leader is required to determine the non-productive hours of each job class while orienting to a specific clinical setting. Non-productive hours for orientation are defined as those hours where the employee is not given an independent assignment. This can vary by department or specialty. For example, a med-surg RN may require 6 weeks (240 hours) of non-productive orientation time to their unit of assignment, as compared to an ICU RN, who may require 12 weeks (480 hours) of non-productive orientation time. **TABLE 5.4** demonstrates an example of the number of education, meeting, and orientation hours a nurse leader may allot for each job class in specified clinical settings. Remember, these are examples and may differ from your organization's requirements.

Facility Overview

Establishing a Facility Overview is a helpful step in defining key components of the department that stand to influence staffing and budgeting. **TABLE 5.5** represents the information required to complete the facility overview.

Facility—This is the name of the facility.

Time Period—This number should represent the fiscal year for which you are planning your staffing budget. If the organization's fiscal year begins September 1 and ends on August 31 of the following year, that period will generally be referred to by the year in which the fiscal year ends.

Cost Center—The accounting number provided by the Department of Finance that incorporates the unit's budget parameters and associated expenses.

Unit Type—This section represents the clinical setting (ICU, Med/Surg, Pediatrics, etc.).

ADC—The average daily census. This can also represent the average number of patient visits expected in an emergency department, outpatient clinic, etc.

Total Patient Days—The average daily census multiplied by days of the year that the clinical entity is operational. For example, clinical entities that are open 7 days per week, 24 hours per day (365 days), multiply 365 by your average daily census to obtain the annualized total patient days (Total Patient Days = ADC × Number of Operational Days per Year). Units open Monday through Friday, such as recovery rooms and operating rooms, multiply the average number of daily visits by 260 days. The number 260 represents the number of days that a 5-day-per-week clinical entity is operational in a year (5 days per week multiplied by 52 weeks = 260). For those clinical entities that do not provide services on holidays, subtract 8 hours per holiday from 260 hours. For example, in a case where a hospital does not schedule surgery on Thanksgiving, Christmas Eve,

TABLE 5.4 Education and Orientation Summary

Skill Mix		Required Education and Meetings (hours)			Orientation (hours)		
Title	Abbreviation	Med/Surg	Stepdown	ICU	Med/Surg	Stepdown	ICU/ED
Manager	MGR	Exempt	Exempt	Exempt	Exempt	Exempt	Exempt
Asst. Nurse Manager	ANM	Exempt	Exempt	Exempt	Exempt	Exempt	Exempt
Charge Nurse	CHG	36	52	76	240	320	480
Registered Nurse	RN	36	52	76	240	320	480
Licensed Vocational Nurse	LVN	20	20	20	240	320	N/A
Nursing Technician/ Nursing Assistant	NT/NA	8	8	8	80	80	80
Monitor Tech	MT	8	8	8	80	80	80
Unit Secretary	US	8	8	8	80	80	80

ED, emergency department; ICU, intensive care unit.

Christmas Day, New Year's Eve, New Year's Day, Memorial Day, Labor Day, and 4th of July, the nurse leader subtracts 64 holiday hours from 260 to obtain the total number of patient days of 196.

PTO—Represents the percent of average paid time off per FTE. This figure is usually provided by the Finance Department or Human Resources.

Incidental Overtime—The percent of total work hours worked in an overtime capacity.

TABLE 5.6 represents a breakdown of nursing job classes in the clinical entity's budget and their corresponding abbreviations. We will use these abbreviations as we progress through developing our staffing plan.

▶ Building a Staffing Model

With the necessary historical and projective data collected, we can begin to build a staffing model for the department. **FIGURE 5.4** represents an example of a staffing model template. This template will be referred to as Schedule 1 of 4.

Notice the top left-hand corner of Schedule 1. Information from the Facility Overview is listed here, including the facility name, time period, unit

TABLE 5.5 Facility Overview

Facility:	St. Elsewhere
Time period:	2017
Unit name:	Urgent Care Clinic
Cost center:	1000
Unit type:	ED
	Volume
ADC:	24
Total patient days:	8,760
PTO%	10.0%
Incidental overtime	5.0%

© 2005 Gary J. Eubank, all rights reserved.
ADC, average daily census; ED, emergency department; PTO, personal time off.

TABLE 5.6 Job Classes with Abbreviations

Skill Mix Name	Abbreviation
Manager	MGR
Asst. Manager	ANM
Charge Nurse	CHG
RN	RN
LVN	LVN
NT/NA	NT
Monitor Tech	MT
Unit Secretary	US
Other	OTH

Schedule 1: Staffing by ADC

Facility: St. Elsewhere	Unit name: 2West
Time period: 2010	Cost center: 1000
Unit type: Med/surg	

| Using ADC (midnight census) |
| ADC: 24 | Total pat days: 8,760 | Direct HPPD: |

| Using conversion factor (what goes into PLUS) |
| Total USO: | Direct Hrs/UOS: |

Shift distribution

Days	Eve	Night

SKILL MIX TABLE

	MGR	ANM	CHRG	RN	LVN	NT	MT	US	Other	TOT
FTEs	-	-	-	-	-	-	-	-	-	-
%										

7A-7P, 7A-3P	SUN 8HR 10HR 12HR	MON 8HR 10HR 12HR	TUE 8HR 10HR 12HR	WED 8HR 10HR 12HR	THU 8HR 10HR 12HR	FRI 8HR 10HR 12HR	SAT 8HR 10HR 12HR	ALL SHIFTS 8HR 10HR 12HR	TOT HRS 8, 10, 12	FTE 8, 10, 12
Manager								- - -	-	-
ANM								- - -	-	-
Charge nurse								- - -	-	-
RN								- - -	-	-
LVN								- - -	-	-
NT/NA								- - -	-	-
MT								- - -	-	-
Unit secretary								- - -	-	-
								- - -	-	-
TOTAL	- - -	- - -	- - -	- - -	- - -	- - -	- - -	- - -	-	-

3P-11P	SUN 8HR 10HR 12HR	MON 8HR 10HR 12HR	TUE 8HR 10HR 12HR	WED 8HR 10HR 12HR	THU 8HR 10HR 12HR	FRI 8HR 10HR 12HR	SAT 8HR 10HR 12HR	ALL SHIFTS 8HR 10HR 12HR	TOT HRS 8, 10, 12	FTE 8, 10, 12
Manager								- - -	-	-
ANM								- - -	-	-
Charge nurse								- - -	-	-
RN								- - -	-	-
LVN								- - -	-	-
NT/NA								- - -	-	-
MT								- - -	-	-
Unit secretary								- - -	-	-
								- - -	-	-
TOTAL	- - -	- - -	- - -	- - -	- - -	- - -	- - -	- - -	-	-

7P-7A, 11P-7A	SUN 8HR 10HR 12HR	MON 8HR 10HR 12HR	TUE 8HR 10HR 12HR	WED 8HR 10HR 12HR	THU 8HR 10HR 12HR	FRI 8HR 10HR 12HR	SAT 8HR 10HR 12HR	ALL SHIFTS 8HR 10HR 12HR	TOT HRS 8, 10, 12	FTE 8, 10, 12
Manager								- - -	-	-
ANM								- - -	-	-
Charge nurse								- - -	-	-
RN								- - -	-	-
LVN								- - -	-	-
NT/NA								- - -	-	-
MT								- - -	-	-
Unit secretary								- - -	-	-
								- - -	-	-
TOTAL	- - -	- - -	- - -	- - -	- - -	- - -	- - -	- - -	-	-

| UNIT TOTAL | - | - | - | - | - | - | - | | - | - |

FIGURE 5.4 Staffing model

type, unit name, and cost center (or department identification number). Additionally, the average daily census and the annual total patient days are transferred to this document. While not required to be included on the staffing template, it is helpful to have this information available on a single page.

Our next step will be to determine the job classes that will be required on each shift. Abbreviations for each job class are listed along the left column. Three rows of columns, referred to herein as "shift sets," are provided in this example, allowing for day, evening, and night shift staffing patterns. Depending on the clinical setting and hours of operation, only one or two shift sets may be required.

The nurse leader should next determine the number of licensed staff necessary to provide the standard of care for a selected patient population. The number and type of UAP should then be determined to assist licensed staff in meeting patient care needs.

Scenario: We are required to have one RN (not classified as Charge Nurse) during all clinic hours (12 hours/day). Additionally, we have a manager who works 8 hours per day Monday through Friday, and two LVNs working 12 hours per day Monday through Friday. Fill in the staffing pattern template below using these known staffing resources. In each appropriate box, enter the number of staff allocated to each job class utilized. Focus only on the shaded areas at this time.

	SUN 8HR	SUN 10HR	SUN 12HR	MON 8HR	MON 10HR	MON 12HR	TUE 8HR	TUE 10HR	TUE 12HR	WED 8HR	WED 10HR	WED 12HR	THU 8HR	THU 10HR	THU 12HR	FRI 8HR	FRI 10HR	FRI 12HR	SAT 8HR	SAT 10HR	SAT 12HR	ALL SHIFTS 8,10,12	TOT HRS 8,10,12	FTE 8,10,12
Manager																								
ANM																								
Charge Nurse																								
RN																								
LVN																								
NT/NA																								
MT																								
Unit secretary																								
TOTAL																								

	SUN 8HR	SUN 10HR	SUN 12HR	MON 8HR	MON 10HR	MON 12HR	TUE 8HR	TUE 10HR	TUE 12HR	WED 8HR	WED 10HR	WED 12HR	THU 8HR	THU 10HR	THU 12HR	FRI 8HR	FRI 10HR	FRI 12HR	SAT 8HR	SAT 10HR	SAT 12HR	ALL SHIFTS 8,10,12	TOT HRS 8,10,12	FTE 8,10,12
Manager				1			1			1			1			1								
ANM																								
Charge nurse																								
RN			1			1			1			1			1			1			1			
LVN						2			2			2			2			2						
NT/NA																								
MT																								
Unit secretary																								
TOTAL																								

With the information provided, your scheduling template should look similar to the one below. Notice that, at a glance, the nurse leader can quickly determine the number and skill mix of licensed staff working each day, as well as the number of hours each job class is scheduled. In the following chapter, we will calculate total FTEs and hours per shift and show how these numbers stand to impact the organization from a financial perspective.

PTO, Education, and Orientation

When nursing staff is required to attend educational offerings, they are being relieved of their direct patient care obligations. Therefore, time away from the bedside must be anticipated and allotted for in the budget. **FIGURE 5.5** shows Schedule 2 of 4.

In Schedule 2, we need to calculate the FTEs necessary to allow for budgeting secondary resources to offset the loss of productive time due to PTO, orientation, and education. The first section deals with Replacement FTEs. Using Schedule 1 as a reference, determine the number of FTEs that are essential for each shift. Those FTEs are reflected in the subtotal PTO line. Remember that the PTO percentage has already been identified on the Facility Overview. This is the percent of time an average FTE is paid to take paid benefit time away from the workplace. In most institutions, an average FTE receives benefit time equating to approximately 10% of their regularly scheduled hours. This number is reflected in the Hours section. The FTE multiplied by the hours gives the total hours. Total hours reflect the number of hours that employees will be away from the workplace during the year.

Recognizing that there are seasonal fluctuations in the census (higher than average in winter, lower than average on holidays and during summer), the nurse leader must project what percent of those hours are necessary to be replaced. To determine the number of replacement hours that are necessary, multiply the replacement percent by the total hours.

Refer to the Education and Orientation Summary previously completed to determine the hours of required education and attendance

Schedule 2: PTO, Education, and Orientation

Facility: St. Elsewhere	Unit name: 2West
Time period: 2010	Cost center: 1000
Unit type: Med/surg	
Using ADC (midnight census)	
ADC: 24	Total pat days: 8,760
Using conversion factor (what goes into PLUS)	
Total USO:	-

Replacement FTEs	FTEs	Hours	Total hours
Subtotal PTO		208.57	-
PERCENT (%) OF REPLACEMENT			
Subtotal PTO replacement	-		-

Education/meetings	FTEs	Hours	Total hours
Manager			
Asst. manager			
Charge nurse			
RN			
LVN			
NT/NA			
Monitor tech			
Unit secretary			
Other			
Subtotal education/meeting	-	-	-

Orientation	Head count	Hours	Total hours
Manager			
Asst. manager			
Charge nurse			
RN			
LVN			
NT/NA			
Monitor tech			
Unit secretary			
Other			
Subtotal orientation	-	-	-

FIGURE 5.5 PTO, Education, and Orientation

at meetings. Document this in the Education/Meeting section by job class.

In the Orientation section, estimate the number of new employees that will be hired in the fiscal year. Consider historical turnover rates and

Education						
Skill mix	Job title	Hourly wage	FTE	Total hours	FTES annualized	Total wages
Manager	Manager		.	.	.	$.
Asst. manager	Asst. manager		.	.	.	$.
Charge nurse	Charge nurse		.	.	.	$.
RN	RN		.	.	.	$.
LVN	LVN		.	.	.	$.
NT/NA	NT/NA		.	.	.	$.
Monitor tech	Monitor tech		.	.	.	$.
Unit secretary	Unit secretary		.	.	.	$.
Other	Other		.	.	.	$.
Subtotal education/meeting			-	-	-	$ -

Orientation						
Skill mix	Job title	Hourly wage	FTE	Total hours	FTES annualized	Total wages
Manager			.	.	.	$.
Asst. manager			.	.	.	$.
Charge nurse			.	.	.	$.
RN			.	.	.	$.
LVN			.	.	.	$.
NT/NA			.	.	.	$.
Monitor tech			.	.	.	$.
Unit secretary			.	.	.	$.
Other			.	.	.	$.
Subtotal orientation			-	-	-	$ -
Total			-	-	-	$ -

Note: Total FTEs include Orientation and Education/Meeting Annualized FTEs.

nursing supply within the community. Referring back to the Education and Orientation Summary, determine the number of non-productive hours an employee will be oriented. Enter this information in the Orientation section by job class.

With Schedule 2 completed, you now have the total number of secondary resources necessary to provide direct patient care in the absence of existing staff.

Productive Hours Overview

With Schedules 1 and 2 completed, it is necessary to determine the financial impact of the staffing model being proposed. **FIGURE 5.6** shows Schedule 3 of 4.

Section 1 requires the nurse leader to list each skill mix along with job title, incumbent's current hourly rate of pay and any forecasted increases (projected market factor increases, pay for performance, etc.), and the number of FTEs allotted per job class. These FTEs per job class must be a mirror image of the numbers arrived at in Schedule 1. For each job class, calculate the total hours. The total hours multiplied by the hourly wage gives the total wages per job class. Complete these steps for each job class. Added together, these will provide the total FTEs, Hours, and Wages. These numbers must match the totals from Schedule 1.

Section 2 addresses Bonus Pay. If your organization provides bonus pay, the skill mix, job title, and hourly wage should be completed in this section. The hourly wage section should only reflect the differential, not the total hourly

Schedule 3: Productive Hours Overview

Facility: St. Elsewhere		Unit name: 2West			
Time period: 2010		Cost center: 1000			
Unit type: Med/surg					
Using ADC (midnight census)					
ADC: 24		Total pat days: 8,760			
Using conversion factor					

Regular					
Skill mix	**Job title**	**Hourly wage**	**FTE**	**Total hours**	**Total wages**
Manager				-	$ -
Asst. manager				-	$ -
Charge nurse				-	$ -
RN				-	$ -
LVN				-	$ -
NT/NA				-	$ -
Monitor tech				-	$ -
Unit secretary				-	$ -
				-	$ -
				-	$ -
				-	$ -
				-	$ -
				-	$ -
				-	$ -
Subtotal regular			-	-	$ -

FIGURE 5.6 Schedule 3

wage. For example, if the incumbent earns $15 per hour and the bonus is $2 per hour, only enter $2 in the hourly wage column. Complete this for each effected job class to obtain the total hours and wages for this section.

Section 3 (Other Pay) is directing the nurse leader to project incidental overtime based on historical and anticipated occurrences. Financial statements will have a line item for overtime, usually provided in hours and dollars. Review the previous year's actual overtime and make projections for the upcoming year. Also take into consideration the number of existing and projected vacancies when calculating the overtime hours. Document the total annualized hours for overtime. Convert those hours to FTEs by dividing by 2,080 and place this number in the FTE column. To determine the hourly wage for overtime, one method is to use the RN rate

of pay. Another method is to average the rate of pay for all job classes. If the nurse leader chooses to use the first method, and an RN earns $35 per hour, then the hourly rate is half of that figure ($35/2 = $17.50). This figure is placed in the hourly wage column. The rationale behind this is that the regular time has already been calculated in Section 1. Section 3 requires the half pay. Therefore, you have accounted for time-and-one-half. Take the hourly wage $\times$ total hours = total wages for incidental overtime. If using the average method, take the sum of each skill mix with the propensity of working overtime, and then divide by the number of affected job classes.

The next element in Section 3 is calculating the charge pay. If the organization pays a differential for the nurse to be in charge, this is where you would put that amount.

Contract labor/bonus pay					
Skill mix	**Job title**	**Hourly wage**	**FTE**	**Total hours**	**Total wages**
				-	$ -
				-	$ -
				-	$ -
				-	$ -
				-	$ -
				-	$ -
				-	$ -
Subtotal contract labor/bonus pay			-	-	$ -
Other pay					
Skill mix	**Job title**	**Hourly wage**	**FTE**	**Total hours**	**Total wages**
Bonus pay	Incidental overtime		-	-	$ -
Bonus pay	Charge differential			-	$ -
Bonus pay	On call			-	$ -
Bonus pay	Call back			-	$ -
Subtotal other pay			-	-	$ -

Replacement FTE					
Skill mix	**Job title**	**Hourly wage**	**FTE**	**Total hours**	**Total wages**
Total from schedule 2			-	-	$ -
RN	PRN			-	$ -
RN	Bonus			-	$ -
RN	Agency			-	$ -
				-	$ -
Subtotal replacement FTEs			-	-	$ -

For those nurses who are required to be on call and return to the physical site on demand, most organizations determine what their on-call differential is, and that amount should be entered in the hourly wage section. The number of FTEs that are on call should be multiplied by 2,080 and documented in the total hour column. Those total hours multiplied by the hourly wage will give the total wages for on call.

Callback hours are hours where the nurse is actually called back to the physical site while they are on call. Wages are usually time-and-one-half during callback, but this can vary.

Replacement FTEs

Section 4 addresses data that have been pulled from Schedule 2, Section 1. The nurse leader must now determine from which resource pool these FTEs will be worked. Some organizations have internal float pools, PRN (*pro re nata*, as needed) pools, and some rely heavily on supplemental staffing from nurse agency companies.

Of the FTEs calculated from Schedule 2, the nurse leader must determine how to allocate these FTEs based on secondary resources available. For example, if the organization has a float pool and contracts with freestanding nurse agency companies, the nurse leader will estimate the number of FTEs from each entity needed to meet secondary resource needs.

The hourly rate for each secondary resource is entered into the Hourly Wage column, alongside the FTE for that resource. The FTEs need to be converted to total hours by multiplying by 2,080. Hourly wage multiplied by total hours will give the Total Wages. The total replacement FTEs in Section 4 of Schedule 3 must be the same number as calculated in Section 1 of Schedule 2.

Replacement FTE					
Skill Mix	**Job Title**	**Hourly Wage**	**FTE**	**Total Hours**	**Total Wages**
		Total from Schedule 2	**1.76**	**3,669.12**	
RN	PRN Pool			-	$ -
RN	Float Pool			-	$ -
RN	Agency		1.76	3,660.80	$ -
				-	$ -
	Sub Total Replacement FTEs		**1.76**	**3,660.80**	**$ -**

FTE, full-time equivalent.

Section 5 factors the education and meeting expenses that were determined in Section 2 of Schedule 2. Place the hourly wage by the appropriate skill mix, allocating the hours and FTEs.

Section 6 calculates the financial impact of orientation identified in Section 3 of Schedule 2 by entering the hourly wage of each skill mix.

We will now see the total financial impact of the staffing model you established (see **FIGURE 5.7**).

Schedule 4 of 4 provides totals of key areas of impact and are all carried over from Schedule 3.

Productive Time

- Subtotal Regular includes subtotals of Section 1 of Schedule 3.
- Subtotal Bonus Pay is taken from Section 2 of Schedule 3.

Education						
Skill Mix	**Job Title**	**Hourly Wage**	**FTE**	**Total Hours**	**FTEs Annualized**	**Total Wages**
Manager	Nurse Manager		1.00	-	-	$ -
RN	RN	$ 35.00	14.70	529.2	0.25	$ 18,522
Nurse Tech	Nurse Tech	$ 15.00	10.50	84.0	0.04	$ 1,260
Dept. Secretary	Dept. Secretary	$ 14.00	2.10	16.8	0.01	$ 235
Sub Total Education/Meeting			**28.30**	**630.00**	**0.30**	**$ 20,017**

Schedule 4: Summary

Facility: St. Elsewhere	Unit name: 2West
Time period: 2010	Cost center: 1000
Unit type: Med/surg	

Using ADC (midnight census)	
ADC: 24	Total pat days: 8,760

Categories	FTEs	Total hours	Total wages
Subtotal regular	-	-	$ -
Subtotal other pay	-	-	$ -
Total direct care FTEs	-	-	$ -
Subtotal replacement FTEs	-	-	$ -
Subtotal bonus pay	-	-	$ -
Subtotal education/meeting	-	-	$ -
Subtotal orientation	-	-	$ -
Total	-	-	$ -

Note: other pay is not included in schedule 3 categories

NHPPD

Total worked hours per patient day	-
Productive houes per patient day	
Paid Hours	-

FIGURE 5.7 Schedule 4

Orientation						
Skill Mix	**Job Title**	**Hourly Wage**	**FTE**	**Total Hours**	**FTEs Annualized**	**Total Wages**
Manager	Nurse Manager	-	-	-	-	$ -
RN	RN	$ 55.00	2.00	240.00	0.12	$ 13,200
Nurse Tech	Nurse Tech				-	$ -
Dept. Secretary	Dept. Secretary		-	-	-	$ -
Sub Total Orientation			2.00	240.00	0.12	$ 13,200

- Subtotal of Other Pay is derived from Section 3 of Schedule 3, *which only reflects the overtime calculations* because regular hours worked plus overtime hours worked equals total **direct care hours or FTEs.**

Non-Productive Time

- Subtotal Replacement FTEs is taken from Section 4 of Schedule 3.
- Subtotal Bonus Pay is taken from Section 2 of Schedule 3.

- Subtotal of Education and Meeting is taken from Section 5 Schedule 3.
- Subtotal of Orientation is taken from Section 6 Schedule 3.
- Add up the bottom lines that reflect TOTAL PAID HOURS, FTEs, and WAGES.

Calculating Nursing Hours Per Patient Day

Take total direct care hours and divide by annualized patient days (shown as Total Patient Days at the top of Schedules 1–4).

Total paid hours per patient day (HPPD) is calculated by dividing total hours by total patient days. This figure is the direct HPPD plus all budgeted non-productive hours (replacement FTEs, Bonus Pay, education/meeting and orientation).

The direct nursing hours per patient day (NHPPD) is also listed at the top of Schedule 1 as Direct HPPD.

Summary

Creating a staffing model and corresponding budget is a complex process that requires consideration of multiple influencing factors. This chapter was intended as an overview, an opportunity to gain exposure to key terminology and calculation methods. In the following chapter, we will design staffing plans and budgets for two different types of clinical settings: inpatient and outpatient. While these examples will not cover all of the types of nurse department budgeting you might encounter, with each exercise your ability to build these models will improve and your understanding of each component will expand. Using the same templates (Facility Overview and Schedules 1–4), you will gain familiarity with the flow of the staffing model development process.

Discussion Questions

1. Why is it important for the nurse leader to provide a reasonable and fair operation budget?

2. Although budget figures are estimates of future projections, why and how should nurse leaders be prepared to explain short-term variations?

3. Nurse leaders have many responsibilities when it comes to the development of the budget. What issues would be considered most important for the nurse leader in this process?

4. How should a nurse leader prepare to handle minimum staffing requirement costs in the budget process in case this is challenged?

5. Besides a department budget approach, what other alternatives are available in the budgeting process?

Glossary of Terms

Breakeven when the costs of operations exactly equal the revenues; there is no profit or loss.

Capital Budget covers the purchase of land, buildings, and long-lived (at least 2 years) equipment.

Direct Labor the labor that actually turns direct materials into a finished product.

Fixed Costs costs that stay the same regardless of the level of activity.

Full-Time Equivalent (FTE) unit of measurement that represents a person or people working 40 hours a week and 2,080 hours a year.

Hours per Patient Day (HPPD) the number of nursing staff hours needed to provide care to an inpatient in 24 hours.

Indirect Labor those persons who do not actually turn direct materials into a finished product; part of overhead.

Minimum Staffing needing at least two staff members on duty at all times to staff a unit.

Non-Productive Time time when an employee is paid but is not working, such as holidays, sick time, vacation time, and/or paid time off (PTO).

Nursing Workload the volume of work performed by nursing caregivers; better presented as NHPPD or HPPD.

Operating Budgets cover the day-to-day costs of a unit, including such things as wages for regular and temporary workers, medical and office supplies, equipment rental, repair and maintenance, travel and education, and dues and subscriptions. Like all budgets, operating budgets represent the "best guess" for costs over a coming period.

Productive Time actual time worked.

Revenues charges made to patients or other clients.

Staff Mix marketing term that specifies which kind of direct care staff will provide care.

Unit of Service used by healthcare organizations to measure specific services a patient uses within a specific time frame that is, minutes, hours, days, visits, births, treatments, operations, or other patient encounters.

Variable Costs those costs that change depending on the level of volume.

CHAPTER 6

Budget Development and Evaluation

Paul Brown, MSN, RN, and **Gary Eubank** MSN, RN, and **J. Michael Leger**, PhD, MBA, RN

OBJECTIVES

- Demonstrate a working knowledge in the development of a staffing budget.
- Calculate budgeted FTEs, replacement FTEs, and indirect work hours (orientation and education).
- Understand the impact that incidental overtime hours can have on a department's budget.

▶ Introduction

In Chapter 5, you were presented with an overview of the budget responsibilities for the nurse leader. In addition, the budgeting process, along with an introduction to budgeting terms, was provided. This chapter will continue to explain the development of a staffing budget based upon the principles introduced in the previous chapter. This chapter will provide you with two case studies of an inpatient and an outpatient clinical setting. You will use the same Schedules introduced in Chapter 5 to build upon your budgeting knowledge.

▶ Case Study #1—Inpatient Setting

St. Elsewhere is preparing to open a new 30-bed Med/Surg unit in 2017. The Cost Center established for this new unit is 1001, with a designated internal name "Inpatient." Anticipated average daily census (ADC) based on comparison of similar units within the area is 24. The staffing is based on 12-hour shifts/7 days per week. The community standard for nurse–patient ratio is 1:6 on day shift and 1:8 on night shift. The ratio for unlicensed nurse assistants, which our organization classifies as a "nurse tech" (NT), is commonly 1:8 on the day shift and 1:10 at night. The organization has provided the following information and tasked you with building a nursing staffing model and budget for the new Med/Surg unit.

- Historical incidental overtime: 5%
- Employee personal time off (PTO) 10%
- Current registered nurse (RN) agency costs: $55/hr
- Approved job classes:

Skill Mix Name	Abbreviation
Manager	MGR
Registered nurse	RN
Nurse tech	NT
Unit secretary	US

Established replacement factors in the organization by ADC:

Replacement Factors		
Unit Type	ADC	% Replaced
Med/Surg	<14	100%
Med/Surg	≥14	70%
Stepdown	<7	100%
Stepdown	≥7	80%
ICU	<5	100%
ICU	≥5	100%

ADC, average daily census; ICU, intensive care unit.

Average turnover by job class:

Job Class	Turnover Last Fiscal Year
Manager	0
Registered nurse	2
Nurse tech	2
Unit secretary	0

Budgeted hourly rate of pay by job class:

Job Class	Hourly Rate of Pay
Manager	$39.21
Registered nurse	$35
Nurse tech	$15
Unit secretary	$14

Established education and meeting hours by job class:

Education and Orientation Summary

Skill Mix		Required Education and Meetings			Orientation		
Title	Abbreviation	Med/surg	Stepdown	ICU	Med/surg	Stepdown	ICU/ED
Director	DIR						
Manager	MGR						
Charge nurse	CHG	36	52	76	240	320	480
Registered Nurse	RN	36	52	76	240	320	480
Licensed Vocational Nurse	LVN	20	20	20	240	320	
Nurse Technician / Nurse Assistant	NT	8	8	8	80	80	80
Unit secretary	US	8	8	8	80	80	80
Monitor tech	MT	8	8	8		80	
Dept secretary	OTH	8	8	8	80	80	80

▶ Data Collection

Let's begin by completing the facility overview discussed in the previous chapter. Here, we will begin to collect the essential data needed to formulate staffing and budgeting for the new unit. Total Patient Days can be calculated by multiplying the ADC by 365.

Once completed, your facility overview should mirror the following:

Facility overview

	Reserved
Facility:	
Time period:	
Unit name:	
Cost center:	
Unit type:	
	Volume
ADC:	
Total pat days:	
PTO%	
Incidental overtime	

Facility overview

	Reserved
Facility:	St.Elsewhere
Time period:	2017
Unit name:	Inpatient
Cost center:	1001
Unit type:	Med/surg
	Volume
ADC:	24
Total pat days:	8,760
PTO%	10.0%
Incidental overtime	5.0%

▶ Schedule 1—Staffing Matrix

With the facility overview established, we can begin to develop a staffing plan to meet the patient care needs of our new unit. Keeping in mind funded job classes and recommended patient ratios for licensed and unlicensed staff, establish a work matrix for day shift.

	SUN			MON			TUE			WED			THU			FRI			SAT		
7A-7P, 7A-3P	8HR	10HR	12HR	8HR	10HR	12HR	8HR	10HR	12HR	8HR	10HR	12HR	8HR	10HR	12HR	8HR	10HR	12HR	8HR	10HR	12HR
Manager																					
ANM																					
RN																					
LVN																					
Nurse tech																					
Monitor tech																					
Unit secretary																					
Total	-	-	-	-	-	-	-	-	-	-	-	-	-	-	-	-	-	-	-	-	-

First, our manager is an 8-hour Monday-through-Friday position. (Depending on budget and acuity levels, an organization may also have an Assistant Nurse Manager and/or charge nurses for each shift. In our case, these job classes are not available.)

Next, you will recall that the anticipated ADC for our new unit was 24 and the patient ratio for licensed staff on day shift was 1:6. Dividing the ADC by 6 reveals that we will need to staff four RNs per day shift (24/6 = 4).

Using this same approach, let's calculate the staffing needed for unlicensed nurse assistants. Divide the ADC (24) by 8 (remember that NAs have a 1:8 staffing ratio on the day shift). This calculation reveals the need to staff three NAs per day shift (24/8 = 3).

Finally, your new unit will require a unit secretary (US). For this example, plan to have one US scheduled for 12 hours per day, 7 days per week on the day shift. (Note: depending on the organization, the US may not be on the nursing budget. In this scenario, the US is being funded from the nursing budget and must, therefore, be accounted for in staffing and budgeting plans.)

Now that you have a basic scheduling matrix established, add together the total hours for each day in the bottom row titled "TOTAL." With the matrix complete, your schedule should look similar to the following.

	SUN			MON			TUE			WED			THU			FRI			SAT		
7A-7P, 7A-3P	8HR	10HR	12HR	8HR	10HR	12HR	8HR	10HR	12HR	8HR	10HR	12HR	8HR	10HR	12HR	8HR	10HR	12HR	8HR	10HR	12HR
Manager				1.00			1.00			1.00			1.00			1.00					
ANM																					
RN			4.0			4.0			4.0			4.0			4.0			4.0			4.0
LVN																					
Nurse tech			3.0			3.0			3.0			3.0			3.0			3.0			3.0
Monitor tech																					
Unit secretary			1.0			1.0			1.0			1.0			1.0			1.0			1.0
Total	-	-	8.0	1.0	-	8.0	1.0	-	8.0	1.0	-	8.0	1.0	-	8.0	1.0	-	8.0	-	-	8.0

Using the same approach as earlier, establish a staffing pattern for the night shift. Keep the following in mind:

- Nurse-to-patient ratio for the night shift is 1:8 in your community.

- NT–to-patient ratio at night is 1:10.
- The organization does not allocate a US position for the night shift.

Your completed matrix should result in a total of three RNs and two NTs for each 12-hour shift.

7P-7A, 11P-7A	SUN			MON			TUE			WED			THU			FRI			SAT		
	8HR	10HR	12HR	8HR	10HR	12HR	8HR	10HR	12HR	8HR	10HR	12HR	8HR	10HR	12HR	8HR	10HR	12HR	8HR	10HR	12HR
Manager																					
ANM																					
RN																					
LVN																					
Nurse tech																					
Monitor tech																					
Unit secretary																					
Total	-	-	-	-	-	-	-	-	-	-	-	-	-	-	-	-	-	-	-	-	-

Note: At this point it is important to reinforce that while community standards for nurse-to-patient ratios serve as a valuable guideline, any number of circumstances may exist at your facility that warrant a higher or slightly lower ratio. Integration of standards of care with personal insight and knowledge is critical to accurately developing a staffing plan that is sufficient to meet the specific patient care needs of your unit.

We will now calculate the total full-time equivalents (FTEs) and hours by job class required to meet this staffing pattern. To calculate the total hours per job class, per shift, a simple formula to remember is

Total shifts per week × Hours per day × 52 = Total hours of job class

This formula breaks down as follows: First, we must identify the total number of shifts per week. In the example of the RN, we allocated four employees for each day shift **7** days per week. If we multiply 4 × 7, we see that we have 28 total shifts per week for this job class. Next, we multiply this total by the hours worked per day. Because the RNs will be on 12-hour shifts,

multiply 28 (total shifts per week) by 12 (hours per day).

336 × 52 = 17,472 total hours per year for this job class

This reveals 336 total hours worked per week. To find the annual total hours, we now simply multiply the total hours per week (336) by the number of weeks in a year (52).

Let's break down the remaining job classes using this formula:

Day Shift
Manager

Total shifts per week: **5** (1 employee working Monday through Friday)

Hours worked per day: **8**

5 × 8 × 52 = **2,080** hours

RNs (previous example)

Total shifts per week: **28**

Hours worked per day: **12**

28 × 12 × 52 = **17,472** hours

	SUN			MON			TUE			WED			THU			FRI			SAT		
7P-7A, 11P-7A	8HR	10HR	12HR	8HR	10HR	12HR	8HR	10HR	12HR	8HR	10HR	12HR	8HR	10HR	12HR	8HR	10HR	12HR	8HR	10HR	12HR
Manager																					
ANM																					
RN			3.0			3.0			3.0			3.0			3.0			3.0			3.0
LVN																					
Nurse tech			2.0			2.0			2.0			2.0			2.0			2.0			2.0
Monitor tech																					
Unit secretary																					
TOTAL	-	-	5.0	-	-	5.0	-	-	5.0	-	-	5.0	-	-	5.0	-	-	5.0	-	-	5.0

NTs

Total shifts per week: **21**

Hours worked per day: **12**

$21 \times 12 \times 52 =$ **13,104** hours

USs

Total shifts per week: **7**

Hours worked per day: **12**

$7 \times 12 \times 52 =$ **4,368** hours

Using this same approach, calculate the total hours per job class for the night shift. Totals should match the following:

RNs – **13,104** hours (21 shifts × 12 hours × 52)

NTs – **8,736** hours (14 shifts × 12 hours × 52)

▶ Calculating FTEs from Total Hours

You may recall from Chapter 5 that one FTE is considered the equivalent of 2,080 hours worked per year. Now that we know the total annual hours of scheduled work for each job class, we can calculate the FTEs by simply dividing total hours by 2,080.

Day Shift

Manager

2,080/2,080 = 1 FTE

RNs

17,472/2,080 = 8.4 FTEs

Continue this formula for the remainder of the day shift.

NTs

_____/_____ = _____ FTEs

US

_____/_____ = _____ FTEs

Combined, the established staffing plan calls for a total of 17.8 FTEs to provide day shift coverage. Repeat these steps to calculate the night shift FTEs.

RN

_____/_____ = _____ FTEs

NTs

_____/_____ = _____ FTEs

Your calculations should result in a total of 10.5 FTEs for night shift coverage (6.3 RN and 4.2 NT). Combined with day shift FTEs, we have a total of 28.3 FTEs (17.8 day shift and 10.5 night shift) in Nursing Services to provide 24-hour care at a staffing level consistent with community standards.

▶ Schedule 2— Determining Replacement FTEs

Staffing challenges are an inevitability of managing Nursing Services. Turnover, medical leave, vacation, and sick leave all result in unfilled slots on a scheduling matrix. Replacing these lost hours of work using overtime and supplemental agency services can add significant costs to the bottom line of an organization. The nurse leader must be diligent in identifying which positions are essential to meeting patient care needs and, therefore, must be replaced. Generally, licensed nurse positions are considered essential because the department is unable to operate without licensed staff. One exception may be the manager who, while licensed, is an exempt (salaried, not hourly) employee working in a managerial role. It is crucial that the nurse leader carefully consider standards of care and anticipate patient acuity in planning replacement factors. For our purposes, we will assume that the new Med/Surg unit will not require replacement of the unit manager or unit secretaries, but that all other positions, including the NT, will be included in our replacement factor.

We will now complete calculations for our replacement factors. To begin, calculate the number of FTEs to be replaced and subtract the non-essential FTEs (those that will not be replaced) from the total FTEs allocated for the unit.

Total FTEs: **28.3**
Nonessential FTEs: (unit manager) – **1**, USs – **2.1**
Remaining (essential) FTEs: **25.2**

Replacement FTEs	FTEs	Hours	Total Hours
Subtotal PTO	25.20		-
Percent (%) of replacement			
Subtotal PTO replacement	-		-

Next, calculate the hours that will be replaced. This is accomplished by multiplying the PTO % that we established at the beginning of this chapter (10%) by 2,080.

$$0.1 \times 2,080 = 208$$

Replacement FTEs	FTEs	Hours	Total Hours
Subtotal PTO	25.20	208.00	-
Percent (%) of replacement			
Subtotal PTO replacement	-		-

Now, calculate the total hours by multiplying the FTEs (25.2) by the hours (208).

$$25.2 \times 208 = 5,241.6$$

Replacement FTEs	FTEs	Hours	Total Hours
Subtotal PTO	25.20	208.00	5,241.60
Percent (%) of replacement			
Subtotal PTO replacement			

Next, identify the percent of replacement. This number was provided to us by the organization (see Case Scenario at the beginning of this chapter). A Med/Surg unit with an ADC exceeding 14 qualifies for a 70% replacement.

Replacement FTEs	FTEs	Hours	Total Hours
Subtotal PTO	25.20	208.00	5,241.60
Percent (%) of replacement		70%	
Subtotal PTO replacement			

With this information, we can calculate our Subtotal PTO Replacement. For Total Hours, multiply the Total Hours of Subtotal PTO (5241.6) by the Percent of Replacement (70%):

$$5,241.6 \times 0.7 = 3,669.12$$

Replacement FTEs	FTEs	Hours	Total Hours
Subtotal PTO	25.20	208.00	5,241.60
Percent (%) of replacement	70%		
Subtotal PTO replacement			3,669.12

For FTEs, divide the Subtotal PTO Replacement (3,669.12) by 2,080:

$$3,669.12 / 2,080 = 1.76$$

Replacement FTEs	FTEs	Hours	Total Hours
Subtotal PTO	25.20	208.00	5,241.60
Percent (%) of replacement	70%		
Subtotal PTO replacement	1.76		3,669.12

▶ Education and Meeting Hours

We will now identify Education and Meeting Hours by job class. Refer to the Education and Orientation Summary provided in the case scenario. In the first column of the table that follows, enter total FTEs for each job class (remembering to include both day and night shift). In the second column, enter the appropriate hours from the Education and Orientation Summary. Under Total Hours, multiply the total FTEs for each job class by the hours allotted.

Education/Meetings	FTEs	Hours	Total Hours
Manager			
ANM			
RN			
LVN			
Unit secretary			
Nurse tech			
Dept secretary			
Subtotal education/meeting			

Your completed table should mirror the following:

Education/Meetings	FTEs	Hours	Total Hours
Manager			
ANM			
RN	14.70	36.0	529.2
LVN			
Nurse tech	10.50	8.0	84.0
Dept secretary	2.10	8.0	17
Subtotal education/meeting	27.30	52.0	630.0

Referring again to the Education and Orientation Summary, identify the orientation hours required for essential staff. Here, we will be estimating the number of staff that will be hired in the fiscal year. Recall that the organization provided us with the Average Turnover by Job Class based on the previous fiscal year. Use this data, along with the Education and Orientation Summary, to complete the following. Leave blank positions that are not expected to turn over.

Orientation	Head Count	Hours	Total hours
Director			
Manager			
RN			
LVN			
Nurse tech			
Dept secretary			
Subtotal orientation			

Once completed, your table should look like this:

Orientation	Head Count	Hours	Total Hours
Director			
Manager			
RN	2.00	240.0	480
LVN			
Nurse tech	2.00	80.0	160
Dept secretary			
Subtotal orientation	4.00	320.0	640.0

We have now compiled all necessary data to determine the financial impact that our staffing model will have on the organization.

▶ Schedule 3—Financial Impact

The next step in our process is to predict the financial impact that our proposed staffing will have on the unit's budget. Let's begin with establishing expected Regular Pay, the wages each job class is projected to cost based on FTEs, and scheduled hours. Hours are calculated by multiplying the FTE for each job class by 2,080.

Review this simple formula for the manager, and then complete the calculations for each job class:

Manager: FTEs (1) $\times$ 2,080 = 2,080 Total Hours

RN: (FTE) 14.7 $\times$ 2,080 = _____ Total Hours

NT: (FTE) 10.5 $\times$ _____ = _____ Total Hours

Secretary: (FTE)
_____ $\times$ _____ = _____ Total Hours

Once completed, the Total Hours of Regular Pay for our department is 58,864. This is the number of regular hours expected to be worked in the department by all job classes.

Regular					
Skill Mix	**Job Title**	**Hourly Wage**	**FTE**	**Total Hours**	**Total Wages**
Manager	NURSE MANAGER	$39.21	1.00	2,080.00	
RN	RN	$35.00	14.70	30,576.00	
NT/NA	NT	$15.00	10.50	21,840.00	
Unit secretary	US	$14.00	2.10	4,368.00	
		Subtotal regular	28.30	58.864 .00	$ -

To calculate Total Wages, multiply the hourly rate (provided by our organization in the case scenario) by the Total Hours you just calculated for each job class.

Adding the Total Wages for each job class, we find that we will spend $1,540,469 on Regular Pay.

Manager: $39.21 $\times$ 2,080 = $81,557 Total Wages

RN: $35.00 $\times$ 30,576 = _____ Total Wages

NT: $15 $\times$ _____ = _____ Total Wages

Secretary: _____
$\times$ _____ = _____ Total Wages

Regular					
Skill Mix	**Job Title**	**Hourly Wage**	**FTE**	**Total Hours**	**Total Wages**
Manager	NURSE MANAGER	$39.21	1.00	2,080.00	$ 81,557
RN	RN	$35.00	14.70	30,576.00	$1,070,160
NT/NA	NT	$15.00	10.50	21,840.00	$ 327,600
Unit secretary	US	$14.00	2.10	4,368.00	$ 61,152
		Subtotal regular	28.30	58.864 .00	$1,540,469

Next, we will calculate projected overtime costs. Our organization's policy is that only RNs are qualified for overtime. While this could impose limitations on our ability to meet patient care needs, we are bound by organizational policy. As such, we must anticipate the financial impact of RN overtime. To make this calculation, multiply our Total FTEs for the department (28.3) by the Incidental Overtime figure provided in the case scenario (5%). This provides us with an anticipated overtime FTE of 1.42, meaning that we will need an additional 1.42 FTEs of RNs just to cover overtime.

$$28.3 \times .05 = 1.42 \text{ FTEs}$$

Next, we will calculate the total hours of overtime by multiplying the known FTEs of 1.42 by 2,080.

$$1.42 \times 2,080 = 2,953.6 \text{ total hours}$$

$$\$35 / 2 = \$17.5 \times 2,943.2 = \$51,506$$
$$\text{total wages}$$

Finally, take half the established hourly RN salary of $35 (overtime = 1.5 of hourly rate) and multiply it by the total hours to determine the cost of this overtime.

Overtime					
Skill Mix	Job Title	Hourly Wage	FTE	Total Hours	Total Wages
RN	RN	$17.50	1.42	2,953.60	$51,688
				-	$-
				-	$-
				-	$-
				-	$-
				-	$-
				-	$-
		Overtime	1.42	2,953.60	$51,688

Supplemental Resources

We anticipate that not all hours will be covered by overtime. Inevitably, our staff will need PTO. This will require us to pool resources from outside our department in order to maintain our required nurse-to-patient ratios. Our organization does not have an established PRN or Float Pool available, so we will be depending on outside staffing agencies.

In Schedule 2, we have already calculated a PTO replacement (1.76) and total hours of PTO (3660.8). We can now simply multiply the total PTO replacement hours by the hourly wage for agency nurses provided to us by the organization ($55).

$$3660.8 \times 55 = \$201,344 \text{ Total Projected}$$
$$\text{Agency Costs}$$

Replacement FTE					
Skill Mix	Job Title	Hourly Wage	FTE	Total Hours	Total Wages
	Total From Schedule 2		1.76	3,669.12	
RN	PRN pool			-	$-
RN	Float pool			-	$-
RN	Agency	$55.00	1.76	3,660.80	$201,344
				-	$-
	Subtotal replacement FTEs		1.76	3,660.80	$201,344

Now, let's calculate costs for Education. Refer to Schedule 2 where we have already calculated the total hours of education for each job class. Multiply the hourly wage by the total hours to obtain the cost of training by job class. In total, you will see that we project an additional $20,017 in education costs.

Education						
Skill Mix	**Job Title**	**Hourly Wage**	**FTE**	**Total Hours**	**FTE Annualized**	**Total Wages**
Manager	Nurse manager		1.00			$-
RN	RN	$35.00	14.70	529.2	0.25	$18,522
Nurse tech	Nurse tech	$15.00	10.50	84.0	0.04	$ 1,260
Dept secretary	Dept secretary	$14.00	2.10	16.8	0.01	$ 235
	Subtotal education/meeting		**28.30**	**630.00**	**0.30**	**$20,017**

The final step before we look at our total financial impact is to calculate the cost of orientation. Average Turnover by Job Class provided by the organization revealed that we can anticipate replacing two RNs and two NTs during the fiscal year. Knowing this, we can project the costs of orientation for our department by multiplying the hourly replacement wage for each job class by the established orientation hours in the Orientation and Education Summary. Recall that we replace RNs only, and that the cost of agency is $55/hr.

RN: $55 $\times$ 240 = $13,200 Total
Wages to Cover Orientation for RNs

Orientation						
Skill Mix	**Job Title**	**Hourly Wage**	**FTE**	**Total Hours**	**FTE Annualized**	**Total Wages**
Manager	Nurse manager		-	-	-	$-
RN	RN	$55.00	2.00	240.00	0.12	$13,200
Nurse tech	Nurse tech				-	$-
Dept secretary	Dept secretary		-	-	-	$-
	Subtotal orientation		**2.00**	**240.00**	**0.12**	**$13,200**

With all of our calculations completed, it is time to have a look at the total financial impact of our staffing model.

▶ Schedule 4

Throughout this chapter, we have been building a model in pieces and sections. Each step has brought us closer to determining the complete financial picture of the department. In this final step, we will develop a summary of the Nursing Department Financials using the information previously collected.

Beginning with Regular Pay from Schedule 3, fill in the Subtotal Regular FTEs, Total Hours, and Total Wages. Complete the same columns for all rows except Total Direct Care FTEs and Total which we will calculate in the next steps.

Categories	FTEs	Total Hours	Total Wages
Subtotal Regular			
Overtime			
Total Direct Care FTEs			
Subtotal Replacement FTEs			
Subtotal Education/Meeting			
Subtotal Orientation			
Total			

Now, sum each row for Subtotal Regular and Overtime to determine the Total Direct Care FTEs.

Categories	FTEs	Total Hours	Total Wages
Subtotal Regular	28.30	58,864.00	$ 1,540,469
Overtime	1.42	2,953.60	$ 51,688
Total Direct Care FTEs			
Subtotal Replacement FTEs	1.76	3,660.80	$ 201,344
Subtotal Education/Meeting	0.30	630.00	$ 20,017
Subtotal Orientation	0.12	240.00	$ 13,200
Total			

Finally, compile the total for each column in the bottom row beginning with the Total Direct Care FTEs row.

Categories	FTEs	Total Hours	Total Wages
Subtotal Regular	28.30	58,864.00	$ 1,540,469
Overtime	1.42	2,953.60	$ 51,688
Total Direct Care FTEs	**29.72**	**61,817.60**	**$ 1,592,157**
Subtotal Replacement FTEs	1.76	3,660.80	$ 201,344
Subtotal Education/Meeting	0.30	630.00	$ 20,017
Subtotal Orientation	0.12	240.00	$ 13,200
Total			

We now have a complete succinct representation of the financial impact of our staffing plan and budget. FTEs, hours, and wages are all represented with breakdowns for overtime, replacement, education, and orientation. Armed with this information, we are prepared to enter into discussions with the Chief Financial Officer with information necessary to defend and justify our staffing plan.

Categories	FTEs	Total Hours	Total Wages
Subtotal Regular	28.30	58,864.00	$ 1,540,469
Overtime	1.42	2,953.60	$ 51,688
Total Direct Care FTEs	**29.72**	**61,817.60**	**$ 1,592,157**
Subtotal Replacement FTEs	1.76	3,660.80	$ 201,344
Subtotal Education/Meeting	0.30	630.00	$ 20,017
Subtotal Orientation	0.12	240.00	$ 13,200
Total	**31.89**	**66,348.40**	**$ 1,826,718**

▶ Case Study #2— Outpatient

North American Health Systems (NAHS) is a national healthcare organization that operates hospitals and outpatient clinics. The organization has tasked you with identifying the nursing department cost associated with opening a 12-hour minor care outpatient clinic. A prime corner lot in a major metropolitan area has been secured and the organization is anticipating a high volume of patients at this location. As a result, they are budgeting to have three physicians working seven-day-per-week rotations. Monday through Thursday, two physicians will be available to see patients but on Friday, Saturday, and Sunday of each week, all three physicians will be onsite for patient visits. Each physician is expected to spend 20 minutes per patient and will work from 7 am to 7 pm. Clinic traffic is projected to average 60 patients per day Monday through Thursday and approximately 90 patients each day on Friday, Saturday, and Sunday.

Due to budgetary restrictions, supplemental agency staffing will not be approved for use at the outpatient clinic. You will, however, be approved to use float pool nursing staff from NAHC's local hospital to cover PTO and orientation. Additionally, the organization has committed to providing relief staff from another clinic to cover education commitments. In each case, you will be responsible for paying wages for coverages at the employee's current rate of pay. A US will be provided Monday through Friday but will not be part of the nursing budget. The Chief Financial Officer (CFO) has provided the following organizational information to assist you in your budget planning:

NAHS Minor Care Clinic (Doing Business as "Bumps-N-Bruises")			
Cost Center 601			
Allowable Incidental Overtime	5%	Employee PTO	12%
Supplemental Agency Budget	$0	PRN Pool Availability	No
Float Pool Cost Per Hour – RN	$55	Anticipated Annual Turnover – Director	0
Float Pool Cost Per Hour – LVN	$40	Anticipated Annual Turnover – RN	0
Float Pool Cost Per Hour – NT	$31	Anticipated Annual Turnover – LVN	1
Average Annual Rate of Pay – Director	$70,000	New Employee Orientation Hours – All Job Classes	16
Average Annual Rate of Pay – RN	$64,000	Annual Education / Meeting Hours – All Job Classes	12
Average Annual Rate of Pay – LVN	$33,000	Education coverage cost per hour – RN	$30.77
		Education coverage cost per hour – LVN	$15.87

▶ Data Collection

Following the same process that we used in the Inpatient model, begin by completing a Facility Overview with the information we have available. Because we are working with an Outpatient model, for ADC use the average number of clinic visits projected for each day. To do this, add the number of visits expected each week and divide by seven, rounding to the nearest whole, then calculate Total Patient Days by multiplying the ADC by 365.

ADC = 510 / 7 = 72.86 or 73 visits/day
× 365 = 26,645

Facility:	
Time period:	
Unit name:	
Cost center:	
Unit type:	
	Volume
ADC:	
Total pat days:	
PTO%	
Incidental overtime	

Your completed Facility Overview should be as follows:

Facility:	Minor care clinic
Time period:	2017
Unit name:	Bumps-N-Bruises
Cost center:	601
Unit type:	12hr
	Volume
ADC:	73
Total pat days:	26,645
PTO%	12.0%
Incidental overtime	5.0%

▶ Schedule 1—Staffing Pattern

Next, we will establish a staffing model aimed at meeting the anticipated patient care needs of our clinic. If we were taking over an existing clinic, we would look at historical data such as current staffing models, previous year's clinic visits, secondary staffing resource utilization, and any seasonal predictors for budget overruns. Because this is a new clinic, we will need to look at the information that can be attained from similar clinics within the community and do our best to determine how these will compare to our operations.

For our purposes, there are two smaller but similar clinics operating in our community. One averages 20 patients per day and is staffed with one physician, one RN, and one LVN that is responsible for lab work and administrative scheduling duties. The other clinic is slightly larger, averaging close to 40 patients per day and is staffed with one MD, one mid-level provider, one RN, and two LVNs. Each clinic provides minor care similar to what is planned for Bumps-N-Bruises. With no other information available, how might we anticipate the scheduling and staffing needs of our clinic?

Let's begin with known comparables. We have identified the staffing that is currently being used by similar clinics and we have an idea of the number of daily clinic visits for similar care needs of patients. Because we will anticipate averaging significantly more clinic visits per day, we must adjust our staffing model for this to be addressed. Additionally, we know that all three physicians will be seeing patients on Thursday, Friday, and Saturday of each week, so we can anticipate higher clinic appointment numbers on those days. What we do not know is the rationale for the skill mix of each clinic. In an outpatient setting, skill mix is not a simple matter of nurse-patient ratios. The acuity of the patients will certainly play a role, but determining skill mix really comes down to the level of nursing care each patient requires, defined practice parameters of the RN versus LVN by a state's board of nursing, and the budgetary funding available. While we anticipate higher numbers of clinic visits than the comparable clinics, the level of care provided will be similar. Therefore, let's plan to staff one RN each day. Because the larger clinic averages 40 patients per day and we are anticipating 60–90 per day, it will be wise to add an additional LVN to our staffing model. We must also plan for the heavy clinic days (Thursday–Saturday), so an additional LVN on these days may be necessary. Complete the staffing model with the aim of addressing each of these variables (and be sure to include your 8-hour Monday–Friday Director so that you will have someone present to manage the clinic).

7A-7P, 7A-3P	SUN			MON			TUE			WED			THU			FRI			SAT		
	8HR	10HR	12HR	8HR	10HR	12HR	8HR	10HR	12HR	8HR	10HR	12HR	8HR	10HR	12HR	8HR	10HR	12HR	8HR	10HR	12HR
Director																					
Charge nurse																					
RN																					
LVN																					
Nurse tech																					
Monitor tech																					
Unit secretary																					
Total	-	-	-	-	-	-	-	-	-	-	-	-	-	-	-	-	-	-	-	-	-

Once complete, your staffing plan should look similar to the following:

7A-7P, 7A-3P	SUN			MON			TUE			WED			THU			FRI			SAT		
	8HR	10HR	12HR	8HR	10HR	12HR	8HR	10HR	12HR	8HR	10HR	12HR	8HR	10HR	12HR	8HR	10HR	12HR	8HR	10HR	12HR
Director				1.00			1.00			1.00			1.00			1.00					
Charge nurse																					
RN		1.0			1.0			1.0			1.0			1.0			1.0			1.0	
LVN		3.0			3.0			3.0			3.0			4.0			4.0			4.0	
Nurse tech																					
Monitor tech																					
Unit secretary																					
Total	-	-	4.0	1.0	-	4.0	1.0	-	4.0	1.0	-	4.0	1.0	-	5.0	1.0	-	5.0	-	-	5.0

Notice that we planned for our Director to work 8 hours per day, Monday–Friday. This is typically when the majority of management business will be conducted. We also have one RN and three LVNs Sunday through Wednesday, with a fourth LVN staffed on our projected heavy days.

▶ Calculating Total Hours per Job Class

To determine the number of employees required to meet this staffing pattern, we need to calculate the FTEs for each job class. We must first, however, calculate the total hours projected annually for each job class. Use the following formula to calculate total hours:

Total shifts per week × Hours per day × 52 = Total hours of job class

Let's begin with the Director. This position works 5 days per week, 8 hours each day. Using the formula above, we calculate total hours as follows:

5 (shifts per week) × 8 (hours per day) × 52 = 2,080 total hours

Now, apply the same formula to each remaining job class.

▶ Calculating FTEs from Total Hours

Now that we have the total hours for each job class, we can calculate the required FTEs required to meet the proposed staffing pattern by dividing Total Hours by 2,080.

Director: 2,080 / 2,080 = 1 FTE
RN: 4,368 / 2,080 = _____ FTEs
LVN: 14,976 / 2,080 = _____ FTEs

Your calculations should return **2.1** FTEs for the RN and **7.2** FTEs for the LVN job class. All totaled, we have identified 10.3 FTEs required to meet the staffing needs of this clinic based on our projections of clinic visits and workload.

RN

7 (shifts per week) × _____ (hours per day) × **52** = _____ total hours

LVNs

___ (shifts per week) × ___ (hours per day) × _____ = _____ total hours

Total hours for the RN are 4,368 (7 × 12 × 52).
Total hours for the LVNs are 14,976 (24 × 12 × 52).

▶ Schedule 2— Replacement FTEs

It is important to remember that the FTEs we have identified for each job class represent a perfect world where no one calls in sick or takes vacation, turnover does not exist, and nurses are never required to attend training or orientation that takes them away from their clinic duties. Knowing that this will not be the case, we must plan for these eventualities and budget replacement FTEs to supplement our workforce staffing.

Having established the FTEs needed, we must identify those positions which will be essential to clinic operations—that is, the minimal acceptable staffing that the clinic will require to meet operational needs. Generally speaking, licensed nurses are considered essential, with the exception of the Director whose managerial duties will not directly impact the ability to

open and operate the clinic on a given day. Non-licensed employees, such as secretaries, are usually classified as non-essential.

Our clinic will classify all licensed non-managerial staff as essential. Begin by calculating the total number of essential FTEs (those we will need to replace).

RNs 2.1
LVNs 7.2
Total 9.3 FTEs

Replacement FTEs	FTEs	Hours	Total Hours
Subtotal PTO	9.30		
Percent (%) of replacement			
Subtotal PTO replacement			

Next, calculate the hours of projected PTO by multiplying the PTO % obtained in our clinic scenario by 2,080.

PTO 12% × 2080 = 249.6 hours

Replacement FTEs	FTEs	Hours	Total Hours
Subtotal PTO	9.30	249.6	
Percent (%) of replacement			
Subtotal PTO replacement			

Now, multiply the FTEs (9.3) by the hours (249.6) to obtain total hours.

9.3 × 249.6 = 2,321.28 total hours

Replacement FTEs	FTEs	Hours	Total Hours
Subtotal PTO	9.30	249.6	2,321.28
Percent (%) of replacement			
Subtotal PTO replacement			

With hours established, we must now determine what percent of our essential staff we anticipate replacing each year. Healthcare appointments can vary by month or season. Generally, winter months see higher clinic visits due to influenza and other viruses common in colder months. Summer, however, can also be busy for a minor care clinic as injuries occur related to recreational activities. It is important to consider the annual fluctuations that may occur in a clinic setting when planning replacement factors. For our clinic, let's anticipate replacing 80% each year, with the expectation of lower clinic visits in the spring.

Replacement FTEs	FTEs	Hours	Total Hours
Subtotal PTO	9.30	249.6	2,321.28
Percent (%) of replacement	80%		
Subtotal PTO replacement			

Now calculate the Subtotal PTO Replacement beginning with Total Hours. Multiply Total Hours by Replacement percent to obtain this figure.

$$2{,}321.28 \text{ (Total hours)} \times 80\%$$
$$(\text{Replacement percent}) = \mathbf{1{,}857.02}$$

Replacement FTEs	FTEs	Hours	Total Hours
Subtotal PTO	9.30	249.6	2,321.28
Percent (%) of replacement	80%		
Subtotal PTO replacement			1,857.02

Finally, let's find out how many FTEs will be required to fill the 1,857.02 replacement hours. To determine this, simply divide the Subtotal PTO Replacement Hours by 2,080.

$$1{,}857.02 / 2{,}080 = 0.89 \text{ FTEs}$$

Replacement FTEs	FTEs	Hours	Total Hours
Subtotal PTO	9.30	249.6	2,321.28
Percent (%) of replacement	80%		
Subtotal PTO replacement	0.89		1,857.02

So what is the purpose of this exercise? Consider the information we now have. We know that we have 9.3 FTEs that we have identified as "essential." Our annual PTO will amount to 249.6 hours per employee, or a total of 2,321.28 hours for our essential workforce. Of those hours, we intend to replace 80%, or 1,857.02 hours. To accomplish this, we will require 0.89 in additional FTEs.

Education and Meeting Hours

In addition to replacing PTO, a nurse leader must also anticipate and plan for replacement of staff attending required education and meetings. The data provided by the organization in our case scenario shows that orientation for all job classes is 16 hours and that each employee is expected to spend 12 hours each year in education and meetings. This is time away from the clinic that we will want to substitute with agency nurses for our essential employees.

Beginning with education, identify the FTEs, hours, and total hours for each job class. Total hours will be calculated by multiplying the hours by the FTEs. Remember that the Director has been identified as non-essential. Total each column in the Subtotal Education/Meeting row.

Education/Meetings	FTEs	Hours	Total Hours
Director			
RN			
LVN			
Subtotal education/meeting			

Your completed table should mirror the following data:

Education/Meetings	FTEs	Hours	Total Hours
Director			
RN	2.10	16.0	33.6
LVN	7.20	16.0	115.2
Subtotal education/meeting	9.30	32.00	148.80

The process for identifying orientation hours is similar. Here, however, you will be counting individuals instead of FTEs. We are looking for the number of employees we anticipate hiring each year by job class. Refer to the information provided in the case scenario and complete the following table.

Orientation	Head Count	Hours	Total Hours
Director			
RN			
LVN			
Subtotal orientation	-	-	-

In reviewing the case scenario, you will note that we anticipate only one LVN turnover annually at this clinic. This means we should plan to hire and orientate one LVN. All new employees receive 16 hours of orientation.

Orientation	Head Count	Hours	Total Hours
Director			
RN			
LVN	1.00	16.0	16
Subtotal orientation	1.00	16.0	16.0

With this information completed, we are now prepared to begin calculating the costs associated with our staffing plan.

▶ Schedule 3—Financial Impact

Our first step in this section will be to establish Regular Pay. Regular Pay represents the wages that are expected to be paid based on the number of FTEs and scheduled annual hours of work.

Regular					
Skill Mix	Job Title	Hourly Wage	FTE	Total Hours	Total Wages
Director	Manager				
RN	RN				
LVN	LVN				
	Subtotal regular				

The wage section requires an hourly rate of pay for each job class. The information provided by our organization for average rate of pay gives us the projected annual salaries. To ensure that we understand this process, however, let's do the calculations in this section.

To identify the hourly rate, divide the annual salary by 2,080.

Director – $70,000 / 2,080 = $33.65
RN – $_____ / 2,080 = $_____
LVN – $_____ / _____ = $_____

Regular					
Skill Mix	Job Title	Hourly Wage	FTE	Total Hours	Total Wages
Director	Manager	$33.65			
RN	RN	$30.77			
LVN	LVN	$15.87			
	Subtotal regular				

In the FTE column, list the total number of FTEs that were established per job class not including replacement FTEs. This calculation was completed under Schedule 2 in the section titled Calculating FTEs from Total Hours. Add the FTEs to ensure they equal 10.3 total FTEs.

Regular					
Skill Mix	**Job Title**	**Hourly Wage**	**FTE**	**Total Hours**	**Total Wages**
Director	Manager	$33.65	1.00		
RN	RN	$30.77	2.10		
LVN	LVN	$15.87	7.20		
		Subtotal regular	10.30		

We have already determined total hours in the section titled Calculating Total Hours per Job Class using the formula Shifts per Day × Hours per Shift × 52. Another approach to determining total hours is FTEs × 2,080.

Calculate the Total Hours for each job class.

Director – 1 FTE × 2080 = _____ Hours

RN – ___ FTEs × 2080 = _____ Hours

LVN – _____ FTEs × _____ = _____ Hours

Your calculations should result in 2,080 Director hours, 4,368 RN hours, and 14,976 LVN hours. Note that these calculations match the numbers you identified in the Calculating Total Hours per Job Class section. Total the hours for each job class in the Subtotal Regular row.

Regular					
Skill Mix	**Job Title**	**Hourly Wage**	**FTE**	**Total Hours**	**Total Wages**
Director	Manager	$33.65	1.00	2,080.00	
RN	RN	$30.77	2.10	4,368.00	
LVN	LVN	$15.87	7.20	14,976.00	
		Subtotal regular	10.30	21,424.00	

With these sections completed, we can now calculate the total wages per job class. The formula for calculating wages is Hourly Wage × Total Hours.

Director – $33.65 × 2,080 = $69,992

RN – $30.77 × _____ = $_____

LVN – $_____ × _____ = $_____

Calculations should match the following. All totaled, we are budgeting $442,064 in wages for regular pay.

Regular					
Skill Mix	**Job Title**	**Hourly Wage**	**FTE**	**Total Hours**	**Total Wages**
Director	Manager	$ 33.65	1.00	2,080.00	$ 69,992
RN	RN	$ 30.77	2.10	4,368.00	$ 134,403
LVN	LVN	$ 15.87	7.20	14,976.00	$ 237,669
		Subtotal regular	10.30	21,424.00	$ 442,064

▶ Overtime

With regular pay established, we will now calculate projected overtime. This projection will be based on the incidental overtime percentage provided by the organization in the case scenario.

RN – $30.77 × 0.5 = $_____

LVN – $_____ × 0.5 = $_____

Overtime					
Skill Mix	Job Title	Hourly Wage	FTE	Total Hours	Total Wages
Director	Manager				
RN	RN				
LVN	LVN				
	Overtime				

Our Director will be an exempt employee, and, therefore, not susceptible to overtime. For the remaining job classes, we determine the hourly overtime wage, which will be time and a half. Here, we will calculate the 0.5.

Overtime					
Skill Mix	Job Title	Hourly Wage	FTE	Total Hours	Total Wages
Director	Manager				
RN	RN	$15.39			
LVN	LVN	$ 7.93			
	Overtime				

To determine the FTE, we will multiply Incidental Overtime (5%) by the total FTEs for the job class.

RN – 5% × 2.1 = _____

LVN – 5% × _____ = _____

Overtime					
Skill Mix	Job Title	Hourly Wage	FTE	Total Hours	Total Wages
Director	Manager				
RN	RN	$ 15.39	0.11		
LVN	LVN	$ 7.93	0.36		
	Overtime		0.47		

Totaled, we have 0.47 FTEs.
For total hours, we will multiply the FTE by 2,080.

Overtime					
Skill Mix	Job Title	Hourly Wage	FTE	Total Hours	Total Wages
Director	Manager			-	
RN	RN	$ 15.39	0.11	228.80	
LVN	LVN	$ 7.93	0.36	748.80	
	Overtime		0.47	977.60	

To complete this section, calculate the Total Overtime Wages by multiplying the Hourly Wage by the Total Hours.

Totaled, we have identified $9,459 in additional expenses projected from overtime.

RN – $15.39 × 228.8 = _____

LVN – $_____ × _____ = _____

RN – 0.11 × 2,080 = _____

LVN – _____ × 2,080 = _____

Overtime					
Skill Mix	**Job Title**	**Hourly Wage**	**FTE**	**Total Hours**	**Total Wages**
Director	Manager			-	$ -
RN	RN	$15.39	0.11	228.80	$ 3,521
LVN	LVN	$ 7.93	0.36	748.80	$ 5,938
		Overtime	**0.47**	**977.60**	**$ 9,459**

▶ Replacement FTE

If the facility had established the rates of pay and expectations of charge nurse duties, on-call, or call back, those costs would need to be calculated as well. Because our clinic will not utilize those classifications, we will move on to determining Replacement FTE costs.

Replacement FTE					
Skill Mix	**Job Title**	**Hourly Wage**	**FTE**	**Total Hours**	**Total Wages**
		Total from schedule 2	0.89	1,857.02	
RN	Float pool				$ -
LVN	Float pool				$ -
		Subtotal replacement FTEs			$ -

Let's begin with our known variables. In Schedule 2, we calculated our Subtotal replacement of 0.89 and total hours of 1,857.02. The hourly rate for float pool nurses is provided in our clinic scenario.

Replacement FTE					
Skill Mix	**Job Title**	**Hourly Wage**	**FTE**	**Total Hours**	**Total Wages**
		Total from schedule 2	0.89	1,857.02	
RN	Float pool	$55.00			
LVN	Float pool	$40.00			
		Subtotal replacement FTEs			

We must now determine what percentage of those replacement figures we estimate to go to each job class.

If we were dealing with a single replacement option, we could simply multiply the PTO hours by the hourly wage to obtain replacement costs. In our situation, however, we will need to replace both RN and LVN job classes at different rates of pay. We have a total of 9.3 essential FTEs. The majority of FTEs are LVN. We can determine the percentage of LVN FTEs with a simple formula:

7.2 (LVN FTEs) / 9.3 (Total FTEs) = 77%,

so we know that approximately three quarters of our replacement FTEs will be LVNs.

We can validate our number by applying the same formula to the RN FTEs.

2.1 (RN FTEs) / 9.3 (Total FTEs) = 23%, or roughly 1/4th of replacement FTEs. 77% + 23% = 100%.

With an approximation of job class percentage established, let's divide up the 0.89 replacement factor. To do this, simply divide 0.89 by 4, rounding to the third decimal.

$$0.89 / 4 = 0.222$$

We now know that 0.222 FTEs will be RN, and 0.666 (0.222 × 3) FTEs will be LVN.

Replacement FTE					
Skill Mix	Job Title	Hourly Wage	FTE	Total Hours	Total Wages
		Total from schedule 2	0.89	1,857.02	
RN	Float pool	$55.00	0.222		
LVN	Float pool	$40.00	0.666		
		Subtotal replacement FTEs	0.89		

To calculate total hours, multiply the FTE by 2,080.

RN: 0.222 × 2,080 = 461.76
LVN: 0.666 × 2,080 = 1,385.28

Totaled, we have 1,847.04 replacement hours.

Replacement FTE					
Skill Mix	Job Title	Hourly Wage	FTE	Total Hours	Total Wages
		Total from schedule 2	0.89	1,857.02	
RN	Float pool	$55.00	0.222	461.76	
LVN	Float pool	$40.00	0.666	1,385.28	
		Subtotal replacement FTEs	0.89	1,847.04	

To complete the replacement factor calculations, multiply Hourly Rate by Total Hours.

RN: 55 × 461.76 = $_____
LVN: 40 × _____ = $_____

Once completed, we have our replacement FTE Hours and Costs.

Replacement FTE					
Skill Mix	Job Title	Hourly Wage	FTE	Total Hours	Total Wages
		Total from schedule 2	0.89	1,857.02	
RN	Float pool	$55.00	0.222	461.76	$25,397
LVN	Float pool	$40.00	0.666	1,385.28	$55,411
		Subtotal replacement FTEs	0.89	1,847.04	$80,808

▶ Education

An important distinction to remember between education and orientation is that education is reoccurring, whereas orientation only applies to new employees and is generally only incurred during the first few weeks of their employment. For this reason, it is crucial that we calculate them separately.

Education						
Skill Mix	**Job Title**	**Hourly Wage**	**FTE**	**Total Hours**	**FTEs Annualized**	**Total Wages**
Director	Nurse manager		-	-	-	$ -
RN	RN					
LVN	LVN					
Subtotal education/meeting						

We will not calculate education costs for the Director because that position will be exempt. For the RNs, and LVNs, all will be required to participate in education hours, so we will account for all essential FTEs. You may recall that our organization has agreed to provide coverage from another clinic for education hours. The hourly wages of each job class was provided in the case scenario. Total Hours for Education was calculated in Schedule 2.

Education						
Skill Mix	**Job Title**	**Hourly Wage**	**FTE**	**Total Hours**	**FTEs Annualized**	**Total Wages**
Director	Nurse manager			-	-	$ -
RN	RN	$30.77	2.10	33.6		
LVN	LVN	$15.87	7.20	115.2		
Subtotal education/meeting			9.30	148.80		

Because we are reviewing annual hours and costs throughout this process, it can be beneficial to know the annualized FTEs of these education hours. To calculate Annual FTEs, simply divide the Total Hours for each job class by 2,080.

RN: 33.6 Total Hours / 2,080 = _____

LVN: _____ Total Hours / 2,080 = _____

Education						
Skill Mix	**Job Title**	**Hourly Wage**	**FTE**	**Total Hours**	**FTEs Annualized**	**Total Wages**
Director	Nurse manager			-	-	$ -
RN	RN	$30.77	2.10	33.6	0.02	
LVN	LVN	$15.87	7.20	115.2	0.06	
Subtotal education/meeting			9.30	148.80	0.07	

Lastly, we calculate Total Wages for Education by multiplying the Hourly Wage for each job class by the Total Hours.

RN: $30.77 × 33.6 = $_____

LVN: $15.87 × _____ = $_____

Education						
Skill Mix	**Job Title**	**Hourly Wage**	**FTE**	**Total Hours**	**FTEs Annualized**	**Total Wages**
Director	Nurse manager			-	-	$-
RN	RN	$30.77	2.10	33.6	0.02	$1,034
LVN	LVN	$15.87	7.20	115.2	0.06	$1,828
	Subtotal education/meeting		**9.30**	**148.80**	**0.07**	**$2,862**

With this process completed, we see that we can anticipate $2,862 annually in costs associated with Education.

▶ **Orientation**

Newly hired nurses will be expected to attend a 16-hour orientation. During this time, we will need to supplement our staffing pattern. As outlined in the case scenario, we will rely on float pool nurses for this purpose. Annual turnover only projects one LVN and no RN separations in an average year. The hourly wage for our calculations will be based on the hourly replacement cost of a float pool nurse.

We have already calculated the information we need for FTE and Total Hours in Schedule 2, Section "Orientation."

Orientation						
Skill Mix	**Job Title**	**Hourly Wage**	**FTE**	**Total Hours**	**FTEs Annualized**	**Total Wages**
Director	Nurse manager		-	-		
RN	RN		-	-		
LVN	LVN	$40.00	1.00	16.00		
Dept secretary	Dept secretary		-	-		
	Subtotal orientation		**1.00**	**16.00**	**-**	**$ -**

Annualize the FTEs by dividing total hours by 2,080.

LVN: 16 / 2,080 = 0.01

Orientation						
Skill Mix	**Job Title**	**Hourly Wage**	**FTE**	**Total Hours**	**FTEs Annualized**	**Total Wages**
Director	Nurse manager		-	-	-	
RN	RN		-	-	-	
LVN	LVN	$40.00	1.00	16.00	0.01	
Dept secretary	Dept secretary		-	-	-	
	Subtotal orientation		**1.00**	**16.00**	**0.01**	**$ -**

Calculate total wages multiplying Hourly Wage by Total Hours.

LVN: $40 × 16 = $640

Orientation						
Skill Mix	**Job Title**	**Hourly Wage**	**FTE**	**Total Hours**	**FTEs Annualized**	**Total Wages**
Director	Nurse manager		-	-	-	$ -
RN	RN		-	-	-	$ -
LVN	LVN	$40.00	1.00	16.00	0.01	$640
Dept secretary	Dept secretary		-	-	-	$ -
	Subtotal orientation		**1.00**	**16.00**	**0.01**	**$640**

With the replacement costs of orientation established, we have now accounted for all staffing cost factors.

▶ Schedule 4—The Big Picture

We can now take the calculations we have made throughout this process and create a financial overview of the cost breakdown of our planned operations.

Refer to your calculations in Schedules 1–3 to fill in the FTE, Total Hours, and Total Wages columns that follow. Sum Regular and Overtime columns to obtain the Total Direct Care FTEs information for section.

Categories	FTEs	Total Hours	Total Wages
Subtotal Regular	10.30	21,424.00	$ 442,064
Overtime	0.47	977.60	$ 9,459
Total Direct Care FTEs	**10.77**	**22,401.60**	**$ 451,524**
Subtotal Replacement FTEs	0.89	1,847.04	$ 80,808
Subtotal Education/ Meeting	0.07	148.80	$ 2,862
Subtotal Orientation	0.01	16.00	$ 640
Total	**11.74**	**24,413.44**	**$ 535,834**

Finally, total each column and you will have a representation of the total financial impact of our staffing plan, with detailed information on hours and wages for regular pay, overtime, replacement, education, and orientation.

We would be remiss here not to emphasize the importance of the nurse executive expectations of the nurse leader. These expectations are critical to overall organizational success. In the budget evaluation process, the nurse executive should expect monthly variance reports (see Chapter 8) and annual evaluations of each cost-center budget from the nurse leader. The reports should include recommendations and rationales for any budget changes needed for each cost center.

The budget calculations presented in this chapter have additional uses. These data provide objective evidence to determine and compare staff workloads, to measure outcomes, and to provide quality or research data. In addition, these data could be compared with benchmark data from other organizations.

Summary

In this chapter, you have learned the basic steps of developing a staffing budget for an inpatient (30-bed Medical/Surgical) unit and an outpatient (12-hour minor care clinic) clinical setting. You have been provided with the tools you will need to build a nurse staffing model including projecting for the appropriate number of FTEs which includes the budget for indirect / non-productive work hours as well as the best staffing mix for your model and calculation of replacement hours. As you likely recognized by the end of this chapter, although there are some differences between what an inpatient and outpatient staffing mix and model look like, the process for determining the necessary figures is similar for both.

Discussion Questions

1. How does "minimum staffing" impact your ability to meet your budgeted numbers?

2. This chapter deals with specific units of service for nursing workload requirements. What role should the nurse leader play and how should the leader interact with the finance department for a standard definition of measurement?

3. As a nurse leader, you have to set up a new patient service budget. What sources of information do you need to build the budget?

4. How should a nurse leader use a patient classification (acuity) system to justify nursing hours per day/staffing mix/nurse-to-patient ratios for budget purposes that would be understood by the finance department?

CHAPTER 7

Budget Variances

J. Michael Leger, PhD, MBA, RN, **Paul Brown**, MSN, RN, and
Norma Tomlinson, MSN, RN, NE-BC, FACHE

OBJECTIVES

- Recognize the value of budget variance analysis as a tool for nurse leaders to control costs
- Identify methods to respond to budget variances
- Analyze the impact of unbudgeted overtime, contract labor, or orientation hours on the salary budget

▶ Introduction

Unlike physician services, a nursing department is considered a cost center, not a revenue source. This is a crucial distinction for the nurse leader to understand when working with departmental budgets. Whereas expenses of revenue-generating departments can be weighed against income, the nursing department generally operates under an established budget. Failure to stay at or under budget creates a financial burden for the organization.

▶ Budget Variance

Despite the best efforts to accurately budget and staff a clinical setting, unforeseen circumstances often impact expense projections. These projections, or **forecasts**, are generally based on a combination of historical data and future predictions. Differences between budget and actual expenditures are referred to as **variance**. An unfavorable variance reflects actual expenses that exceed the amount budgeted. A favorable variance, by contrast, is seen when actual expenses are at or lower than the amount budgeted.

TABLE 7.1 represents two simple budget variance examples.

In the first example, actual costs exceeded budgeted expenses, resulting in an unfavorable variance of $2,000. Note the parenthesis around the unfavorable variance, indicating a negative variance. In the second example, actual costs were lower than the budgeted expenses amount, leaving a surplus, or favorable, variance of $7,000.

▶ Analyzing History to Predict the Future

To some degree, variances can be anticipated based on historical evidence and anticipated future influencers. Review of year-over-year data can provide valuable insight into future performance. Consider this example (shown in **TABLE 7.2**): As the new nurse leader, you are reviewing the past 3 years of staffing financials for your department. What trends can we immediately identify from this year-over-year data?

Obviously, the department consistently runs overbudget. Also, despite changes in the budgeted funding, actual expenses consistently run between $10,000 and $13,000 more than the amount that is budgeted for each year. Also notable is that year after year the variance increases. Based on this known historical information, what can we assume about the department's finances in the coming year? It is likely that, excluding unknown variables, the organization can expect to overspend by roughly the same amount in Year 4, if not slightly more, unless modifications are made. Knowing this information in advance gives the nurse leader insight into the need to adjust finance strategies to meet organizational expectations.

With known historical trends established, the nurse leader must next consider current challenges and changes that the department may be undergoing. Reductions in departmental budgets, difficulties in recruiting and retaining nursing talent, and expansions or decreases in average daily census are just a few examples of influencers that stand to impact

TABLE 7.1 Examples of Budget Variance			
	Budgeted Expenses	**Actual Expenses**	**Variance**
Example 1	$100,000	$102,000	($2,000)
Example 2	$250,000	$243,000	$7,000

TABLE 7.2 Salary Variance Report

Year	Budget	Actual	Variance
Year 1	$100,000	$110,000	($10,000)
Year 2	$150,000	$162,000	($12,000)
Year 3	$138,000	$151,000	($13,000)

TABLE 7.3 Detailed Salary Variance Report

Year	Budget	Actual Scheduled Dollars	Actual Overtime Dollars	Actual Agency Dollars	Variance
Year 1	$100,000	$97,000	$3,000	$10,000	($10,000)
Year 2	$150,000	$144,500	$3,500	$14,000	($12,000)
Year 3	$138,000	$132,000	$4,000	$15,000	($13,000)

the financial solvency of a department through either decreases in budgeted funds or increases in actual expenses.

▶ Clarity through Details

In the preceding example, we looked at expenses from a global aspect of total dollars available and total dollars spent. While this general information gives some indication of past performance, a more granular look into the specifics of budgeted and actual expenses is necessary to identify specific challenges to meeting fiscal goals.

Let's break down the preceding example in more detail in **TABLE 7.3**.

We now have a clearer picture of how the actual expenses are being utilized to staff this department. What trends do you see occurring in the year-over-year data? It is clear that this department relies heavily on supplemental agency nursing versus overtime to cover shortages. It is also clear that agency expenditures continually rise each year regardless of fluctuations in budgeted funding. Of course, there may be valid reasons for the year-over-year agency expense increases, validating that even further research into trends and influencers is needed.

▶ Causative Factors of Variance

A nurse leader must continually question what is driving expenses and seek specificity in order to develop an action plan to offset identified variances. Whether these variances are related to staffing, equipment and supplies, or other departmental expenditures, it is crucial that underlying causative factors be identified and that controllable variances be addressed.

Understand that not all variances from budgeted funding may be under the nurse leader's authority or the nurse leader's ability to influence. Changes in hospital policy, such as an increased nurse–patient ratio requirement in the mid–fiscal year, may negatively impact the nursing department's budget if the organization does not allocate additional funding to offset the increase in expenditures. For our purposes here, we will focus on controllable variance, where the nurse leader has the authority to identify and address variance.

Supply Costs

If the nurse leader is fiscally responsible for supply costs utilized in the nursing department, it will be important to establish a mechanism for the tracking and utilization of supplies, as well as supply costs. Costs can vary significantly by vendor and securing favorable contracts stands to save the department considerable costs over time. Monitoring the appropriate utilization of unit supplies is also the responsibility of the nurse leader. Whether the supplies are used for direct patient care (minor equipment, patient nonchargeable items, such as admission kits and syringes) or to support clinical staff (ink cartridges for printers, pens, paper for copier/printer), these non-salary expenses can quickly add up if use is not supervised. **FIGURE 7.1** provides an example of a monthly non-salary expense report including variances.

Staffing

Nursing services often has one of the largest footprints in an organization in regard to the size of the workforce. As a result, staffing is often the largest expenditure for a nurse leader, who must balance fiscal usage of overtime and agency staffing with the organization's scheduled hours of operation and commitment to high-quality care. Accurately projecting and budgeting for these secondary resources, as outlined in Chapter 5, helps to minimize variance, but unforeseen or unplanned for circumstances can have serious financial consequences. Excessive or prolonged vacancies in licensed staff that must be replaced with overtime or agency nurses can quickly deplete budgeted funds for the fiscal year. This being said, the organization's mission and commitment to patient care must remain at the center of fiscal decision making. Compromises in quality of care to meet financial goals can have longstanding consequences for the integrity and reputation of the organization. While every effort should be made to ensure a fiscally responsible usage of funds, the nurse leader has an obligation to stand firm in the commitment to quality patient care.

Man-Hours Budget

Because staffing is usually the most expensive resource in the provision of care, the amount and type of man-hours expensed to a nursing unit is very critical. The monthly operations report usually does not break down the man-hours by job classification, such as registered nurse (RN), licensed practical/vocational nurse (LPN/LVN), nursing assistant, and unit clerk. That information is normally provided in biweekly reports that show individual employee hours and/or man-hours or full-time equivalents (FTEs) by job classification (**TABLE 7.4**).

Although biweekly reports may not correspond to the exact days, or the month, covered by the operations report, they provide good data to monitor if your mix of staff corresponds to that budgeted. Man-hours are usually broken down into contract, productive, paid time off (PTO), overtime, education, orientation, and other.

Contract labor is usually the most expensive man-hours. Contract staff can be through local agencies or the more expensive "travelers" who are agency personnel assigned for several weeks or months at a time and usually live in local temporary housing. Although they may provide for better continuity of care than local agency staff, their costs include, at a minimum, hourly rate, rent, food, travel, and car rental.

Department Non-Salary Expense Report for the period ending 11/30/200_ Main 7								
MONTH					**YTD***			
Actual	Budget	Var%	Prior	Non-salary Expense	Actual	Budget	Var%	Prior
0	0	0.0%	0	**Purchase Professional**	250	0	0.0%	0
30,934	11,858	(160.9)%	14,338	**Patient Nonchargeable**	92,458	60,656	(52.4)%	59,995
0	32	(100.0)%	0	**Drugs**	0	165	100.0%	0
975	790	(23.4)%	1,068	**Food Service**	5,252	4,313	(21.8)%	4,736
0	68	100.0%	0	**Medical Supplies**	0	349	100.0%	0
2,038	1,866	(9.2)%	2,472	**Department Supplies**	9,668	9,546	(1.3)%	6,429
197	245	19.6%	264	**Forms and Paper**	1,024	1,254	18.3%	1,204
959	1,134	15.4%	47	**Minor Equipment**	5,148	5,670	9.2%	1,529
0	216	100.0%	0	**Equipment Rental**	0	1,080	100.0%	0
0	1	100.0%	0	**Dues & Membership**	0	5	100.0%	0
136	46	(195.7)%	0	**Books & Publications**	225	46	(389.1)%	40
228	207	(10.1)%	470	**Travel**	567	1,058	46.4%	1,325
0	82	100.0%	0	**Other Expenses**	0	410	100.0%	37
35,467	16,545	(114.4)%	18,659	**Total Non-Salary Expense**	114,592	84,552	(35.5)%	75,295

FIGURE 7.1 Example of a Monthly Report of Non-Salary Expense for a Surgical Nursing Unit

* YTD = Year-to-date

TABLE 7.4 Example of a Biweekly FTE Report

Pay Period xx		1/13/XX–1/26/XX			
Name	Classification	Productive FTE	Non-productive FTE	Overtime FTE	Total FTE
T. Moore	Manager	1.0	0	0	1.0
Subtotal	**Manager**	**1.0**	**0**	**0**	**1.0**
A. Todd	Charge RN	1.0	0	0.1	1.1
S. Shaw	Charge RN	1.0	0	0	1.0
Subtotal	**Charge RN**	**2.0**	**0**	**0.1**	**2.1**
R. Barry	RN	1.0	0	0.2	1.2
J. Brown	RN	0.45	0.45	0	0.9
C. Collins	RN	0.9	0	0	0.9
R. Dix	RN	0.9	0.1	0	1.0
E. Fisher	RN	0.6	0	0	0.6
J. Robinson	RN	0.9	0	0	0.9
R. Smith	RN	0.45	0.45	0	0.9
Subtotal	**RN**	**5.2**	**1.0**	**0.2**	**6.4**
J. Edwards	LPN	0.9	0	0	0.9
R. Falls	LPN	0	0.9	0	0.9
E. George	LPN	0.9	0	0	0.9
T. Hall	LPN	0.6	0.3	0	0.9
Subtotal	**LPN**	**2.4**	**1.2**	**0**	**3.6**
J. Adams	PCT	0.9	0	0	0.9

Name	Classification	Productive FTE	Non-productive FTE	Overtime FTE	Total FTE
N. Coates	PCT	0.6	0	0	0.6
T. East	PCT	0.9	0	0	0.9
Subtotal	**PCT**	**2.4**	**0**	**0**	**2.4**
A. Thomas	Unit Clerk	1.0	0	0	1.0
S. Vender	Unit Clerk	1.0	0	0	1.0
Subtotal	**Unit Clerk**	**2.0**	**0**	**0**	**2.0**
TOTAL		**15.0**	**2.2**	**0.3**	**17.5**

Note: These are fictitious names.
LPN, licensed practical nurse; PCT, patient care technician; RN, registered nurse.

Productive man-hours are those hours where employed staff members provide care for patients. In the case of direct caregivers, such as RNs, LPNs, and patient care technicians, this is the time they are assigned on the nursing unit actually providing hands-on care to patients. For indirect caregivers, such as unit clerks, it includes the time they spend on the nursing unit providing their specific indirect services.

Non-productive man-hours include PTO, such as vacation, holidays, jury duty, sick time, and any other time off where the employee is paid by the organization but does not actually work during that paid time. It is an employee benefit. PTO may be expensed (charged) to the cost center at the time it is earned or at the time it is taken.

The time at which PTO is expensed is important to know when analyzing the unit costs for the month. If it is expensed to your department *at the time it is earned*, you will see it charged as an expense against your department based on the hours worked during that month. In this case, it goes into a "bank" that the employee draws against when it is taken. Your department is not charged for it again when the employee takes the time off because it was already expensed to you once. You will see it in the detail of what was paid to the employee on your biweekly report.

However, those dollars are not added to the total on your monthly report. If you need to replace the employee to cover the man-hours required to care for the volume of patients, you will be charged only for the hours worked by the replacement employee. If, on the other hand, PTO is charged to your budget *only when taken* by the employee, you will see it included in the total on the monthly report. If, because of volume, you had to replace the employee to cover the man-hours required to care for the volume of patients, you will be charged for that employee's hours as well.

In most organizations, PTO is earned based on the hours worked. If you use part-time staff members more than their allocated FTE, they will earn PTO on those hours as well. That will increase the non-productive time and dollars expensed to your department.

Overtime is the time worked over 40 hours in a week if on a 40-hour workweek. It can include, at the discretion of the organization, hours worked over a scheduled 8-, 10-, or 12-hour shift

	MONTH					YTD*			
Actual	**Budget**	**Var%**	**Prior**	**Statistic**	**Actual**	**Budget**	**Var%**	**Prior**	

Department Man-Hours Report for the period ending 11/30/20XX Main 7

Actual	Budget	Var%	Prior	Statistic	Actual	Budget	Var%	Prior
344	315	(9.2)%	258	**Man-Hours Contract**	1,840	1,575	(16.8)%	284
5,759	5,267	(9.3)%	5,291	**Man-Hours Productive**	28,469	26,893	(5.9)%	26,860
611	570	(7.2)%	573	**Man-Hours PTO**	2,883	2,912	1.0%	2,988
192	270	28.9%	363	**Man-Hours Overtime**	1,117	1,380	19.1%	1,627
764	750	(1.9)%	667	**Man-Hours Ed/Orient/ Etc.**	3,392	3,825	11.3%	3,933
7,670	7,172	(6.9)%	7,152	**Total Man-Hours**	37,701	36,585	(3.1)%	35,692
44.86	41.95	(6.9)%	41.83	**Total FTEs**	43.24	41.96	(3.1)%	40.94

FIGURE 7.2 Example of a Monthly Report of Man-Hours for a Surgical Nursing Unit

*YTD = Year-to-date

even if less than 40 hours are worked in a week. It can also include time designated as overtime at the discretion of the organization, such as any hours called in and hours worked when on-call. Although discretionary overtime pay can be a positive retention tool, it is also an added expense. It is important to know what the policy is in your organization regarding the designation of overtime.

On-call pay is a minimal hourly rate paid to staff who are not at work but who have committed to be available to work on short notice. It is important to know whether in your organization on-call pay hours stop when the individual is called into work. Some organizations stop on-call pay at the time the employee clocks into work. In

this case, if employees clock out before the end of their time on-call, the on-call pay picks up again when they clock out. Some organizations continue to pay the on-call pay in addition to any hours worked while on-call.

Education and orientation hours are those spent learning and meeting the competencies required for the employee's position. With implementation of electronic medical records and new regulatory rules, many hours of mandatory education are being added to the cost of staffing to ensure that all employees are educated about the changes.

In **FIGURE 7.2**, the data demonstrate a large increase in contract labor that has been utilized

| Department Salary Report for the period ending 11/30/200_ Main 7 | | | | | | | | |
| MONTH | | | | | YTD* | | | |
Actual	**Budget**	**Var%**	**Prior**	**Salary Expense**	**Actual**	**Budget**	**Var%**	**Prior**
85,670	76,243	(12.4)%	80,107	**Salaries Productive**	424,059	381,320	(11.2)%	399,027
9,125	7,601	(20)%	8,567	**PTO**	43,208	38,826	(11.3)%	42,621
4,547	6,701	32.1%	9,611	**Salaries Overtime**	22,283	34,237	34.9%	42,610
18,319	8,734	(109.7)%	13,939	**Contract Salaries**	95,318	43,670	(118.3)%	15,357
900	2,070	56.5%	251	**Salary/ Lump-Sum/ Retent**	1,982	5,988	66.9%	3,251
8,279	9,184	9.9%	7,119	**Ed/Orient/ On-Call/Etc.**	39,699	46,838	15.2%	48,424
126,840	110,533	(14.8)%	119,594	**Total Salary Expense**	626,549	550,879	(13.7)%	551,290

FIGURE 7.3 Example of a Monthly Report of Salaries for a Surgical Nursing Unit

* YTD = Year-to-date

both for the month (344 hours) and year-to-date (YTD) (1,840 hours). YTD in the prior year shows only 284 hours of contract labor was used for the month.

Salary Budget

Salaries are normally the largest expense for a cost center. Salaries are broken down into the same categories as man-hours. The percentage of variance in salaries not only reflects the number of man-hours used to care for a particular volume of patients, but also reflects the mix of staff

providing that care, such as RNs, LPNs, nursing assistants or patient care technicians, and unit clerks. Salaries for the department usually include the unit manager. If nursing education is decentralized, it may include a nursing educator for the unit. If the unit has a clinical nurse specialist, that salary may be charged to the unit as well.

In **FIGURE 7.3**, productive salaries are higher for the month ($85,670) than budgeted ($76,243), with the variance percentage being 12.4% overbudget for the month. The same is true YTD ($424,059 actual against a budget of $381,320 and 11.2% overbudget).

▶ Dissecting the Variance Report

A basic variance report will outline the basic components of budget, actual, and variance similar to the examples provided earlier in this chapter. Each organization will have their own method for presenting this information, but the commonalities are in these essential key components.

As the nurse leader, you are provided with the variance report for your department, shown in **TABLE 7.5**.

As discussed earlier, this report gives a global perspective but very little insight into causative factors. What it does provide, however,

is information into which aspect of expenses are overbudget. In this case, the department is managing equipment and supply costs within budget, but labor costs are exceeding budgeted funding. We know at this point that labor costs are where we need to focus. What further information would you obtain or request based on this report? Detailed variance information related specifically to labor costs would likely provide further needed information.

TABLE 7.6 is the detailed variance report for labor costs provided by the finance department.

As we delve deeper into the details, we begin to see specifically where we are overspending. Note that productive time appears to be on budget, but virtually every other expense has

TABLE 7.5 Outpatient Clinic YTD Variance Overview Report – Nursing Services, December, 2016

Expense	Budget	Actual	Variance
Labor	$1,200,000	$1,650,000	($450,000)
Equipment	$2,600,000	$2,400,000	$200,000
Supplies	$450,000	$400,000	$50,000

YTD, year to date.

TABLE 7.6 Detailed YTD Variance Report—Labor Costs—Nursing Services, December, 2016

Expense	Budget	Actual	Variance
Productive time	$1,050,000	$1,050,000	($0)
Non-productive time	$60,000	$180,000	($120,000)
Overtime	$40,000	$166,000	($126,000)
Agency	$50,000	$175,000	($125,000)
Other	0	$79,000	($79,000)

YTD, year to date.

TABLE 7.7 Non-Budgeted Expenses YTD Variance Report—Nursing Services, December, 2016			
Expense	**Budget**	**Actual**	**Variance**
Charge differential	$0	$50,000	($50,000)
On-call time	$0	$14,000	($14,000)
Callback	$0	$15,000	($15,000)

YTD, year to date.

an unfavorable variance. Non-productive time is $120,000 over budgeted costs. What might be driving that number? This could be related to personal time off, excessive required educational offerings, or any number of factors that take the licensed nursing staff away from the bedside. This high unfavorable non-productive variance is likely driving the expenses in overtime and agency. And what about the "Other" category? What does that $79,000 in costs encompass? Clearly, we need to delve further into the details to determine the true causative factors behind these numbers.

TABLE 7.7 offers a deeper detailed report that gives insight into the "Other" category.

We now see that we have expenses that are not budgeted, thereby negatively impacting our financials. The reason for these expenses not

being budgeted could be due to operational changes that occurred after the beginning of the fiscal year or due to a failure to plan and budget. In any case, the key to overcoming unfavorable variance is to seek out the causative factors in as much detail as possible. The purpose of this exercise was to encourage you to seek out the details of the causative factors driving expenses.

▶ Identifying Variance Early

Up to this point, we have been focusing on uncovering the causative factors of variance during the review of reports. The challenge with this approach, however, is that you are always reacting

RN	**Monday**	**Tuesday**	**Wednesday**	**Thursday**	**Friday**	**Saturday**	**Sunday**
White	X	O	O	O	O	X	X
Smith	X	X	X	O	O	O	O
Green	O	O	O	X	X	X	X
Jones	O	R	R	R	R	O	O

X = Schedule work rotation
O = Regular Day Off
R = Requested Day Off

to the variance rather than preventing it. Ideally, you want to identify causative factors as they occur, or even beforehand, and take steps to prevent the issue before it shows up on a financial report.

Predicting variance requires astute attention to the daily utilization of resources. Staffing, supplies, and all replenishable resources must be monitored closely, and any variation from scheduled utilization must be accounted for. In doing so, variances from the budget can be anticipated and, in many cases, avoided.

Take, for example, a registered nurse, RN Jones, who is on a 12-hour rotation and informs you that she will need to be off the following week. She has four scheduled rotations that will need to be covered. You are required to have two RNs on each rotation. What options can you identify from the following scheduling matrix?

Obviously, you can modify the schedule to have the other nurses work overtime, but can you identify a possibility for covering the schedule with less or, ideally, no overtime?

One solution may be to request that Jones work her regularly scheduled days off, switching work days with an employee working opposite her. (This may pose overtime issues as well, but is worth exploring.) While this approach does not work in every situation, the point is to seek out creative solutions to variance. Recognizing that Jones' request will potentially result in an unfavorable variance gives the nurse leader the opportunity to develop and enact corrective action measures to mitigate negative budget impact.

So how might this approach work with anticipating supply variances? Beyond monitoring supply usage for changes in real time, which is certainly beneficial, how might we utilize available data to anticipate the increases in advance?

One approach is to anticipate supply utilization based on average daily census. As census increases, a corresponding increase in the utilization of certain supplies can be anticipated. While those increases may not be avoidable,

there are opportunities to reduce overall costs, especially with predictable increases. For example, if the organization averages a 20% increase in average daily census over the summer months, opportunities for increased savings through larger bulk purchases of certain supplies may allow for increased savings on a per-patient basis that is not necessarily justifiable during times when the average daily census is lower. The key is to think creatively and explore options to control costs while maintaining high-quality patient care. What other opportunities can you think of that may allow for anticipating and offsetting variance?

Summary

The annual budget is based on assumptions based on experiences from the previous year and what is expected to occur in a given department or cost center during the coming fiscal year. The difference between the budget and what happens is called the variance. When you compare the budget to what actually occurred each month and YTD and analyze the variance, you have powerful data to understand what is happening on your unit. Given the multiple departments that can charge items to a given cost center, it is happening on your unit. Given the multiple departments that can charge items to a given cost center, it also allows for review and accountability to ensure that items are charged correctly or credited in a timely manner. This also maintains the integrity of the data for future budgeting purposes.

Budget variance analysis that uses a line-item-by-item approach to determine cost per unit of service puts the information into an understandable context. It reflects the impact of volume and staff mix changes, new technology changes, and other variables experienced throughout the year. Translating and sharing that information with unit staff allows for planning and implementation of measures to creatively manage fiscal resources required for excellence in patient care.

Discussion Questions

1. What is it important for a nurse leader to understand variance reporting? How does this reporting become a valuable tool?

2. Because staffing is usually the most expensive resource in the provision of care, what reports would provide you with valuable information for this expense?

3. Contract labor is usually the most expensive man-hours. Why?

4. In your man-hour analysis, why it is important to keep track of education and orientation hours?

5. The monthly distribution register for your department's expenses should be carefully monitored. Why?

Glossary of Terms

Benefit Expense includes retirement, group health, flex benefits, and FICA

Non-productive Man-Hours include paid time off (PTO) which includes vacation, holidays, jury duty, sick time, and any other time off

Productive Man-Hours hours where employed staff members provide care for patients

Variance Analysis includes finding all the pieces of the puzzle, which include the various reports that you are sent by the finance, materials management, and human resources departments

Variance Report summary of the major exceptions to the budget that are experienced during a given time frame and an explanation of why the exceptions occurred

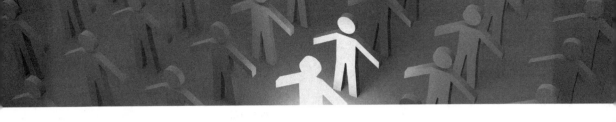

CHAPTER 8

Comparing Reimbursements with Cost of Services Provided

J. Michael Leger, PhD, MBA, RN, and **Patricia M. Vanhook**, PhD, MSN, RN, FNP-BC

OBJECTIVES

- Determine areas within the nurse leader's control that influence profitability.
- Recognize whether a service is profitable.

▶ Note to the Reader

1. This process is most effective when completed as a collaborative inter-departmental effort.
2. The information in this section only provides an example. You need to find out current information when actually following these procedures. It is also important to reevaluate the data as conditions/reimbursement/costs change.

▶ Introduction

One very important question the nurse leader needs to answer is *whether the overall unit expense budget falls within the reimbursement amount*. The evaluation activity described in this chapter helps the nurse leader to recognize whether a service line is profitable and determine areas within the nurse leader's control that influence profitability. To accomplish this, the nurse leader needs to have a clear understanding of the different mechanisms of cost accounting used to reflect both services and reimbursement. This chapter explains and provides examples of cost and reimbursement for acute care, hospital outpatient, ambulatory surgery, skilled care, and home health. It is imperative the nurse leader be well-versed on this topic in order to understand and respond appropriately to cost and reimbursement questions generated from the departmental operations reports produced by finance.

▶ Reimbursement

Over the past 20 years, hospitals, healthcare agencies, and primary care providers have moved from a retrospective cost reimbursement system to a prospective payment system (PPS) where the payer determines the cost of care before the care is given. Under prospective payment, the organization is paid a set fee regardless of the amount of resources used to provide the service, or level of care. This type of payment system creates some financial risk for the provider of services and keeps costs under control for the insurer (payer), while also providing financial rewards to the provider for services provided at a lower cost. If the organization can deliver services under cost and under the prospective payment reimbursement fee, the difference equates to profit. However, if services cost more than the reimbursement amount, it results in a monetary loss. Therefore, prospective payment is an attempt to control rising healthcare costs through improved efficiency within the healthcare agency.

In prospective payment, rates are negotiated between the provider and the insurer under a contractual agreement for a specific period of time: routinely one year. Reimbursement rates may be for all services offered or for one specific service area, called a "carve-out," such as laboratory or pharmacy. Within the healthcare setting, financial administration under this type of reimbursement model requires critical financial management and knowledge of the payers.

This transition in reimbursement methods has been compounded by the change from a volume-based reimbursement system to a value-based reimbursement system "focused on outcomes, population health management and a patient-centered, coordinated care-delivery approach" (Health Research and Educational Trust, 2013, p. 4). In this new environment, reimbursement can be lost when certain specified care is not received, when never events occur (e.g., hospital-acquired pressure ulcers), and when patients are readmitted within 30 days of discharge. *Nurse leaders have a key role in avoiding this lost reimbursement.* Organizational performance on quality measures is used from year to year to determine reimbursement amounts that can be lowered when quality is not achieved.

Thus, it is important that the nurse leader understands the various healthcare payers to appreciate the diversity of billing and reimbursement methods. The two types of payers for healthcare services are public and private. Federal and state are public payers and include Medicare and Medicaid. The insured and uninsured are considered private payers, which are various insurance plans, indemnity insurance, and self-pay. (Refer to Chapter 2 for reimbursement sources.)

Costs

Hospital cost determination mirrors other businesses and industries with the exception that hospitals have high fixed costs (administration, depreciation, utilities, maintenance, etc.) and must attempt to cover these costs by increasing inpatient volume, adding services, using stringent contract management, and investing in capital to attract more business. Costs are calculated as direct or indirect, and fixed or variable. *The nurse leader should consider himself or herself both the chief executive officer and chief financial officer of his or her nursing unit or department and develop a good understanding of costs and revenue.*

Hospital outpatient service payments, under the Ambulatory Patient Classification (APC) system, were based on historical average costs. Here, relative payment weights were assigned by calculating the APC median cost of a midlevel cardiovascular clinic visit (that was found to be the most common outpatient service) and assigned a numerical value of 1.0. The assignment of each APC group relative payment rate was determined by dividing the median cost of each APC by the median cost for the midlevel cardiovascular visit.

There are two significant items the nurse leader must understand from this discussion. First, comparison of the relative relationship of one APC to another, by knowing the median payment weight is 1.0, and understanding the reimbursement will be less or greater, is based on the variation from 1.0. Second, the hospital is reimbursed separately for each APC billed. Therefore, a patient may have radiological and endoscopy procedures on the same day, with each procedure reimbursed independently.

The concept of Resource Utilization Groups (RUGs) is that there are conditions that require similar resources and services, and therefore, costs can be calculated based on the resources used by the skilled nursing facility patient. Direct and indirect costs include routine services, such as room, board, administrative services, nursing care, and therapy services that are the components of the RUG.

Home health cost determination varies somewhat from inpatient services. The home health agency manager considers different types of visit costs that are provided by a service line that includes nursing care, therapy services, and nursing assistance. The average cost per visit is calculated, much the same as acute care, by applying direct and indirect costs, and allocating for special fees such as accreditation services and other intermittent expected fees. The costs are averaged for the Medicare Cost Report, and charges are set at an amount greater than the cost to recoup costs from high-level-care patients and provide an established level for contract negotiations for private carriers that ensure costs are reimbursed.

▶ Clarifying the Cost Issue

Defining Costs, Charges, and Payments

It is a common fallacy that the terms *cost* and *charges* can be used interchangeably. *Costs* and *charges* are not interchangeable terms, and the nurse leader needs to understand the difference.

- *Costs* are determined by the organization's financial accounting system, which takes into account actual costs of supplies, manpower, facility, and administration for services provided.
- *Charges* are determined by the allocation of costs to the revenue-producing centers and then are used to project an amount needed to recover all the costs.

■ *Payment* is the amount the healthcare agency actually receives for the services provided. All payers pay differing amounts for the same service depending on the type of payer and the contractual agreement between the agency and the insurer.

Projection of reimbursement is calculated by a payment-to-cost ratio that indicates the percentage of costs that are covered by reimbursement. Healthcare organizations use the private-payer reimbursement as a cushion to offset the reimbursement from Medicare and Medicaid because it does not cover the full cost of the services provided. As less is received from all sources, it becomes harder to stay solvent.

The manager must remember that each private payer negotiates fees contractually with the healthcare agency, and payment *may or may not* cover costs. **FIGURE 8.1** demonstrates a fictional example of charge, payment, and cost of a hospitalization. The hospital calculated the costs of care to be $7,250 and determined the charge to be $9,500 to capture any extended costs that may occur, as well as to recoup losses that may be experienced from Medicare and Medicaid reimbursement. Contract negotiations between the hospital and the health maintenance organization (HMO) and preferred provider organization (PPO) agreed on the reimbursement for the hospitalization to be $8,250. The last column represents the prospective payment

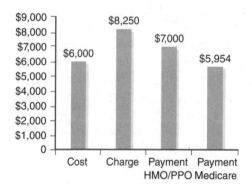

FIGURE 8.1 Comparison of Cost to Charge and Payment*

*The Y axis represents whole dollars, and the X axis is the cost, charge, and payment information.

from Medicare, which equals approximately 99.4% of the actual costs incurred.

Cost of Service Versus Reimbursement

What if more money is being spent on providing the service than is brought in by the reimbursement? In this case, the executive team needs to determine an effective way to do one of the following:

■ Provide the service and cut the overall budget.
■ Decide to take a loss on the service.
■ Stop providing the service.

It is possible that we cannot answer this question because we do not know how much a service costs, nor the actual revenue amount that is realized. This section provides some helpful suggestions that can lead us to finding some answers.

The key financial question is, *Are we spending less than the reimbursement amount to provide the specified service?* A *yes* answer is desired. However, if the answer is that we are spending more than the reimbursement amount—or worse, that we do not know—*immediate action* needs to be taken by the entire management group—including the nurse leader.

Calculating the answer to this question is complicated because most often many cost centers—that is, nursing, pharmacy, laboratory, dietary, medical records, therapies—have been involved in providing the service. So, to answer this question, the interdisciplinary team needs to figure all the actual costs expended to provide the specified service. This activity is sometimes called *costing a service*. This costing exercise should take place for all major services provided within the healthcare organization. Let's break this down into priority levels for the nurse leader. The first issue is determining cost.

Cost Determination Methods

Four distinct methods of cost determination are used in health care today (Udpa, 2001). The first method is the *cost-to-charge ratio (CCR)*. Medicare specified this method be used to report annual costs. Thus, most healthcare organizations today use this ratio as the primary source of all hospital costs and cost accounting information (Magnus & Smith, 2000). This report, called the *Medicare Cost Report*, is used by the Centers for Medicare and Medicaid Services (CMS) to calculate and update reimbursement rates. Nationwide data are available as public information from the Healthcare Cost Report Information System, or HCRIS (at www.cms.gov), and healthcare agencies use this information to benchmark their costs and performance.

Cost-to-Charge Ratio. The information contained in the *Medicare Cost Report* includes CCRs for inpatient, outpatient, departments, and functions such as medical education, utilization data, and financial statement data. The report is required for all Medicare-certified hospitals, skilled nursing facilities, home health agencies, and renal facilities. The ratio is determined by dividing the costs by the charges. **BOX 8.1** demonstrates the CCR calculation. A ratio under 1.0 (equal costs and charges) is positive and indicates that the organization is making money on the service. A ratio over 1.0 indicates the organization is experiencing a loss—the costs are more than the charges (expected reimbursement). In the first example, the service is making money. In the second example, the service is losing money.

Using the CCR, it is assumed that reimbursement (revenue) reflects the intensity of care, and therefore indirect costs (overhead) are assigned accordingly. This method of cost determination does not allow for a full assessment of the true revenue production of a service because all service areas are considered profitable if the healthcare agency as a whole is profitable. In addition, this means that the higher the revenue generation, the higher the proportional allocation of overhead regardless of actual resource utilization. The nurse leader should be aware that CCR could lead to misrepresentation of cost when evaluating the profitability of a service.

Volume-Based Measures. The second method of cost accounting is *volume-based measures*, which is much like it sounds. Here, the indirect costs are assigned according to the volume (which may be visits, admissions, nursing hours per patient day) or machine hours (in radiology and the laboratory). A typical example of this measure is demonstrated (**BOX 8.2**) when the patient volume increases by 15% on a nursing unit, while the nursing hours remain the same. The allocation of indirect cost is increased by 15%. Nursing hours did not increase to accommodate an increase of patient volume, yet the department is allocated higher overhead. It is difficult for the nurse leader to demonstrate increased productivity under this method of cost assignment. The nurse leader must understand the method of allocation of indirect costs to explain variation.

Per Diem Approach. The third approach to cost allocation is the *per diem approach*. This approach accumulates the indirect costs, divides by the number of patient days to determine per diem costs, and allocates the indirect cost equally to all the nursing units. This method considers all patients the same regardless of intensity of

---

BOX 8.1 Calculation of Cost-to-Charge Ratio

Cost ÷ charge = cost-to-charge ratio

Examples:

1. If costs are $50 and charges are $100:
   $50 ÷ $100 = 0.5 cost-to-charge ratio (in the black)
2. If costs are $100 and charges are $50:
   $100 ÷ $50 = 2.0 cost-to-charge ratio (in the red)

BOX 8.2 Volume-Based Cost Calculation

For an average daily census of 18:

- Budgeted direct cost (salaries and benefits) for average daily census of 18 = $18,331
- Budgeted indirect costs (professional fees, depreciation, and utilities) for nursing unit for average daily census of 18 = $5,781

For an average daily census of 21:

- Average unit census per day for month X = 21
- Actual direct costs for census of 21 = $18,331
- Actual indirect costs for nursing unit for census of 21 = $6,648

---

care. In a facility that cares for various types of patients, such as intensive care and obstetrics, this method of costing may also distort departmental costs. For example, in 1 month a 10-bed cardiovascular intensive care unit has 100% occupancy and the 30-bed obstetric unit occupancy rate is 55%. The indirect costs are distributed equally to the units when the per diem method of cost allocation is used. This means the departmental operations reports for the obstetric unit and the cardiovascular intensive care unit have the same dollar amount for indirect expenses even though the obstetric unit had fewer patient days.

Balanced Scorecard and Activity-Based Costing. The last method, *balanced scorecard (BSC) and activity-based costing (ABC)*, became a part of the industry in the 1980s but quickly lost favor because of the resources required to initiate and maintain this process (Easier Than ABC, 2003). Over time, the advancement of healthcare management software technology has allowed health care to use ABC as a means of identifying true patient costs. This method of costing is more closely aligned with the true costs of caring for the patient (Ross, 2004; Udpa, 2001; Young, 2007). ABC methodology also resembles performance improvement methods as processes and outcomes are evaluated. The complexity of "procedures and tests involved, the intensity of nursing care, the duration of an activity, and the intricacies

of operative and postoperative care" identify the true costs (Udpa, 2001, p. 36). In this method, all areas and processes of patient interaction are identified and costs are allocated to the activity center.

The BSC adds the quality dimension to cost and reimbursement data. For instance, cost drivers outside the system, such as patient satisfaction and hospital-acquired conditions, can be measured and reflected in the overall scorecard. In this example, by combining these tools the nurse leader has an excellent overview of the financial aspects from cost, reimbursement, and quality perspectives.

Nurse Leader's Role in Cost Control

The nurse leader usually has access to information that assists with identification of overall organization costs. Cost drivers that increase healthcare costs include salaries and wages, bad debt expense, depreciation and interest, supplies, and direct fringe benefits (an example is given in **FIGURE 8.2**). While the nurse leader has little control over cost drivers other than salaries, in addition to wages and supplies, it is important to have an understanding of the relationship of these drivers to the total operating revenue. This knowledge provides guidance for the nurse leader who can identify cost areas

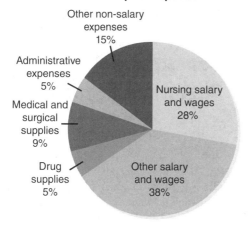

Health care cost drivers: where do hospitals spend?

FIGURE 8.2 Healthcare Cost Drivers

Data from Centers for Medicare and Medicaid Services. Retrieved from www.cms.gov.

Kane and Siegrist (2002) reported aggregated cost data for inpatient and outpatient care. *Nursing comprised 33% of the outpatient cost and approximately 50% of the inpatient cost.* In 2002, salaries of healthcare workers increased by 6.1% as a result of a workforce shortage (Carpenter, 2003). However, reimbursement rates did not increase to accommodate this increase in cost of providing care. Kane and Siegrist (2002) noted that small increases in nursing costs have a tremendous impact on the overall cost of hospitalization. The manager must be aware of this impact and thus plan the budget to accommodate annual performance evaluation raises.

Is the nurse leader able to control bad debt, depreciation, interest, or liability insurance? Of course not. Areas of cost the nurse manager cannot control need to be understood but are not the nurse leader's responsibility. Instead, the executive team must be concerned with these costs. Utilities, equipment expense, maintenance, and administrative costs are fixed costs that do not change as volume changes. (Of course, if the administrative team decides to take actions that decrease costs in these areas, the fixed cost amounts can change.) During the budget period, the manager may be responsible for projecting

within his or her control. In this example, the median cost per hospital discharge was $5,619 (Nursing Leadership Academy, 2003). **FIGURE 8.3** demonstrates the contribution of each cost component to the overall total cost for one hospitalization episode.

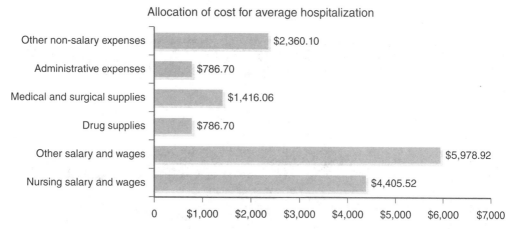

FIGURE 8.3 Allocation of Cost for One Hospitalization*

Data from McMahon, P. (2012). Worldwide price survey puts U.S. medical, hospital costs at top. Los Angeles Times. Retrieved from http://articles.latimes.com/2012/mar/06/business/la-fi-mo-u.s.-medical-prices-high-20120306

* The Y axis represents direct and indirect drivers of cost, while the X axis represents the cost of expense in whole dollars.

Average cost per hospitalization = $15,734.

these costs, or they may be supplied from the finance department. Whether the manager is given this responsibility or the fixed costs are supplied by the finance department, the manager must ensure allocations are made for unusual seasonal or billing issues that may increase or decrease the expense that has been noted by historical data.

For example, fees associated with accreditation may occur only once every 2 to 3 years, and the cost of this service may be distributed among the nursing units under professional services. Another example is the expense of rental equipment such as ventilators. The nurse leader is aware of increased use during the winter months because of the increase in volume of respiratory disease patients requiring ventilators. The astute manager, being a clinician, will not only ensure this information is supplied to finance during the budgeting processes but also will be able to provide sound rationale for the requested increased allocation.

Costs within the realm of nursing administrative control are variable costs. These costs vary in direct relationship to volume. Examples of variable costs include nursing hours, patient care supplies, and dietary services. Variable costs per patient day are calculated by dividing the patient days for the month into the total variable expense. Knowledge of the costs per patient day assists the nurse leader to improve control of the variation and be fiscally astute.

BOX 8.3 demonstrates how the nurse leader can calculate the variable (controllable) costs per patient day.

▶ Departmental Operations Report

When you begin work as a new manager, how do you determine the cost of care on your unit? The most efficient process is to determine the average daily census and review the departmental operations report from finance. **TABLE 8.1** is part of a departmental operations expense report for November 20*XX* from nursing unit 5 North.

How do you, the new manager, analyze this information? This is shown in **BOX 8.4**. The actual and budgeted average daily census can be calculated by dividing the actual or budget expenses total amount by the actual or budget per unit amount. The actual average daily census (this might also be called the average patient volume per day) was 12.7, whereas the budget had projected an average daily census of 16.7 patients. Although the total expenses were 18% less than budgeted (−18% variance that was favorable), the cost per individual patient was higher by 7.8% (7.8% variance that was unfavorable). The contributors of these variances may be linked to employee

---

BOX 8.3 Calculation of Variable Costs

Cost per unit of service equals total variable expense divided by patient days.

($450,000 variable expense ÷ 500 patient days = $900 per patient day)

TABLE 8.1 Departmental Operations Expense Report

Nov 20XX 5 North	Actual	Budget	Variance	Variance %	Favorable/ Unfavorable
Expenses total	87,121	106,305	−19,184	−18	F
Per unit	229.27	212.61	16.66	7.8	U

BOX 8.4 Calculation of Average Daily Census from Departmental Expense Report

Actual expenses total ÷ actual expenses per unit ÷ 30 (days in the month) = actual average daily census

$87,121 ÷ $229.27 ÷ 30 = 12.7 actual average daily census

Budget expenses ÷ budget expenses per unit ÷ 30 (days in the month)

= budgeted average total daily census

$106,305 ÷ $212.61 ÷ 30 = 16.66 budgeted average daily census

---

costs, supply costs, and how overhead is allocated to the department. The manager would need to investigate each possible contributing factor to identify opportunities to reduce expenses or to explain the variation that may in fact be the result of a higher patient acuity, requiring increased nursing staff to provide safe, good quality care.

Now, what if you do not have an operations report? Unfortunately, in many healthcare organizations costing does not take place at this level of detail. A usual mode of practice is to examine the overall bottom line for the organization or to examine costing of a major service, represented by a product line or group of designated cost centers (i.e., cardiology or women's health). Here, the total reimbursement is compared with the total expenditures. In this case, if there is an overexpenditure for one group of patients or services, there needs to be a savings accrued by another group of patients or services because the overall goal is that the bottom line is "in the black" (**TABLE 8.2**).

The problem with this method is that the *organization may not be aware that one service is losing money and another service is saving money*. Using the hospital example, one DRG may be delivered over cost (losing money), whereas another DRG is costing less than the DRG (profit). So, in a time when the reimbursements are not what were anticipated, services may be asked to cut back equally, even though the services for one DRG may have been efficient, while another was not. The nurse leader can use these data as an argument as to why cuts should not apply to the unit (or units) coming in under costs. The following DRG examples are used to further explain actual costs and reimbursement.

DRG Costing Examples

Let's examine a hospital DRG to determine whether we are spending more or less than the reimbursement amount to provide the specified service.

You are a hospital nurse manager/director/nurse executive responsible for an orthopedic cost center. A typical service provided on this cost center is DRG 209: Major Joint/Limb Reattachment Procedure, Low Extremities—No Complications (for Total Hip Replacement) and the Medicare reimbursement for this DRG

TABLE 8.2 Comparison of Revenue and Costs of Two Strategic Service Units

Strategic Service Unit	Revenue (Actual)	Departmental Cost (Actual)	Variance	Variance %	Favorable/ Unfavorable
Cardiology	$706,313	$650,980	$55,333	8.5%	F
Women's health	$309,687	$325,987	−$16,299	5%	U

is $9,269. Do you actually know how much you are expending to provide medical care services for that DRG?

In this particular DRG, there is a further complication: The costs of the prosthesis and direct supplies needed to do the total hip replacement may expend more than 50% of the reimbursement dollars. So, the amount of money left to provide all other services this patient requires from admission to discharge must be low enough to stay within approximately 50% ($4,600) of the reimbursement amount. The question then is whether the service provided to a patient utilizing DRG 209 is more or less than $4,600. If the cost is more than the estimated $4,600, the organization is losing money on each patient having a total hip replacement. *With profit margins as tight as they currently are in health care, it is very important that the nurse leader—as well as the executive team—know the actual costs of the services provided.*

Using the total hip replacement example, figuring out costs is further complicated because the reimbursement amount includes services and supplies delivered from several cost centers (i.e., operating room, laboratory, pharmacy, radiology, physical therapy (PT), and the orthopedic inpatient unit). So, if the orthopedic nurse leader is working on the cost of this DRG, other cost center managers need to provide their departmental costs of service assigned to each hip replacement patient to calculate the total DRG cost. (Interdepartmental collaboration is very important. This is a good example that portrays the importance of department managers working together effectively.)

As a nurse leader figures nursing costs on the orthopedic inpatient unit, she or he will need to figure out the cost of the nursing care provided, as well as the cost of materials and supplies, pharmaceuticals, and other expenses incurred while on this unit. If the nurse leader takes a typical patient and works out costs incurred with that patient, this can provide a basis for determining costs associated with the DRG. When examining nursing time spent with the patient, if there is a patient classification system

in place, this can be used. If this is not available, there is a way to cost out the direct and indirect nursing time spent for this patient. (An example can be found in Finkler, Jones, & Kovner, 2013.)

The following provides a specific patient example to demonstrate a case scenario for a patient admitted for a total hip replacement.

Jill Anderson is a 78-year-old woman with severe degenerative arthritis of the right hip. She has been evaluated by the orthopedic surgeon, who recommends a total hip replacement. Ms. Anderson agrees to the surgery and is scheduled for the procedure 1 week from the office visit. **TABLE 8.3** is a representation of the hospital costs incurred for a 3-day length of stay for a total hip replacement (DRG 209).

As the manager can see, the cost of providing this service is greater than the reimbursement by $1,668 ($10,937 actual cost – $9,269 reimbursement = $1,668 actual loss), and an average caseload of 500 total hips for the year would cost the hospital $834,000.

How can this procedure be profitable for the hospital? First, the interdisciplinary team must work aggressively to transfer the patient to another level of care, such as skilled care, as soon as medically indicated. The hospital also generates additional revenue from the other services the orthopedic surgeon orders for the patient, such as the surgical procedure, outpatient radiology studies, outpatient PT, and referrals to a skilled nursing unit housed within the facility. By standardization of the hip prosthesis being used, the hospital can negotiate a contract with a supplier to be the vendor of choice and thereby decrease costs. Also, the hospital may opt to purchase a prosthesis that costs less money. In addition, the volume of patients can be an important factor. We know that excellent patient satisfaction leads to the patient using the facility as his or her hospital of choice. As the manager can see, many global issues are reviewed by management in deciding to provide a service line.

Now, let's take the same patient admitted to the skilled nursing unit. As you recall, the skilled units are reimbursed by RUGs consisting of the

TABLE 8.3 Costs for DRG 209 Total Hip Replacement

Day	Med Surg	OR	Pharmacy	Pharmacy IV	Implants	Pathology	Lab	Supplies	Blood	Physical Therapy	Total
1 (Adm)	480	2,800	253	120	4,600	54	380	217	175	0	9,079
2	480		384				32			175	1,071
3	480		64				21			126	691
4 (D/C)			22	42			32				96
Total	**1,440**	**2,800**	**723**	**162**	**4,600**	**54**	**465**	**217**	**175**	**301**	**10,937**

DRG, Diagnosis-related group; OR, operating room.

costs for administration, room and board, nursing service, and therapy services. The length of stay on the skilled unit for Ms. Anderson is 11 days.

Ms. Anderson's RUG category is "ultrahigh" because her admission assessment indicated her need for nursing care, PT, and occupational therapy (OT) (U.S. General Accounting Office, 2002). In the ultrahigh category, therapy must demonstrate Ms. Anderson received a total of 720 minutes of services in 7 days (Medicare SNF-PPS Indices, 2003). The reimbursement and cost for the ultrahigh category is noted in **TABLE 8.4**. As you can see, the skilled care facility is losing $800 per day of care and services provided to Ms. Anderson. In addition, as her therapy and nursing care requirements decrease as she improves, the reimbursement also decreases. After her 7-day assessment, the reimbursement for her care decreases to $296.15 per day.

How does a healthcare agency afford to care for patients like Ms. Anderson? Van der Walde and Lindstrom (2003) report that freestanding skilled nursing facilities have fewer Medicare and more private pay patients, whereas a skilled nursing facility in an acute care facility admits a higher percentage of Medicare patients. As their report indicates, the freestanding skilled nursing facilities are profitable, whereas skilled nursing facilities in an acute care setting are not profitable. Many hospitals have closed their skilled nursing facilities because of the continued financial drain on the organization's bottom line.

The next two examples demonstrate costs and reimbursement for a home health and same-day surgery patient. It is probable that The Patient Protection and Affordable Care Act (ACA) will change the available days, but this scenario presents a way to approach the costing exercise for home health. As you recall, home health came under prospective payment in October 2000, and outpatient surgery also began to be reimbursed by APCs in 2000. The following case scenario is provided to explain the method used for a scenario about home care.

Mr. Harold James is a 78-year-old diabetic, hypertensive patient with new onset atrial fibrillation who has survived a right hemispheric stroke (DRG 14). His deficits include left hemiparesis and speech difficulties, and he is discharged from a skilled nursing facility to home with a home health referral. Home health skilled nursing care includes medication management for diabetes and anticoagulation, in addition to medication education. The following additional services will be used: PT three times a week, speech therapy twice a week, and certified nursing assistant (CNA) visits three times a week. As Mr. James

TABLE 8.4 RUG III Reimbursement for Ultrahigh Level of Care

Category	Nursing Care	OT, PT, Speech	Room, Board, and Administration	Total Rate per Day
Ultrahigh*	$142.32	$186.01	$55.88	$384.21
Actual costs	$444.03	$574.30	$165.77	$1,184.10
Difference	−$301.71	−$388.29	−$109.89	−$799.89

*Difference in RUG rates obtained from https://www.cms.gov/medicare/medicare-fee-for-service-payment/pcpricer/snf.html. Actual costs calculated from historical data from a skilled nursing facility.
OT, occupational therapy; PT, physical therapy; RUG, resource utilization groups.

continues to improve, the CNA visits will be discontinued and OT will begin services three times a week. Medicare covers 60 days of home health service, and a total of 66 home visits will be made during the 60-day period (www.cms.gov/).

Because home health for this patient is primarily labor-intensive, the manager can predict the cost of care by calculating the salaries and benefits for each team member, adding supplies and overhead, multiplying by number of visits, and finally multiplying this number by two (average hours spent in the home by each caregiver). **TABLE 8.5** demonstrates this calculation.

Under prospective payment, our patient reimbursement is $6,098. Because the total cost for Mr. James is $6,428.80, the agency will lose $330.80 for this patient (i.e., $6,428.80 total cost − $6,098 reimbursement = $330.80). For this reason, many home health agencies have limited the complex cases they enroll in their service (van der Walde & Choi, 2003).

In the present scenario, the home health manager is also faced with the issue of the short-term home health admission. For example, a new diabetic may be ordered to receive home health visits for teaching. The visits are limited to three. The cost of admitting the patient to the service is $200 due to the time and intensity of the assessment as well as completion of Outcome and Assessment Information Set (OASIS). Our previous calculation indicates the cost of the two remaining visits (plus supplies of $25) is $155.10. The payer reimburses only $90 for each visit ($270 total), and the agency again loses $85.10. Although the manager may believe this is a small amount, over time the agency will not be self-sustaining as a result of losses from complex patients and short-term admissions. Therefore, the home health manager must be creative and identify areas of savings such as decreasing supply costs that are not reimbursable and set budget expenditures based on historical data that provide insight into payer reimbursements, as well as the types of patients admitted to the agency.

The same-day surgery patient, under prospective payment, receives services reimbursed by APC codes. These are based on relative value units (RVUs), which are a measure of time and resources that are bundled into hundreds of assigned categories (van der Walde & Choi, 2002). Many outpatient services have benefited from the APC process of reimbursement, more so from the private payers than Medicare. **TABLE 8.6** shows a comparison of costs and reimbursement for a

TABLE 8.5 Projection of Home Healthcare Costs for 60 Days of Care

Salary/hr × benefits (20%) + supplies + overhead × no. visits × average time/visit = costs						
RN costs	= ($18.79/hr × 0.2)	+ $37.45	+ $30	× 12	× 2	= $2,160.00
PT costs	= ($19.50 × 0.2)	+ $0	+ $30	× 16	× 2	= $1,708.80
CNA costs	= ($8.50 × 0.2)	+ $20.00	+ $30	× 16	× 2	= $1,926.40
OT costs	= ($19.00 × 0.2)	+ $0	+ $30	× 6	× 2	= $633.60
Total costs	=					$6,428.80

CNA, certified nursing assistant; OT, occupational therapy; PT, physical therapy; RN, registered nurse.

TABLE 8.6 Same Day Surgery Cost and Reimbursement for Laparoscopic Cholecystectomy

51.23 Laparoscopic Cholecystectomy	Charge Code Units (RVU)	Charges	Actual Payment	Total Direct Costs	Total Indirect Costs	Total Cost
Private Insurance						
1662 Anesthesia	9	$1,658		$240	$77	$317
1665 Same day surgery	29	$4,514		$1,140	$927	$2,067
1710 Central supply	6	$264		$131	$34	$165
1715 Pharmacy	12	$352		$96	$21	$117
1720 Pathology	1	$175		$12	$9	$21
1722 Lab	3	$91		$16	$6	$22
Total Private Insurance	**60**	**$7,054**	**$4,573**	**$1,635**	**$1,074**	**$2,709**
Medicare Patient						
1662 Anesthesia	7	$1,384		$201	$64	$265
1665 Same day surgery	28	$4,546		$1,065	$866	$1,931
1710 Central supply	5	$255		$126	$33	$159
1715 Pharmacy	16	$469		$127	$28	$155
1722 Lab	5	$135		$26	$11	$37
Total Medicare Payment	**61**	**$6,789**	**$1,767**	**$1,545**	**$1,002**	**$2,547**

same-day surgery laparoscopic cholecystectomy. The first example is a 42-year-old woman with private insurance, and the second is a 70-year-old man with Medicare.

From the previous example, the manager has an understanding that the private insurance carriers truly offset the cost of caring for the Medicare patient, although this margin is narrowing as less is received from private payers. The manager, knowledgeable of payer mix, can determine the financial feasibility of the service that is provided by the same-day surgery facility.

Revenue Budget
Nursing Service Does Generate Revenue

In the healthcare organization—whether hospital, long-term care, home care, or ambulatory settings—nursing services provide organizational revenue. If you are a nurse leader on an inpatient unit, you may hear a finance employee say your unit does not generate revenue. Technically, in an inpatient unit you probably do not have a revenue account—unless you have oncology services, operating room, or a service that can be directly billed. Instead, nursing services in inpatient units are most often included in the room rate charge, and the finance department keeps the records of revenues. However, nursing care does generate and contribute to the revenue generation for the DRG payment in hospitals and for the minimum data set (MDS) reimbursement in long-term care.

In this example, revenue becomes muddy because so many disciplines are involved in the patient's care. Remember that patients always come to inpatient units because they need nursing care. Nursing services have traditionally been directly billed in home care as a separate line item. Maine and Maryland, for example, have recognized nursing's contributions to providing inpatient care and have specified that hospitals take nursing service out of the room rate charge and list it as a separate item on the patient's bill. More efforts are being made to get

nursing taken out of the room rate in hospitals, but to date this has not become common practice. This could mean that more inpatient units will be considered profit centers and have a revenue budget.

As noted previously, it is important in the value-based environment that nursing staff give care meeting the reimbursement mandates for protocols, for preventing never events, and for coordinating care so that patients are not readmitted within 30 days. *Nurse Leaders have a key role in making sure revenue is not lost in these instances.*

There may be other services or items that can be directly billed, such as operating room procedures, ambulatory services, home care services, drugs, supplies, educational programs, physical or respiratory therapy, consultation services, or wellness programs. In these programs, nurse leaders usually have a revenue budget, often called a profit center. In this case, the cost center's services are directly billed to patients. In these settings, the revenue budget is used to make sure that the organization/department/clinic remains viable.

Currently, revenues are reported only occasionally on inpatient cost center budgets. If this occurs, the nurse leader must seek information to learn what these figures represent: Are they billed dollars or are these dollars actually received? Are contractual allowances or discounts included in the revenue figures? Is the figure so unreliable that the nurse leader should just ignore it, or does it provide useful data?

When the nurse leader gets a revenue report for billable supplies or services, most often provided by the finance department, the nurse leader should check the accuracy of the figures and then compare costs and revenue. **TABLE 8.7** is an example of a detailed nursing unit operations report that includes revenues for inpatient and outpatient sources. Revenue in this type of financial report does not equal true reimbursement but is a CCR that is used in the *Medicare Cost Report*. The manager can also note from this report the distribution of payers for the department.

TABLE 8.7 Monthly Nursing Departmental Revenue Report by Payer

| | 5 North   Nov-0_ | | | | |
	Actual*	Budget	Variance	Variance %	Favorable/ Unfavorable
Inpatient Revenue					
Medicare	167,519	282,683	−115,164	−40.7	U
Medicaid	22,050	34,802	−12,752	−36.6	U
Managed care	29,578	44,515	−14,937	−33.6	U
Commercial	15,004	9,237	5,767	62.4	F
Self-pay	27,293	5,294	21,999	415.5	F
Other	2,406	3,368	−962	−28.6	U
Total	**263,850**	**379,899**	**−116,049**	**−30.5**	**U**
Per unit	**782.94**	**796.43**	**−14**	**−1.7**	**U**
Outpatient Revenue					
Medicare	16,254	9,624	6,630	68.9	F
Medicaid	5,044	3,994	1,050	26.3	F
Managed care	3,388	6,913	−3,525	−51.0	U
Commercial	627	1,031	−404	−39.2	U
Self-pay	1,533	587	946	161.2	F
Other	627	165	462	280.0	F
Total	**27,473**	**22,314**	**5,159**	**23.1**	**F**
Per unit	**639**	**970**	**−331**	**−34.1**	**U**
Revenue Total	**291,323**	**402,213**	**−110,890**	**−27.6**	**U**
Per unit	**767**	**804**	**−38**	**−4.7**	**U**

* The *Actual* column represents gross revenue times the ratio of costs to charges from the Medicare/Medicaid report.

How is this information interpreted? The first column provides the payer source identified in the CCR. Following the reimbursement are the budgeted dollars expected to be collected. The next column is the variance between actual CCR and what was budgeted, or Actual – Budgeted = Variance. Percent variance follows next. This is the percent deviation between the actual column and the budgeted column. The last column shows whether the variance is favorable (F) or unfavorable (U). As you can tell from this report, the revenue total for both in- and outpatient is below the budgeted amount at an unfavorable 4.7%.

The nurse leader must seek information to explain the variation from budget. For this unit, two areas were identified as reasons for the budget variation. First, the census was lower than expected by the budgeted amount, and second, there was decreased reimbursement from contractual agreements that went into effect in the previous month of October. Although nursing management cannot directly affect contractual agreements, nursing does have a strong influence on the census through providing high-quality, safe care the patient and family value, as well as by building a trusting relationship with physicians, patients, colleagues, and others in the organization. When everyone acts as an effective team, magic happens.

However, this variance is only a piece of the information the nurse leader has to consider. The manager must also compare the same period last year, as well as the year-to-date (YTD) financials to have the total picture of the unit financial performance. **TABLE 8.8** provides the fiscal YTD financial information for 5 North. This nursing unit is generating 5.2% less than budgeted revenue for the fiscal year to date.

The challenge now is for the nurse leader to be knowledgeable not only of employee and supply expenses but also the unit's primary admission diagnoses, length of stay, complication rates, and reimbursement per DRG. The manager should review the DRG historical admission and discharge history of the unit. Then, the nurse leader can evaluate the unit patient population and identify trends or changes in the patient base that may require an expansion of nursing knowledge and skills. In addition, the manager should ask for the following information: length of stay by discharge diagnosis, list of secondary diagnoses, and complications. An analysis of this information will guide the manager to identify areas for improving care to decrease complications (which are costly and are not reimbursed), improve efficiency, decrease supply and manpower costs, and thereby improve the financial performance of the nursing unit.

Another area that affects the financial performance of a nursing unit is the contractual agreements made between the hospital financial management team, a managed care organization, and a preferred price for supplies based on utilization. *Contractual agreements* are negotiations between the healthcare agency and the health insurer or provider of services and supplies. Contracts may range from the amount paid by the insurer for a specific diagnosis to the amount of supply charges based on utilization. The nurse leader does not have control over contract negotiations but plays a significant role in providing information regarding changes in patient care that influence negotiated reimbursement or prices. In addition, the nurse leader must be aware of the dates of contract renewals to recognize shortfalls during the budget planning process.

Currently, two other factors affect payments. First, as the general population is aging, a higher percentage will be on Medicare. But more significantly, because ACA has indicated that everyone will have insurance, there will be a much higher number of patients on Medicaid. The current financial recession also places more people at the poverty level, thus adding to Medicaid numbers.

Table 8.8 demonstrates an example of how changes in patient payers and contractual agreements affect the nursing units' budget. In this example, Medicare admissions decreased, private insurance decreased contractual reimbursement, and there was an increase in self-pay patients, which often contributes to indigent care services, as well as nonpayment

TABLE 8.8 Year-to-Date (YTD) Nursing Department Revenue Report by Payer

	5 North		FYTD		Nov-0_
	Actual *	Budget	Variance	Variance %	Favorable/ Unfavorable
Inpatient Revenue					
Medicare	1,120,051	1,358,542	−238,491	−17.6	U
Medicaid	205,504	167,253	37,801	22.6	F
Managed care	141,956	213,932	−71,976	−33.6	U
Commercial	67,857	44,392	23,465	52.9	F
Self-pay	50,315	25,440	24,875	97.8	F
Other	12,824	16,187	−3,363	−20.8	U
Total	**1,598,507**	**1,825,746**	**−227,689**	**−12.5**	**U**
Per unit	**798.63**	**796.23**	**2.40**	**0.3**	**F**
Outpatient Revenue					
Medicare	88,162	47,653	40,509	85.0	F
Medicaid	18,805	19,776	−971	−4.9	U
Managed care	32,321	34,229	−1,908	−5.6	U
Commercial	3,615	5,106	−1,491	−29.2	U
Self-pay	5,451	2,907	2,544	87.5	F
Other	4,117	817	3,300	403.9	F
Total	**152,471**	**110,488**	**41,983**	**38.0**	**F**
Per unit	**520.38**	**977.77**	**−457.39**	**−46.8**	**U**
Revenue Total	**1,750,978**	**1,936,234**	**−185,706**	**−9.6**	**U**
Per unit	**763.09**	**804.75**	**−41.66**	**−5.2**	**U**

* The *Actual* column represents gross revenue times the ratio of costs to charges from the Medicare/Medicaid report.

issues. The key factor that cannot be seen in the example is that the private insurance contract negotiations occurred after the budget had been set and a lower reimbursement was negotiated by management as a means to increase patient volume by this carrier. The manager needs to continually evaluate admissions by payer to identify whether the negotiated contract actually increased admissions for the nursing unit.

Predicting Financial Success

The case mix index has been used by hospital administrators to predict financial success since prospective payment was instituted. The nurse leader can use this tool to predict financial success at the nursing unit level. DRGs are divided into 25 major diagnostic categories (MDCs) that include the following information: DRG number, narrative description, relative weight, geometric length of stay, arithmetic length of stay, and outlier threshold. The relative weight is an assigned number that is an indicator of the amount of resources needed to care for the patient with that particular disease process and includes all costs related to the hospitalization (Adams, 1996). The nurse leader should understand that the higher the weight, the greater the amount of resources needed to care for the patient. The amount of resources needed to treat a particular disease process is the *relative weight*. A disease requiring many resources, such as total joint replacement, carries a higher weight than atypical chest pain.

From this information, as well as knowledge of supply costs and personnel expense, the nurse leader can be proactive in departmental financial management. Furthermore, the nurse leader can alert the nurse executive and finance department about important reimbursement issues (i.e., lost revenues, higher expenses than revenues). In addition, the nurse leader must realize the hospital's DRG payment rate is also contingent on geographic location, wage index, and patient mix.

The nurse leader should obtain the top 10 DRGs for the nursing unit from the coding department or from the finance department. By knowing this information, the manager can influence reimbursement on the unit by assisting staff and physicians to document thoroughly for accurate coding.

The manager may choose to select one DRG that is costing more than the reimbursement, establish a multidisciplinary team to evaluate processes of care that may affect patient outcomes and increase cost, and strategize to determine less costly ways to deliver the care safely and efficiently. The utilization review/case manager should play an important role in this function of coding.

Nursing Management Decisions Affect Financial Outcomes

The nurse leader must be cognizant of unit expenses, including personnel and supplies. These are two key areas that nursing can affect to ensure a positive bottom line. The flow of patients into and out of a service area determines the staffing and supplies needed. Nursing must have financial savvy and be creative to manage within this environment.

As previously noted, nurse leader involvement is very important in meeting specified protocols, preventing never events, and preventing hospital readmissions within 30 days. These actions can result in revenue not being lost.

In long-term care, reimbursement for Medicaid patients is actually determined by the nurse and depends on how well the nurse has completed the MDS.

Usually, to accomplish a detailed evaluation of cost versus reimbursement, the nurse leader can facilitate an interdisciplinary management team to determine and compare actual costs of the services provided with the reimbursement amount received for those services. The organization and participation on such a team can help all disciplines within the organization to become cognizant of the importance of rectifying systems problems that can contribute significantly to higher costs if left unidentified and unresolved.

Summary

Cost and reimbursement issues are difficult to understand because of the complexity. This is because there are many different ways that costs are calculated and because it is important to know which payer is paying what amount. Hopefully, this chapter has assisted the manager to have an improved understanding of fiscal management for the nursing unit or department and deems himself or herself the chief executive officer and chief financial officer of his or her area, now recognizing the power of the position in determining successful patient outcomes and a positive bottom line. Note that this chapter is concerned only with assisting the nurse leader in the financial aspects, not with other quality and ethical factors involved.

Discussion Questions

1. This chapter discusses the need for an interdisciplinary team approach. Why is this important? Which specific areas/departments should be involved?

2. What is a cost-to-charge ratio? Why should a nurse manager understand this ratio, and how would he or she use it?

3. Finance departments regard nursing units as not being revenue generators. Why do you believe they are inaccurate in their assessment?

4. This chapter hopes to improve your understanding of fiscal management. In your opinion, which factor covered in this chapter would you consider most critical?

5. In the new value-based reimbursement environment, what other measures can a nurse manager take to enhance reimbursement and prevent revenue loss?

Glossary of Terms

Balanced Scorecard and Activity-Based Costing (ABC) this ratio is more closely aligned with the true costs of caring for the patient. ABC methodology also resembles performance improvement methods because processes and outcomes are evaluated. The complexity of procedures and tests involved, the intensity of nursing care, the duration of an activity, and the intricacies of operative and postoperative care identify the true costs. In this method, all areas and processes of patient interaction are identified, and costs are allocated to the activity center. The BSC adds the quality dimension to cost and reimbursement data. For instance, cost drivers outside the system, such as patient satisfaction, can be measured and reflected in the overall scorecard.

Capitation mechanism used by insurers to contain costs by establishing a set payment amount for a population served by a defined healthcare service. Rates are negotiated between the provider and the insurer under a contractual agreement for a year. Reimbursement rates may be for all services offered or for one specific service area, called a "carve-out," such as laboratory.

Charges determined by the allocation of costs to the revenue-producing centers and then projecting an amount needed to recover all the costs.

Costing a Service all the actual costs expended to provide a specified service, as determined by the interdisciplinary team. This costing exercise should take place for all major services provided within the healthcare organization.

Costs determined by the organization's financial accounting system, which takes into account actual costs of supplies, manpower, facility, and administration for services provided.

Cost-to-Charge Ratio (CCR) a ratio determined by dividing the costs by the charges. A ratio under 1.0 (equal costs and charges) is positive and indicates that the organization is making money on the service. A ratio over 1.0 indicates the organization is experiencing a loss— the costs are more than the charges (expected reimbursement). The report is required for all Medicare-certified hospitals, skilled nursing facilities, home health agencies, and renal facilities. The nurse manager should be aware that CCR could lead to misrepresentation of cost when evaluating the profitability of a service.

Operating Payments additional payments to the base DRG reimbursement that vary from large urban (population over 1 million) to other urban and rural hospitals. In 2009, the reimbursement rate for hospitals was tied to their quality performance (Centers for Medicare and Medicaid Services, 2008). These amounts are adjusted for the area market basket update.

Payment amount the healthcare agency receives for the services provided. All payers pay differing amounts for the same service depending on the type of payer and the contractual agreement between the agency and the insurer.

Per Diem Approach a ratio where the indirect costs are divided by the number of patient days to determine per diem costs, and then the indirect costs are allocated equally to all nursing units, which means that the departmental operations report for the obstetric unit and the cardiovascular intensive care unit will have the same dollar amount for indirect expenses even though the obstetric unit had fewer patient days regardless of the actual number of patient days. This method considers all patients the same regardless of intensity of care.

Projection of Reimbursement calculated by a payment-to-cost ratio that indicates the percentage of costs covered by reimbursement.

Volume-Based Environment (first curve) in the past, reimbursement has been determined by the volume of insured patients. Industrial Age organizational design was used.

Value-Based Environment (second curve) presently, reimbursement is changing to include organizational performance mandates. When protocols are not met, and when never events occur, insurers are not paying providers for the event or for the hospital stay. Reimbursement is value-based.

Volume-Based Measures a ratio where the indirect costs are assigned according to the volume (which may be visits, admissions, nursing hours per patient day) or machine hours (in radiology and the laboratory).

References

Adams, T. (1996). Case mix index: Nursing's new management tool. *Nursing Management, 27*(9), 31–32.

Carpenter, D. (2003). Soaring spending: No sign of a slowdown. *H & HN: Hospitals and Healthcare Networks, 77*, 16–17.

Centers for Medicare and Medicaid Services. (2008). Proposed fiscal year 2009 payment policy changes for inpatient stays in general acute care hospitals. Retrieved from http://www.cms.hhs.gov/apps/media/press/factsheet.asp?Counter53045

Easier than ABC: Will activity based costing make a comeback? (2003). *The Economist, 369*, 56.

Finkler, S., Jones, C., & Kovner, C. (2013). *Financial management for nurse managers and executives.* St Louis, MO: Elsevier.

Health Research and Educational Trust. (2013, April). *Metrics for the second curve of health care.* Washington, DC: American Hospital Association.

Kane, N., & Siegrist, R. (2002). Understanding rising hospital costs: Key components of cost and the impact of poor quality. Retrieved from https://www.researchgate.net/profile/Nancy_Kane/publication/265568685_Understanding_Rising_Hospital_Inpatient_Costs_Key_Components_of_Cost_and_The_Impact_of_Poor_Quality/links/55fae1d808aeba1d9f3a0958/Understanding-Rising-Hospital-Inpatient-Costs-Key-Components-of-Cost-and-The-Impact-of-Poor-Quality.pdf

Lane, S., Longstreth, E., & Nixon, V. (2001). *A community leader's guide to hospital finance.* Boston, MA: Access Project.

Magnus, S., & Smith, D. (2000). Better Medicare cost report data needed to help hospitals benchmark costs and performance. *Health Care Management Review, 25*(4), 65–77.

Medicare SNF-PPS Indices [Data file]. (2003). Washington, DC: Centers for Medicare and Medicaid Services. Retrieved from http://www.cms.gov/

Nursing Leadership Academy. (2003). *Fundamentals of nursing finance: A foundation for financial leadership (10889).* Washington, DC: Advisory Board Company.

Ross, T. (2004). Analyzing health care operations using ABC. *Journal of Health Care Finance, 30*(3), 1–20.

Udpa, S. (2001). Activity cost analysis: A tool to cost medical services and improve quality. *Managed Care Quarterly, 9*(3), 34–41.

U.S. General Accounting Office. (2002). *Skilled nursing facilities: Medicare payments exceed costs for most but not all facilities* (GAO-03-183). Washington, DC: Author.

van der Walde, T., & Choi, K. (2002). *Health care industry market update: Acute care hospitals* (Vol. II). Washington, DC: Centers for Medicare and Medicaid Services.

van der Walde, L., & Choi, K. (2003). *Health care industry market update: Nursing facilities.* Washington, DC: Centers for Medicare and Medicaid Services.

van der Walde, L., & Lindstrom, L. (2003). *Health care market update: Home health.* Washington, DC: Centers for Medicare and Medicaid Services.

Young, D. (2007). The folly of using RCCs and RVUs for intermediate product costing. *Healthcare Financial Management: Journal of the Healthcare Financial Management Association, 61*(4), 100–106, 108.

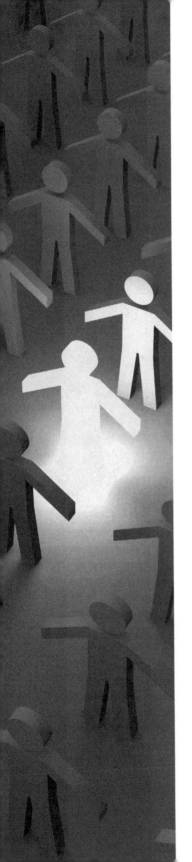

PART III

Financial Strategies and Accounting Issues

CHAPTER 9

Strategic Management: Facing the Future with Confidence

J. Michael Leger, PhD, MBA, RN, and **Sandy K. Diffenderfer**, PhD, MSN, RN, CPHQ

The future ain't what it used to be.

—**Yogi Berra**

OBJECTIVES

- Articulate the evolution of strategic planning to strategic management.
- Describe two approaches to strategic management.
- Compare complexity theory and contemporary strategic management.
- Identify key aspects of traditional strategic management.
- Discuss the strategic management role of the nurse manager.

Effective visioning and decision making are primary tasks of leaders. Teamwork and collaboration are necessary for organizational leaders to make informed decisions and to maintain a viable organization. Seemingly justified by time constraints and the mistaken assessment that issues are minor, nurse leaders often make decisions without essential information. By chance, the nurse leader may be successful in the short run, but in the long run, the use of intuition—without the benefit of systematic input from stakeholders, pertinent data, and careful planning—most often results in calamity.

The delivery of health care devoid of a systematic process for planning forces managers to "fly by the seat of their pants" through reliance on perceptions and experience. The task of strategic planning and management is to generate accurate information for decision making. Forecasting the future with precision, however, is problematic because contemporary healthcare systems are complex, chaotic, and ever changing. Thus, obtaining accurate information can be a challenge in the healthcare environment where the answers and even the questions seemingly change on a daily basis. Strategic planning and management shifts decision making from intuitive information gathering to systematic and objective investigation and action.

In the midst of contemporary healthcare chaos, as the volume and pace of change continue to accelerate, managers may declare they have no choice but to spend time and resources "putting out fires." It is surprising that well-adjusted individuals are overwhelmed by change after years of colliding with it. Notwithstanding, Gelatt (1993) observed that change itself had changed. The author described the chaos found in healthcare organizations as *white water change* because change in health care had become rapid, complex, turbulent, and unpredictable. Years after Gelatt's (1993) description of change, contemporary healthcare leaders bear witness to unparalleled change in the healthcare environment.

Patnaik (2012) defined *strategic planning* as "visualizing the future and making adequate provisions to deal with the same to meet organizational objectives" (p. 27). The dynamic and complex nature of health care mandates that leaders and managers not forsake planning if the organization is to meet key objectives and be positioned for long-term success. The strategic plan must provide an adaptable framework to make ongoing, timely, and dynamic changes to keep pace with the ever-changing healthcare environment. The plan must be designed to be continuous, and thus *adaptable,* because leaders cannot wait until the next planning cycle to decide how to respond to an unanticipated challenge (Greene, 2009). The plan exists to provide direction "not to prophesize by rigidly fixing unalterable boundaries" (Patnaik, 2012, p. 27) for future actions.

In addition to planning, strategic management is needed. *Strategic management* requires monitoring of key organizational metrics, assessment, evaluation, and continuous improvement to sustain the gains. Successful healthcare leaders use strategic management processes to remain informed about the organization, the market, and the competitive arena. The goal of strategic management is early recognition of environmental changes or the need for internal changes to be proactive rather than reactive. Thus, strategic management is fundamental to organizational success in the ever-changing healthcare environment because the processes provide leaders with direction and momentum for change (Ginter, Swayne, & Duncan, 2013).

Mintzberg and Markides (2000) noted that *strategy* is the art of crafting a unique position in the market. Primary strategy does not need to change often; however, when there is a need to rethink the organization's position, the change should emerge from the ideas and actions of the people in the organization. Once again, the focus is on being proactive rather than reactive.

Nurse leaders are in a unique position to recognize the need for a change in strategy because they may be the first stakeholders to recognize when strategies that worked in the past are no longer effective.

Successful organizational leaders understand the need to revise the organization's strategic plan based on feedback from internal as well as external stakeholders. Strategy must be the job of every employee because employees are key internal stakeholders. This is important because the employee's livelihood depends on the success of the organization. In the volatile healthcare market, a flat, fully decentralized, bottom-up organizational structure promotes problem solving and innovation. Innovative strategies are more likely to be formulated if everyone in the organization puts their intellect to the task.

Even though everyone in the organization should be encouraged to come up with new strategic ideas, senior leaders are responsible for the final choices. This is fitting because senior leaders are responsible for the organization's vision. This vision must be congruent with the contemporary healthcare arena. Organizational leaders must determine which ideas will be pursued; otherwise, the result is chaos and confusion. Strategic planning and management enable healthcare leaders to meet the future proactively rather than by responding to the internal and external environment in a haphazard manner. Although strategic planning and management do not eliminate all challenges, the process can drive innovation, integrate the system, and align resources to enable the organization to face the future with confidence.

Strategic planning is a continuous process of revisiting the system and restoring balance. Systematic, objective planning is the key to the development and implementation of plans that drive successful healthcare organizations. Organizational leaders must go beyond large binders with numbers, graphs, charts, and jargon. The data gathered and stored in these binders must be used to improve organizational performance. Often, these valuable data—that took many hours of time and significant money to assemble—are considered during the initial phase of the strategic planning cycle, and then are shelved until the next round of strategic planning. If everyone in the organization does not view the strategic plan as a useful document,

the organization's culture related to the strategic planning process should be explored.

Although many organizations have separate plans for performance improvement (PI), education, finance, operations, recruitment, and retention efforts would be better spent crafting a single document as the outcome of collaborative teamwork among disciplines and workers. The key to successful planning is to make the process a part of the daily operations of the organization rather than a task to be completed during the planning cycle in preparation for the budget.

Healthcare delivery takes place in complex systems sustained by social networks of internal and external stakeholders (Clancy, 2007). Healthcare employees from different departments and facilities must share information and collaborate to ensure the long-term success of the organization. Transparency fosters innovation and synergy because everyone is aligned with the overall strategies of the organization. Lack of transparency results in duplication of efforts, increased costs, poor working relationships, and employees working at cross purposes. The resulting chaos and confusion give an appearance of disorganization to external customers.

Because of the complex nature of health care, "silo mentality" is common. Silo mentality is defined as "a mind-set present in some companies when certain departments or sectors do not wish to share information with others in the same company". Lencioni (2006) described silos as one of the most frustrating aspects of working in an organization. The author stated that these barriers within an organization caused people who are supposed to be on the same team to work against each other and are generally not purposeful but rather the result of leaders failing to provide employees with a compelling purpose for working together. This highlights the importance of the leadership role in creating a common purpose through the organization's mission, vision, goals, objectives, and metrics, all of which are embodied in strategic management.

Healthcare organizational leaders must focus on patient satisfaction as well as patient retention and loyalty. Leaders must know the status of the organization's market share as well as any potential new markets. There may be services that need to be "repackaged" to attract new or evolving markets. These aspects are key factors in competitiveness, profitability, and the success of the organization. Choices made by organizational leaders 3 to 5 years ago may no longer be valid and must be continuously questioned. In the past, being decisive was an essential talent often thought to be reserved for those in administrative positions. The healthcare environment of today has replaced the skill of making up one's mind with a *new essential skill of the future—learning how to change one's mind* (Gelatt, 1993). Technologies, customer preferences, and competitors are ever changing, and the organization must be flexible. Successful organizational leaders *question past choices* to determine whether change is necessary. The heart of strategic planning is to devise a systematic, well-balanced process that allows the organization to fit in the environment.

Strategic planning must be objective. The necessity for objectivity was cleverly stated by the nineteenth-century American humorist Artemus Ward, who said, "It ain't so much what people don't know that hurts as what they know that ain't so" (Creative Quotations, 2009). Thus, the facilitator of the strategic planning process must be detached and impersonal rather than engaged in biased attempts to prove preconceived ideas.

According to Mintzberg and Markides (2000), strategy is nothing more than answering three simple, yet difficult questions:

1. Whom should the organization target as customers and whom should it not target?
2. What should the organization offer these customers and what should it not offer?
3. What is the most efficient way to do this?

If the healthcare team does not have clear answers to these three questions, the organization will drift aimlessly until it eventually fails. Team members need clear parameters to guide their actions; these three dimensions help provide the autonomy they need to focus on the key tasks at hand. Without clarity of these three dimensions, organizational efforts will be disjointed because no common understanding of the strategies, goals, and objectives of the business exists.

Although the term *customer* was not used often in health care until recent years, 21st-century healthcare leaders recognize the primary customer to be *the patient*. Patient-focused and other customer-focused quality efforts lead to customer acquisition, satisfaction, loyalty, referrals, and organizational sustainability that differentiates a healthcare system from its competitors (NIST, 2013). The ultimate test of quality is customer satisfaction. Areas to consider are those important to the patient, such as speed, responsiveness, and flexibility.

In light of the economic forces of healthcare reform, the status quo is not sustainable. *Innovative strategies* are needed for organizations to survive ever-shifting market pressures. Healthcare customers expect **value**, which is a delicate balance between cost and quality. Improvement in work systems contributes to short- and longer-term productivity, cost containment, and the overall well-being of the organization. Finally, organizational and personal learning must be embedded in work systems that are aligned with the organization's strategic plan. This alignment clarifies organizational priorities for employees (NIST, 2013).

Customers of health care are both internal and external to the organization. *Internal customers* include patients and families, physicians, visitors, team members, and volunteers. The employment of physicians has changed physicians from external customers (suppliers of the patients served) to both internal (employees) and external (suppliers) customers. This dual role may conflict when organizational priorities are unclear or when organizational and personal goals are incongruent.

The primary *external customers* of health care are quite complex and consist of suppliers (insurance companies, physicians, labor markets, and donors), consumers (the general public and community), and interfacing organizations (medical profession, teaching and/or other hospitals, boards of directors, health insurances, and drug and supply companies). Additional external influences include licensing, governmental, and regulatory agencies, as well as other healthcare facilities (Bennis & Nanus, 1985). Students who complete clinical assignments in healthcare facilities are also external customers along with faculty and administrators.

Determining the measures customers use when they assess and judge the quality of healthcare services is an important process. Healthcare leaders' perception of quality may be vastly different from customers' perceptions. Nurse managers may believe that achieving zero defects is the priority when, in fact, timeliness is what is most important to the customer. It is important to have multiple listening strategies aimed at assessing how the customer perceives quality. Listening to the customer provides baseline knowledge. Once opportunities to improve are identified, leadership, through strategic planning, must assess and drive improvements.

It is important that healthcare leaders understand why customers choose particular healthcare services. Providing quality care does not guarantee success; customers must perceive added *value*. Healthcare leaders may erroneously perceive that services are superior in design, service, and cost when, in fact, the services are inefficient, outdated, and ordinary. Unless improvements are made, advances in the market will produce customer dissatisfaction rather than satisfaction with services. Customer satisfaction is paramount to the success of the organization, and capturing this information encompasses a major expenditure.

Some healthcare professionals question whether patients and families are qualified to assess healthcare quality. The Internet has eliminated the time-honored adage "We know what is best, after all we have years of education" and has ushered in the age of *informed consumers*. No longer is it acceptable to lecture the patient, "Just do as I say" or "The doctor knows best."

Many patients seek healthcare services after an extensive Internet search on the diagnosis and/or treatment(s) in question. Patients and families often arrive for care with an array of scientific literature—indeed, sometimes they are better informed than the clinician is.

An organization's commitment to performance excellence should not be measured by cost but rather viewed as an *investment*. Organizational leaders purchase equipment to improve processes and cycle times. Leaders who make a similar investment in team members receive a much higher return. Boev (2012) found preliminary support for the relationship between nurses' and patients' satisfaction in adult critical care. Thus, successful healthcare organizations recognize and reward team members. If team members are expected to meet the needs of customers, their needs must be met first. This is important because patient satisfaction is now associated with hospital reimbursement (Centers for Medicare & Medicaid Services, 2011).

A primary concern is cost competitiveness, which is difficult to attain during economic downturns. It is paramount that healthcare leaders remain committed to the facility's mission and values when deciding how to respond to such crises. Operational capabilities such as speed, responsiveness, and flexibility contribute to the organization's competitive fitness. The strategic plan must align work processes with the strategic direction of the organization by embedding improvement and learning in work processes. This alignment ensures that priorities for improvement and learning reinforce the priorities of the organization.

Comprehensive strategic planning establishes the *organization's strategy* (the plan for achieving the desired end result) and *plan of action* (what the organization must do to get there). Of key importance are the deployment of the plan of action to all business units, how strategic management will be operationalized through identification of key results, and how outcomes are measured and sustained.

The healthcare system is undergoing tremendous change. Thus, leaders must determine whether decades of habit related to the strategic planning and management process are appropriate given the current volatile environment. Zuckerman (2006) noted that organizations in stable markets may be able to survive using traditional planning practice; nevertheless, the unstable healthcare environment demands a *flexible, ongoing planning process*. Leaders must decide whether to forge ahead with traditional strategic planning or change to a more fluid compressed cycle strategic planning process. Regardless of the decision, it is most important that the organization's mission, vision, and values guide leaders' actions.

▶ Strategic Planning in Health Care

Although the business sector has successfully used strategic planning for the past 50 years, strategic planning has been used in health care only since the 1970s, and then only sporadically (Zuckerman, 1998). According to Ginter, Swayne, and Duncan (2002), the concept of strategic planning was broadened to strategic management during the 1980s when business transformed planning and budgeting beyond the traditional 12-month operating year and began to understand the importance of strategy implementation and control. Prior to this time, healthcare organizations had little impetus for strategic management because the organizations were autonomous, free-standing facilities with cost-plus reimbursement schemes (Ginter et al., 2013).

Ginter et al. (2013) described the approaches to strategic management as *analytical* and *emergent*. According to the authors, analytical or rational approaches to strategic management involve sequential steps and linear thinking that correspond best with traditional strategic management processes. On the other hand, emergent approaches to strategic management rely on intuitive thinking, leadership, and learning, which correspond with contemporary strategic management processes. Ginter et al.

(2013) declared that both approaches were valid and useful, and that, indeed, both approaches are required. An overview of contemporary and traditional strategic management processes follows.

▶ Contemporary Strategic Management

Complexity theory provides an explanation for the unpredictability that is inherent in strategic planning (Patnaik, 2012). Crowell (2011) described complexity science as "nonlinear, dynamic, often uncertain, and very much relationship-based" (p. 3). The author further stated that complexity leadership ascribes that top-down structures do not necessarily lead to effective outcomes or changed behaviors—in fact, often the reverse. Complexity theory is particularly relevant to healthcare systems because change is the only constant. Thus, traditional strategic management with a goal of forecasting and monitoring future states is inconsistent with the healthcare environment.

Zuckerman (2006) proclaimed that planners and executives who participated in a survey believed that healthcare strategic planning was effective and provided focus and direction for their organizations. The author noted that, in a stable market, traditional strategic planning methods worked well; however, in volatile, ever-changing markets such as health care, a more nimble approach was needed. Furthermore, he identified that healthcare strategic planning was less rigorous and sophisticated than were the planning processes used by organizations outside of health care.

Zuckerman (2006) offered that state-of-the-art strategic planning encompassed some or all of the following qualities:

1. Systematic, ongoing data gathering, leading to use of knowledge management practices
2. Encouragement of innovation and creativity in strategic approaches

3. More bottom-up than top-down strategic planning
4. Evolving, flexible, continuously improving planning processes
5. A shift from static to dynamic strategic planning (p. 8)

Although these characteristics of a state-of-the-art strategic plan are not new, health care has been slow to break the habit of the traditional strategic plan. Turbulent times in health care provide an opportunity to break from the norm and embrace contemporary strategic planning and management processes.

Several contemporary strategic management processes are found in the literature; some are formal processes, some are less so. Recent authors described emerging trends in strategic planning—for example, the use of nonlinear (Crowell, 2011) compressed, flexible cycles for leaders to be able to quickly respond to the ever-changing environments (Dibrell, Down, & Bull, 2007; Greene, 2009; Lazarus, 2011; Patnaik, 2012; Zuckerman, 2006). Dibrell et al. (2007) described *strategic flex points* (p. 28) that allowed quick and effective changes in managers' plans. This planned emergent perspective empowered managers to contact leaders when opportunities or threats were developing to adapt or change the formal strategic plan. The emerging pattern found by these authors was that firms that were able to respond quickly and effectively to external threats and opportunities were more likely to be successful.

Likewise, Greene (2009) described recent seismic events in health care such as the economic crisis, increased market pressures, and healthcare reform as catalysts for change in which decades of habit related to the traditional strategic planning process must be discarded. The author touted the need to address strategy *quarterly* for leaders to ensure that the facility's mission, vision, and values are upheld. A heightened focus on the mission, vision, and values is needed because relentless environmental changes especially related to difficult financial choices may result in a disjoint between the organization's core

purpose and decisions that are made for the organization to remain viable.

Healthcare planners and executives who recognize the need for a more flexible strategic plan place less emphasis on long-term planning because, in such a volatile environment, control is merely an illusion. Rather than standalone strategic plans, the strategic plan is often linked to business operations, including the facility's PI plan (Blatstein, 2012; Lazarus, 2011) and finance and budgeting processes (Blatstein, 2012; Zuckerman, 2006). This decreases silo mentality.

Integrated plans facilitate transparent, focused, and collaborative work among leaders, managers, and team members. Linking the strategic management plan to PI efforts also provides needed metrics to determine the overall state of the organization through the use of a balanced scorecard (BSC) and provides a mechanism for needed improvement through processes such as Lean and Six Sigma.

Ginter et al. (2013) described the use of both analytical and emergent approaches to strategic management as encompassed in three parts: (1) strategic thinking, (2) strategic planning, and (3) strategic momentum management. These authors stated that strategic thinking is the job of all employees because everyone's work must be reinvented to be in tune with the world. Strategic planning encompasses traditional strategic management activities using strategic thinking and is generally the easiest to complete. Finally, strategic momentum is focused on the strategies that are needed to achieve organizational goals. This integrated approach presents an effective strategic management process.

Finally, the complex nature of health care decrees that leaders contemplate systems theory related to strategic planning and management work. Lindberg and Clancey (2010) proclaimed that conventional methods of improvement—for example, Lean and Six Sigma—were under siege because these approaches were not effective in social organizations such as hospitals. Consider the prominence of hospital-acquired infections and the efforts expended toward improvement efforts, yet national statistics document that this patient safety event is pervasive (Reed & May, 2011).

Lindberg and Clancey (2010) proposed that *Positive Deviance (PD)*, which holds that within organizations some individuals or groups have different "deviant" practices that produce better "positive" (p. 152) outcomes. PD holds that staff at the point of care understand what works, what does not work, and what the barriers are to safe practice (bottom-up management). The job is to discover the positive deviant practice, and then through widespread engagement spread this best practice throughout the organization and system. This is contrasted to the traditional PI efforts that are deployed in many healthcare organizations as part of strategic management processes (see the section titled "Strategic Management" later in this chapter). PD is an example of an *emergent strategic management* process that should be considered by leaders in the contemporary healthcare environment for organizations to be competitive in the market.

A final important motivator for hospitals and providers to transition to a contemporary strategic management process was clearly outlined by the American Hospital Association (AHA, 2011) in the seminal work *Hospitals and Care Systems of the Future*. The authors outlined 10 must-do strategies (p. 4) that hospitals must implement in preparation for the future *value-based market* dynamic, termed the "second curve" (p. 3), see **TABLE 9.1**.

▶ Traditional Strategic Management

The traditional strategic management process traces the following map: (1) situation analysis, (2) strategy formation, (3) strategy deployment, and (4) strategic management, which encompasses measurement, evaluation, and PI. **TABLE 9.2** outlines the traditional strategic management process. Blatstein (2012) noted that the real value of the process was not the strategic plan but the

TABLE 9.1 10 Must-Do Strategies for Organizational Strategic Planning	
Strategy 1	Aligning hospitals, physicians, and other providers across the care continuum
Strategy 2	Utilizing evidence-based practices to improve quality and patient safety
Strategy 3	Improving efficiency through productivity and financial management
Strategy 4	Developing integrated information systems
Strategy 5	Joining and growing integrated provider networks and care systems
Strategy 6	Educating and engaging employees and physicians to create leaders
Strategy 7	Strengthening finances to facilitate reinvestment and innovation
Strategy 8	Partnering with payers
Strategy 9	Advancing through scenario-based strategic, financial, and operational planning
Strategy 10	Seeking population health improvement through pursuit of the "triple aim"

Reproduced from American Hospital Association. (2011). *Hospitals and care systems of the future.* Chicago, IL: AHA.

TABLE 9.2 Traditional Strategic Management Process

Situation Analysis	Strategy Formation	Strategy Deployment	Strategic Management
External environmental analysis: ■ Opportunities ■ Threats	Directional strategies: ■ Mission ■ Vision ■ Values ■ Goals and objectives	Culture	Goals and objectives
Internal environmental analysis: ■ Strengths ■ Weakness	Adaptive strategies	Structure	Measurement ■ Balanced scorecard
■ Mission ■ Vision ■ Values ■ Goals	Market entry strategies	Resources	Evaluation standards
	Competitive strategies		Performance improvement

journey that participants take in exploring the future. Such planning reveals future possibilities not previously recognized and helps shape the future for the organization.

Situation Analysis

Situation analysis, the initial stage of strategic planning, is the process of determining the current state of the organization. Although historical data are an asset in determining the current state, leaders should resolve to avoid the trap of focusing on the analysis of past performance. Zuckerman (1998) described this phenomenon as "analysis paralysis," a serious problem that can bog down the strategic planning process. Undue emphasis on past performance can result in loss of focus and momentum. Key players may become disinterested, and buy-in may be lost.

Leaders must focus on *results*, not "busy work." There will always be those in the group who insist on more and better data; however,

profiling key business drivers for the organization should be captured and analyzed on an ongoing basis, thus negating the need for overanalysis of historical data. Rarely are data needed beyond the past 5 years.

Key issues to consider include which factors are within the control or influence of the organization and how external forces affect the competitive position of the organization. Understanding and analyzing the current situation are accomplished through three interrelated processes: external environmental analysis, internal environmental analysis, and the development of the organization's mission, vision, values, and goals. These processes are not separate and distinct but rather overlap, interact with, and influence one another.

External Environmental Analysis

The first process, *external environmental analysis*, focuses on determining the current position of the organization within both the general environment and the healthcare environment. This profile is the beginning of a forward-looking process that considers market trends and forecasts (Zuckerman, 1998). To understand the *external environment*, the organization must look outside its boundaries (beyond itself) to identify and analyze issues taking place outside the organization. These issues represent opportunities and threats and assist in identifying "what the organization should do." This analysis is needed because available resources, competencies, and capabilities influence success in the external environment.

Opportunities and threats influence strategy formation and represent fundamental issues that can directly affect the success or failure of the organization. It is insufficient to simply be aware of these issues; healthcare leaders need to understand the nature of the opportunities and threats before they affect the organization. Organizational leaders must have an effective method for scanning the external environment for pertinent information. **TABLE 9.3** lists the external factors to be considered that have the potential to affect the business (Ginter et al., 2002). Factors to be considered include (Ginter et al., 2002):

Primary market research is completed by focusing on competitive and market changes external to the organization. This information helps to determine the organization's competitive position in the market. Market research is completed through interviews, focus groups, and surveys. Targets of this research include senior leaders of competitor organizations, community leaders, primary employers, and those knowledgeable of the market situation. The primary task is to generate information, thereby decreasing the uncertainty that comes with the managerial art of decision making. Research means literally to "search again," a process whereby one looks at the data to understand all that needs to be known about a subject (Zikmund, 2003). Although caution must be exercised so that this aspect of the process does not take an undue amount of

TABLE 9.3 External Factors that Affect the Business

Legislative & Political Changes	■ Review is necessary to determine any major environmental influences that may affect the future performance of the organization. ■ Major trends should be profiled for the past 3–5 years. ■ Forecasting should be identified with a focus on minimizing negative impacts and maximizing potential benefits.
Economic Modification	■ Forecasts should be exercised with caution; avoid overanalysis. ■ Do not ignore shifts in the national economy.
Demographic Changes	■ Consider the impact of an aging population and increased life span. ■ Population shifts, including social trends, can indicate targets for future market growth. ■ Critical shortages of clinical staff necessitates focus on recruitment and retention efforts.
Technology	■ Needs continue to escalate. ■ Seamless integration is needed. ■ Confidentiality is a major concern.
Competitive Market Changes	■ Identify the organization's current competitive position in the market (interviews, focus groups, surveys).

time and resources and is not overemphasized, leaders must know the market. At times, research reveals information not readily apparent but key to success in the market.

The secret of business is to know something nobody else knows.

—**Aristotle Onassis**

A parallel matrix is helpful when analyzing the external environment. This matrix allows visualization of competitively relevant threats with external opportunities. **TABLE 9.4** provides an example parallel matrix.

Internal Environmental Analysis

Recall that available resources, competencies, and capabilities influence success in the external environment. *Internal environmental analysis* involves an extensive review of internal processes, culture, structure, and technology to reveal strengths and weaknesses. Strengths are those things that the organization does well, not only from the viewpoint of the organization's employees but from the customer's viewpoint (DeSilets & Dickerson, 2008). *Weaknesses* represent organizational vulnerabilities and include processes that are not functioning at the desired level and are in need of PI project work. Nevertheless, resources are finite, and thus targeted projects should link to the organization's strategy.

Shirey (2011) noted that the *influence of organizational culture* when executing strategy cannot be underestimated. Thus, cultural norms must be considered early in the strategic planning process. This is important because culture is enduring and difficult to change (Shirey, 2011). These proclamations are linked to the results of a Wharton School study (Hrebiniak, 2005) that documented that managing change was often the most important factor for successful execution of organizational strategy. Furthermore, Hrebiniak (2005) noted that many leaders in the study held that the ability to change was synonymous with the ability to manage change of the organizational culture. Leaders must consider whether selected strategies that require change have an impact on the culture of the organization. For example, if a strategy is selected by leaders without input from employees in an organization with a history of effective shared governance, the change may not be embraced; thus, execution may be sabotaged and the selected strategy may fail, or the change may not be sustained.

Review of the *structure of the organization* during the internal environmental analysis may reveal strengths or weaknesses. For example, the traditional hierarchical bureaucratic organizational structure continues to be prevalent, especially in large healthcare organizations and systems. Bureaucracies were originally developed to promote efficiency and production during the Industrial Age when divisions of labor and a centralized formal structure promoted production

TABLE 9.4 External Environment Parallel Matrix

Nurse's Heaven Hospital Strategic Plan 20XX Opportunities and Threats	
Opportunities	**Threats**
No competitors offer wound management services.	Increased competition from larger medical center serving the same population.
The hospital owns six vacant physician offices; five new physicians are needed.	Larger medical center recently constructed five new physician offices that are connected to the facility.

(Yoder-Wise, 2010). However, contemporary knowledge workers desire autonomy and the authority to act at all levels of the organization. Thus, flat or participatory management structures and shared governance models demonstrate that leaders trust employees' to act appropriately and that employees embrace accountability. This is important in turbulent environments such as health care where being proactive may facilitate customer satisfaction.

As healthcare systems become internally integrated (radiology, nursing, laboratory, pharmacy, and other ancillary departments), the interface often becomes a logistical nightmare. No one technology system has "one-stop shopping," whereas one system might excel in a key feature but may be deficient in another.

In the internal environmental analysis phase, Gelatt (1993) cautioned against *info-mania*. He described info-mania as the idolizing of information. *Info-maniacs* worship facts. There is sure to be at least one member of the leadership team who demands more and more facts even when the team is drowning in information. Caution is advised because focusing only on facts leaves little time or energy for innovation. Healthcare leaders must understand the competitive relevance of identified issues. Weaknesses require strategies to minimize the vulnerability of the organization, whereas strengths must be optimized to maximize their impact. This information provides a foundation for strategy formulation (Ginter et al., 2002). Plotting strengths and weaknesses on a parallel matrix (**TABLE 9.5**) provides a visual for evaluating the competitive advantages relative to strengths and the competitive relevance of weaknesses.

The real voyage of discovery consists not in seeking new landscapes, but in having new eyes.

—Marcel Proust

Zuckerman (1998) explained that *primary market research* serves to gather information regarding the organization's strengths and weaknesses as it relates to its competitors and to involve leadership in the strategic planning process. Leaders should begin by reviewing any recent market research that is available and gathering information through interviews, focus groups, and surveys. Primary target groups for market research include board members, physicians, health professionals, management staff, and other key stakeholders of the organization.

Many organizations use *focus groups* to solicit *stakeholder input* (Krueger, 1988; Morgan, 1993). Focus groups incur significant cost (time and money); thus, priority is given to key customer groups such as patients, families, team members, community members, and physicians. A focus group consists of a small group of individuals (6–10), usually with similar interests, who participate in an unstructured, free-flowing interview with a skilled facilitator. The facilitator begins by introducing the topic with the goal of uncovering core issues related

TABLE 9.5 Internal Environment Parallel Matrix

Nurse's Heaven Hospital Strategic Plan 20XX Strengths and Weaknesses	
Strengths	**Weaknesses**
Convenient ground level parking	Lack of sufficient parking Monday–Friday
Patient-oriented team members	Team member turnover rate exceeds regional average

to strategic planning. A recorder documents key statements for management to consider in strategy development. Caution must be used, however, because focus groups may not represent the entire population.

Mission, Vision, Values, and Goals

The mission, vision, values, and goals of the organization ultimately affect the strategy that is adopted. A clear understanding by all employees of these foundational underpinnings cannot be overemphasized. MacPhee (2007) stressed that change strategies begin with an analysis of the mission and vision. The mission and vision provide a framework for analysis of personal and organizational values. This is especially important considering the rapid pace of change in the healthcare market where organizations are competitors one day, and the next day, organizations within a merged system.

According to Ginter et al. (2002), the organization's *mission* is the articulation of the external opportunities and threats and the internal strengths and weaknesses. Simply, the mission is the reason the organization exists. The mission of the organization must not be just clichéd words framed on the wall. Likewise, the *vision* is the view of the future based on the understanding of environmental forces. Chapman (2003) described three elements of effective mission and vision statements: clear and easy to remember, a call for dramatic improvement in the lives of others, and proclamation by leaders who, through example, demonstrate a passionate commitment to making the statements come alive.

The core *values* constitute the fundamental truths that the organization holds dear and reflect the philosophy of the organization. Examples include honesty, integrity, customer service, and commitment to excellence. *Goals* specify the major direction of the organization and provide actionable linkage to the mission. The mission, vision, values, and goals are considered a part of the situation analysis because they are

influenced by the results of both external and internal environmental analyses.

Strategy Formation

The first step in the traditional strategic planning process, situation analysis, involves data gathering. *Strategy formation* uses these data for decision making. These decisions are critical to the success of the organization because they become the organization's strategy. Ginter et al. (2013) described four types of strategies: directional, adaptive, market entry, and competitive.

Directional Strategies

Although the mission, vision, values, goals, and objectives are part of the situation analysis, they are also part of strategy formation because they provide the broadest direction for the organization—*directional strategies*. The mission, vision, values, and goals indicate what the organization wants to do. These strategies reflect the critical success factors within the particular service category—in this case, health care. Critical success factors are applicable to all competitors and take into account the external environment. In other words, they define what the organization must accomplish to stay in business. These strategies provide initial direction for the organization and guidance when making key organizational decisions. The reciprocal relationship (adapted from Ginter et al., 2002, p. 177) of directional strategies is shown in **FIGURE 9.1**.

Mission

■ *Articulates the organization's purpose or reason that it exists*

The mission statement describes what makes the organization distinct and reflects the expectations of stakeholders, those who have an interest in the business. In short, the mission defines the organization and describes what it does. The mission statement must be more than

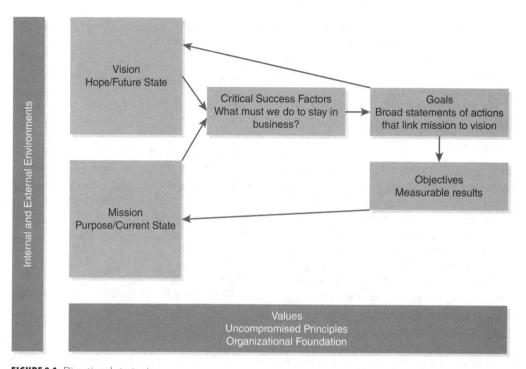

FIGURE 9.1 Directional strategies

Modified from Ginter, P.M., Swayne, L.E., & Duncan, W.J. (2001). *Strategic management of health care organizations* (4th ed.). Malden, MA: Blackwell. Reproduced with permission of Blackwell Publishing, Incorporated.

an attractive wall hanging. The mission must be communicated and lived by all team members in the organization, especially team members who work directly with customers.

Vision

- *Describes the optimal future state of the business*

The vision should create a mental picture of what the organization will be when leaders and team members accomplish their mission. It describes the hope for the future—what should the organization be 5 years from now? Time and effort link the mission (what the organization is today) and vision (what it will be in the future). The vision should be stated in clear, simple terms that provide a challenge and leave no doubt as to the importance of the vision. Stakeholders should be able to understand the vision and commit it to memory. The vision should be inspiring and

is generally not stated in quantitative terms. Though the vision should stand the test of time, it should be constantly challenged and revised when necessary.

Values

- *Represent the basic principles, fundamental beliefs, and tenets of team members, and define what they deem important to the organization*

Values state uncompromised principles that are timeless and do not change with the ever-changing climate of business operations. Some organizations use the terminology "guiding principles" to refer to values. Values guide beliefs, attitudes, and behaviors and provide the foundation for operating the business. Key business decisions should be measured against the values of the organization so that the organization never loses sight of its purpose.

Goals

- *Broad statements that provide direction for team members and link the mission to actions necessary to reach the vision*

Blatstein (2012) stated that goals answer the question, "Where do I want to go?" (p. 33). The author described the importance of a "Big Hairy Audacious Goal (BHAG)" (p. 33), a stretch goal for the organization that is difficult to achieve. The BHAG motivates leaders to consider opportunities and obstacles for the future. During the discussions of the BHAG, as leaders reach common ground related to the goal, leaders gain insight about what motivates and inspires others. This work enables leaders to work together better as a team (Blatstein, 2012). Goals that focus on activities unrelated to the organization's critical success factors have the potential of diverting leadership attention and team member energy. The number of goals should be limited for the same reasons. Goals should be stated in easily understood terms so that team members can readily link what they need to do with the mission and vision for the organization.

Objectives

- *Designed to make each goal operational*

This is an important step because objectives provide a mechanism for quantifiable results or outcomes to measure success. Objectives describe the results to be achieved, when they are to be done and by whom, and they should be measurable. **TABLE 9.6** offers examples of goals and objectives.

The mission, vision, values, goals, objectives, and the external and internal environmental analyses depict the essence of the organization. These entities provide a basis for strategy formation, and thus it is important that this work be completed with careful thought and analysis.

Adaptive Strategies

Whereas directional strategies provide general guidance, *adaptive strategies* are more specific and describe the process for carrying out the directional strategies. Directional strategies are the ends, whereas adaptive strategies are the means. Adaptive strategies describe how the organization will expand, contract, or maintain its scope of services (Ginter et al., 2002). These are the strategies most visible to those outside the organization.

Expansion Strategies

Expansion strategies include diversification, vertical integration, market development, product

TABLE 9.6 An Example of Goals and Objectives	
Goal	**Objective**
1. Expand Women's Services to encompass all key aspects of the business.	1. The director of Women's Health will direct the completion of renovations of the existing unit by December 31, 20XX.
2. Position Nurse's Heaven Hospital as a strong community hospital with a focus on primary care.	2. The Chief Executive Officer will recruit six hospitalists by August 31, 20XX.
3. Develop a comprehensive healthcare system that includes primary care, radiation therapy, skilled nursing facilities, home health, and durable medical equipment.	3. The Chief Nursing officer will recruit/hire 20 team members for the skilled nursing unit by November 30, 20XX.

development, and penetration (Ginter et al., 2002). *Diversification* occurs at the corporate level when markets outside the organization's core business offer the potential for significant growth. Because the organization is venturing outside the core business, diversification is generally considered a risky venture. Diversification is most often seen in health care when there are opportunities in less-regulated markets.

There are two types of diversification (Ginter et al., 2002): related and unrelated. In healthcare organizations, *related diversification (concentric)* includes related products and services such as home health, hospice, or radiation treatment. *Unrelated diversification (conglomerate)* includes businesses in the general environment, such as a laundry, restaurant, or office buildings, and those within the healthcare industry, such as pharmaceuticals, medical supplies, or insurance. Selecting markets and products that complement one another can reduce risk. Nevertheless, unrelated diversification has been found to be generally unsuccessful in generating revenue for healthcare organizations. Ginter and Swayne (2006) warned that unrelated diversification may not be realistic in health care because such organizations have a dominant core business (patient care) that is capital and human intensive, and thus it is difficult for healthcare organizations to be successful outside the core business.

Vertical integration is the second corporate-level expansion of adaptive strategies. The purpose of vertical integration in health care is to enhance the continuity of care while simultaneously managing the channel of demand for healthcare services. Healthcare organizations that use vertical integration grow the business along the channel of distribution of core processes (Ginter et al., 2002). Vertical integration can reduce supply costs and enhance integration. A successful example would be the inclusion of technical education programs for team members in critically short supply, such as nursing assistants and technicians. Vertical integration was the fundamental adaptive strategy of the 1990s. This rapid change was realized as hospitals joined networks or systems in an effort to secure resources, increase

capabilities, and gain greater bargaining power with purchasers and healthcare plans (Ginter et al., 2002). Nevertheless, Ginter and Swayne (2006) recommended caution when considering vertical integration for the same reasons listed earlier regarding unrelated diversification.

Market development occurs at the division or strategic service unit level and focuses on entering new markets with existing products or services. The purpose of this strategy is to add volume through geographic expansion of the service area or by expansion into new market segments within the present geographic area (Ginter et al., 2002). *Horizontal integration* is a type of market development that grows the business by acquiring or affiliating with competitors. Horizontal growth of healthcare systems in the 1980s and early 1990s created multihospital systems. Many of the expected benefits such as reduction of duplication of services, economics of scale, improved productivity, and operating efficiencies did not materialize, and horizontal integration strategies slowed in the late 1990s (Ginter et al., 2002). In addition, Ginter and Swayne (2006) stated that service area limited the market development (expansion) of many services because technologies are often developed by those outside the organization—for example, drug companies and equipment manufacturers.

Product development also occurs at the division or strategic service unit level and involves the introduction of new products or services to existing markets. Whereas related diversification is the introduction of a new product, product development refines, complements, or extends existing products or services, such as women's health or cancer treatment. Product development may be used when customer requirements are changing, technology is changing, or when there is a need to create a differentiation advantage (Ginter et al., 2002).

Penetration strategies, like market and product development, focus on increasing volumes and market share. Market penetration is an aggressive marketing strategy centered on extending existing services. This strategy is used when the present market is growing and expected revenues are high (Ginter et al., 2002).

Contraction Strategies

When the organization needs to decrease the size or scope of operations at either the corporate or divisional level, four *contraction strategies* are considered. Divestiture and liquidation occur at the corporate level, and harvesting and retrenchment occur at the divisional level (Ginter et al., 2002).

When a service unit is viable yet a decision to leave the market and sell an operating unit is made, *divestiture* occurs. Generally, the divested business unit has value and will continue to be operated by the purchasing organization (Ginter et al., 2002). This strategy has become common over the past decade as healthcare organizations carve out noncore business. Examples of noncore healthcare business that may be divested include pharmacy, laboratory, and radiology. Business units may be divested for several reasons, including industry decline, the need for cash to fund priority operations, or marginal performance. Services too far from the core business may be divested in an effort to focus on business at hand, or management expertise for the particular service may not be available within the leadership group.

Liquidation is the selling of assets of an organization that can no longer operate. In contrast to divestiture, liquidation assumes that the operating unit cannot be sold as a viable operation (Ginter et al., 2002). Some assets, of course, may still have value, such as buildings and equipment. Reasons for liquidation include bankruptcy, the need to dispose of non-productive assets, the need to reduce assets, or the emergence of expensive new technology that will make the current technology obsolete.

Harvesting occurs when the market has entered long-term decline or there is a need for short-term cash (Ginter et al., 2002). For example, despite a strong market position, revenues are expected to decline industry-wide over the coming years. The unit will be allowed to generate as much revenue as possible; however, no new resources will be invested in the business. This allows for an orderly exit from the market by planned downsizing. Harvesting has occurred with many small rural hospitals that could not maintain or improve their financial positions because of the lack of physician and community support, an aging population, and the migration of the young to urban areas.

Retrenchment occurs when the market has become too diverse, and there is a decline in profitability as a result of increasing costs (Ginter et al., 2002). Although the market is still viewed as viable, costs are too high. Retrenchment involves redefinition of the market if it is too spread out geographically. Costs such as personnel or facility assets that are marginal or non-productive are reduced.

Recall, however, the role of the organization's mission as related to contraction strategies. Ginter and Swayne (2006) noted that contraction strategies may be limited in healthcare organizations because services may be mandated, needed by the community, or core to the organization's mission.

Maintenance-of-Scope Strategies

When current strategies are appropriate and few changes are needed, the organization may use *maintenance-of-scope strategies* to *maintain* the existing market position. This does not mean that the organization does nothing. It instead pursues either enhancement or status quo strategies (Ginter et al., 2002). Carefully crafting the PI process through direct linkage to resources and performance measures will ensure that processes remain in control or that those that do not perform well are evident to leaders and managers.

When the organization is progressing toward its vision yet still requires improvements, *enhancement strategy* may be used. This may entail quality improvement efforts directed toward improving organizational processes or reducing costs. This is a time for innovation and redesign of timeworn systems. The focus should be on those identified as most important to key customers such as patients and families.

Status quo is based on the assumption of a mature market when growth has ceased. The goal is to maintain the market share. When using the status quo strategy, organizations may attempt penetration or market/product development (Ginter et al., 2002).

Market Entry Strategies

The three major strategies to enter a market include: purchase, cooperation, and development. *Market entry strategies* are not ends in themselves, but rather adaptive strategies that may be used to bring market strategies to fruition (Ginter et al., 2002).

Purchase Strategies

There are three *purchase market entry strategies*: acquisition, licensing, and venture capital investment. *Purchase strategies* enable a healthcare organization to enter the market quickly. Each strategy places different demands on the organization (Ginter et al., 2002).

When healthcare organizations purchase an existing organization, organizational unit, or a product or service, *acquisition entry strategy* is used. Acquisition takes place at the corporate or divisional level. The acquisition may be integrated into existing operations, or it may operate as a separate unit. Acquisitions often flounder because it is difficult to integrate existing culture and operations. Often, it takes several years postacquisition to combine two organizational cultures. Despite the difficulties of integrating cultures, the synergy realized by the creation of a comprehensive healthcare system has demonstrated that acquisition is an effective purchase strategy.

Licensing avoids the time and market risks of technology or product development (Ginter et al., 2002). When licensure is used as a strategy, proprietary technology is usually not purchased, and therefore the organization is dependent on the licensor for support and upgrade. Healthcare organizations frequently use licensing strategies for implementation of clinical documentation systems. This strategy lowers the financial and market risk of technologies outside the core business.

Venture capital investment is a low-risk option whereby healthcare organizations purchase minority investment in a developing enterprise. This provides an opportunity to "try out" and, possibly later, enter into new technology. Examples include life science portals for bioinformatics, home-based healthcare services for elderly adults, and cardiology arrhythmia management companies (Ginter et al., 2002).

Cooperation Strategies

According to Ginter et al. (2002) mergers, alliances, and joint ventures—*cooperation strategies*—were the most popular strategies of the 1990s. Cooperation strategies enable organizations to carry out adaptive strategies.

Although similar to acquisitions, a *merger* involves two organizations combining through mutual agreement to form a single new organization (recall that, in an acquisition, a healthcare organization purchases an existing organization, organizational unit, or a product or service). Merger strategies are used to accomplish horizontal integration by combining two similar organizations, or vertical integration, by creating an integrated delivery system. Reasons for mergers include improving efficiency and effectiveness (combining resources and exploiting cost-reduction strategies), enhancing access (broader services), enhancing financial position (gaining market share), and overcoming concerns of survival (enduring in an aggressive market). As with acquisitions, the major hurdle in a merger is the integration of two separate organizational cultures. Because a new organization is formed, mergers are often more difficult to navigate than acquisitions are. In a merger, a totally new organizational culture must be developed. If mergers are to be successful, work groups must be formed to reformulate the mission, vision, and core values of the new organization.

The merger of two organizational cultures into one takes years to complete (Ginter et al., 2002).

Alliance strategies entail arrangements among existing organizations to achieve a strategic purpose not possible by any single organization. Alliances include federations, consortiums, networks, and systems. Alliances attempt to strengthen competitive position while the organizations maintain their independence. Healthcare organizations often form an alliance to achieve economies of scale in purchasing. Although not a merger or acquisition, alliances have many of the same issues with conflicting cultures.

Joint ventures are used when risks are too high or the project is too large or too expensive to be done by a single organization. In a joint venture, two or more organizations combine resources to accomplish a designated task. The most common healthcare joint ventures are

- Contractual agreements
- Subsidiary corporations
- Partnerships
- Not-for-profit title-holding corporations

In a *contractual agreement*, two or more organizations contract to work together toward specific objectives. *Subsidiary corporations* form a new corporation, usually to operate non–healthcare activities. A partnership is a formal or informal arrangement between two or more parties for mutual benefit of the organizations involved. *Not-for-profit title-holding corporations* form tax-exempt title-holding corporations to provide benefits to healthcare organizations engaged in real estate ventures. The dynamic healthcare environment mandates that organizations engage in joint ventures to lower costs (Ginter et al., 2002).

Development Strategies

In the final stage of strategic formation, a *gap analysis* examines the difference in the current state and the desired state, or the vision for the future. Gap analysis is the process of examining how large a leap must be taken to meet the vision, and what must be done to make the leap.

If organizational leaders set their vision too narrow, they will find their current state meets the vision but lacks incentive to aspire for higher and greater things. Their task is accomplished, and the planning process ends. With this in mind, leaders must communicate the vision in a somewhat revolutionary manner. The vision should inspire team members to perform their best because there is no room for mediocrity in healthcare vision. The desired outcome of the gap analysis is a strategic plan that has a reasonable probability of success. To accomplish this, priorities must be established and resources allocated to narrow the gap between the current state and the desired state. This process establishes the groundwork for the strategies necessary to ensure the desired outcome (Drenkard, 2001).

Planning encompasses stewardship of the organization and its resources. Care must be taken to articulate the core assumptions about the nature of the market, the competitions, and the organization; otherwise, a gap will exist between the aspirations of the organization and the way the organization actually behaves. When what we do day to day is in contrast to what we say we do and hope to be, a paradox exists that leads to team member frustration. For example, does the organization value creativity or discipline? Is the focus on short-term or long-term goals? Quality or the bottom line? Although conflicts occur in every organization, successful organizations meet the challenge and reconcile aspirations and actions as part of the strategic planning process (Solovy, 2002). Decisions regarding resources must be made with the core value—what the patient needs or values and what is best/safest for the patient—as the focal point of the organization. The financial bottom line is a secondary priority to safe care. When the financial bottom line is the priority, money is wasted.

An additional gap can also exist between management's view of the organization and the team members' view. Team members are closer to the core business (patient care), and thus their input must be sought as part of the planning process. A planned process whereby each business unit can share information and seek guidance and clarification facilitates buy-in and avoids duplication of efforts. The alternative, top-down, directive approach may result in a high-quality strategic plan, but team members who have input into planning more readily accept the expected outcomes and so become more vested in work processes. Thus, the process includes a system of notification for team members as to the status of their suggestions and how they were evaluated, or if their ideas were not used, feedback is given to team members as to the rationale.

It is imperative that healthcare leaders understand and focus on their core business. Focusing on the core business provides a clear strategic vision—the big picture—in contrast to scattered plans that steal time and energy with little to show except charts and graphs. Successful organizations focus their strategy on their core rather than on the industry's competitive factors. One method of assessing the health of the organization's strategic planning process is to consider the time spent focusing on the competition. If more time is spent analyzing competitors than focusing on the core business, the process is off task. The primary priorities are the processes and outcomes that the organization must do well to remain in business and those things that the organization does particularly well. Healthcare dollars are scarce. Across-the-board investing often signals that competitors are setting the organization's agenda. Conversely, when an organization's strategy is formed reactively as it tries to keep up with competitors, it loses its uniqueness (Kim & Mauborgne, 2002).

Strategy Deployment

Failure to implement the strategic plan is the most common flaw in the planning process (Zuckerman, 1998). Martin (2010) warned that "a mediocre strategy well executed is better than a great strategy poorly executed" (p. 66). Thus, carefully crafted strategies are useless if sufficient time is not spent developing the plan for *strategy deployment* (Shirey, 2011). Zuckerman (1998) emphasized that team members may be overwhelmed with managing the day-to-day

crises, leaving little time to implement strategic objectives. In addition, if the objectives are not specific, team members may lack the direction needed to meet the established goals. Communication of the strategic plan must be coordinated throughout the entire organization both vertically and horizontally. To provide direction at the work level, goals and objectives must be established for each business unit and ought to link to the overall plan for the organization. This linkage provides guidance and consistency in decision making and enables managers and team members to understand the present and plan for the future. All team members must be able to articulate how "what they do" fits into the overall plan for the organization.

For each goal and objective, *at least one person should be assigned as the primary individual responsible for planning, implementing, and monitoring progress.* This is often a member of senior leadership. Specific target dates are assigned to provide a timeline for expected progress. If realization of goals involves intradepartmental work processes, PI teams may be assigned. Senior leadership should establish specific dates to review progress toward each goal. Accountability is accomplished (and rewarded, or otherwise) through linkage between the goals and objectives of the strategic plan and individual team member evaluation criteria. **TABLE 9.7** provides an excerpt from a strategic planning matrix.

Culture

The *culture* of the organization includes the shared assumptions, values, and behavioral norms of the group. These assumptions and values remain constant over time, even when membership of the organization changes, and are the basis for an informal consciousness (Ginter et al., 2002). This is significant in the current climate of mergers, acquisitions, and buy-outs. The shared values of team members may not reflect the values of the organization. When this occurs, the customary way of doing things (behavioral norms) may sabotage the strategic plan. To ensure congruency, shared assumptions (mission—who we

TABLE 9.7 Sample of Strategic Planning Matrix

	Nurse's Heaven Hospital			Strategic Plan 20XX	
Goal	Objective	Actions	Measure/ Benchmark	Target Date	Responsible Party
Expand Women's Services to encompass all key aspects of the business	Complete renovations of the existing unit by 12/31/XX	1. Monitor progress daily 2. Facilitate weekly construction progress meeting 3. Facilitate monthly medical staff meetings 4. Facilitate biweekly team member meetings	1. Phase I complete by 08/31/XX 2. Phase II complete by 10/31/XX 3. Complete Phase III by 12/31/XX Benchmark: There Medical Center, Anywhere, USA	12/31/20XX	Director of Women's Health

are) must support the organizational vision and goals (what we want to accomplish). If the plan is in conflict with the culture, deployment will be a challenge. Unfortunately, if the culture is in significant conflict with the strategic plan and a strong subculture exists, change will be difficult because team members may prefer to "do things the way we have always done them."

Ginter and Swayne (2006) warn that healthcare organizations have a unique culture related to power. These authors noted that healthcare organizations, and hospitals in particular, have a history of hierarchical power that hampers planning and participation from those closest to the patient. To be cognizant of the assumptions, values, and behavioral norms of team members, successful leaders are involved in the day-to-day operations of the organization. Healthcare leaders must schedule regular visits to each business unit.

In addition, regular visits to all stakeholders are imperative. It is not acceptable to attempt to lead from the office or through computer technology. Email, voice mail, video conferencing, and other technologies do not take the place of face-to-face contact, nor do they reflect a complete picture of the culture of the organization. Insights gleaned from involvement with stakeholders and the day-to-day operations of the organization provide vital insight during the situation analysis. Leaders must assess whether the directional strategies are still appropriate and reflect the culture of the organization. *Considering the organizational culture is perhaps the most crucial aspect in the deployment of the strategic plan.*

It is important to consider strategies that assist in developing a culture that is adaptive to change. Involving stakeholders in the strategic planning process cultivates an environment of trust and respect. Buy-in from those involved in the processes and outcomes of care is worth the extra time necessary to glean these insights. This input is especially pertinent during the shaping of directional strategies—mission, vision, values, and goals. Cultural assessment during the situation analysis may determine that additional implementation strategies are necessary to maintain or change the organizational culture. As previously mentioned, the roles of nurse leaders position them to be acutely aware of the "pulse" of the organization. Nurse leaders must feel comfortable expressing views different from those in senior leadership. An atmosphere of trust encourages risk taking and is necessary for innovation to occur. If trust is absent, personal safety and security become the priority, and the status quo will be maintained despite an elaborate strategic plan. In addition, time and money may be wasted on endeavors that do not reflect current customer needs.

Maintaining a climate of trust and respect, one that encourages risk taking and innovation, is hard work. Leaders must "walk the talk." Saying one thing while doing another (or, even more critical, rewarding another) creates confusion. The directional strategies, mission, vision, values, and goals must be communicated often, both verbally and in writing. The key strategy for maintenance of an organizational culture that is adaptive to change is to live it as reflected in the daily business of the organization.

Structure

Ginter et al. (2002) described three basic organizational structures: functional structure, divisional structure, and matrix structure. Similar to organizational culture, structure must not impede the overall strategy.

Functional organizational structures organize activities around mission-critical functions or processes. This is the most prevalent organizational structure for organizations with a relatively narrow focus such as healthcare organizations. Departments are organized according to their function, such as clinical services, finance,

marketing, or information systems. Organizations that are structured around mission-critical functions may consider clinical services as the center of the functional structure with other sections of the organization organized around clinical processes such as registration, radiology, laboratory, and so forth (Ginter et al., 2002).

Health care is highly specialized, and expertise within the specialty is highly valued. Functional structures can foster efficiency; however, this type of structure can also result in silo mentality. Functional structure slows decision making, makes coordination of work difficult, and inhibits communication as each department looks after its own interest without the realization of how its processes affect others.

Divisional structures are common in healthcare organizations that have grown through diversification, vertical integration, or market or product development (Ginter et al., 2002). Divisional organizations attempt to break down larger, diverse organizations into more manageable and focused sections. This division is especially important when structures of the organization are in different geographic locales, and thus have a different environment and unique customers. Divisional structures have difficulty in maintaining a consistent image and purpose. Divisional structures may additionally require multiple layers of management and duplication of services, thus increasing costs. Organizations that choose divisional structures must carefully coordinate strategic business unit activities.

Matrix structures organize activities around problems to be solved rather than functions, products, or geography (Ginter et al., 2002). The nurse manager may have a dual reporting structure, to the vice president of Women's Health (product) as well as to the vice president of Nursing Services (functional). Thus, the nurse manager is responsible to the vice president of Nursing for nursing care and to the vice president of Women's Health when working on the women's health product line. In some matrix structures, the reporting relationships follow a project or program, and the relationship ends when the project is complete. Matrix structures foster creativity and innovation; nevertheless, they are difficult to manage because priorities can become confused. Thus, matrix structures require expert coordination and communication.

Resources

Deploying the selected strategies uses four key resources: financial, human, information systems, and technology (Ginter et al., 2002). Analysis of *financial resources* was a key factor in the internal environmental analysis. In addition, finance provided key input for strategy formation. Once strategies have been decided, finance is the vehicle to implement them. Leaders should require that major purchase requests be submitted with documented links to the strategic plan. Major projects require capital investment, which generally must be approved by the governing body.

Human resources must be considered before deployment of the strategic plan. There are several questions to consider: Will additional training be required? Are additional team members needed? Will there be a need for team members with different skills and experiences? This is a critical time to complete an organizational learning needs assessment with all team members. This provides a bridge between the strategic plan, education plan, and PI plan. Multiple plans should be consolidated into one master strategic plan. This is less confusing for team members and assists with unified communication of the organization's plan for improvement.

Although *information resources* are crucial to develop the internal and external environmental analysis, they are equally important in the deployment of the strategic plan. As previously mentioned, clinicians can no longer be expected to complete laborious paper documentation. Likewise, leaders must be able to extract data entered into clinical documentation systems with relative ease, thereby negating the need for manual data extraction.

The strategies selected drive the needed technologies. *Strategic technology* is concerned with the type of organization, the sophistication of the equipment, and management of the technology used *within* the organization (Ginter et al., 2002). Healthcare organizations are high-technology organizations. Equipment becomes obsolete as quickly as it is installed. This is an area of increasing concern for healthcare leaders because it represents major expenditures for the organization.

Strategic Management Goals and Objectives

Table 9.7 demonstrates a sample strategic planning matrix. Senior leaders ensure that team members remain focused by assigning specific dates/times for review of the status of each goal and objective. Someone once said, "People respect what you inspect." An additional pertinent adage is, "You are what you measure." Although these statements are poor examples of transformational leadership, the adages unfortunately hold true. Assessment of efforts toward meeting established goals and objectives not only keeps leaders aware of the status of planning efforts, but it also provides team members the opportunity to "show off" their hard work. This personal time and attention by senior leaders demonstrate that the strategic plan is a working document that ebbs and flows with the organization.

Measurement: Balanced Scorecard

Kaplan and Norton (1996) of the Harvard Business School developed scorecards (also known as dashboards, instrument panels, and data display devices) in 1991. The utility of the BSC remains unchanged—the provision of a strategic management and performance management tool. Measurement of key financial, quality, market, and operational indicators provides management with an understanding of performance in relation to established strategic goals and graphically displays a snapshot of the institution's overall health (Health Care Advisory Board, 1999).

As organizations grow increasingly complex, it is critical that leaders have easy access to accurate data that provide a view of overall organizational performance rather than being inundated with mountains of disparate reports. The Health Care Advisor Board (2002) noted in its study of hospital downturns that inadequate performance measurement was the cause of 10% of financial flashpoints—such as unexpected, dramatic declines in total margin and cash flow. This is another reason that supports the importance of selection of critical metrics.

Performance Improvement

PI is a systematic, organization-wide approach to improving the processes and outcomes of the healthcare system. PI shifts the focus from individual performance to the performance of the organization's systems and processes. There are four basic tenets of PI: *customer focus, continuous improvement of processes, team member involvement*, and *use of data and team knowledge to improve decision making*. To be successful, PI effects must be embraced by senior leaders and must involve all departments and team members in clinical as well as nonclinical areas. PI efforts are a part of the strategic planning process, not a separate function orchestrated to comply with regulatory standards.

Cost-Benefit Analysis

Comparison of the benefits and costs of a proposed endeavor is completed through cost-benefit analysis. *Cost-benefit analysis* is a budgeting and an analytical technique that compares the social costs and benefits of a proposed program against the costs of the venture under consideration. If the benefits outweigh the costs, a positive cost-benefit is expected, and it makes sense to spend the money; otherwise, it does not.

The first step in cost-benefit analysis is to determine the goals of the project—what does the organization hope the project will accomplish? What would the community gain if the project comes to fruition? Identifying goals and objectives clarifies the expected benefit for those served.

Once project goals and objectives have been determined, project benefits must be determined. All losses and gains expected to be experienced by society are included, expressed in dollar terms. Losses incurred to some sections of society are subtracted from the gains that accrue to others. The benefits include only those things that are a direct or indirect result of the project. Alternative strategies are considered so as to choose the option with the greatest net benefit or ratio of benefit to cost (Finkler, 2001). Leaders would not include benefits that are a reality whether or not the project is realized.

Costs must be estimated as part of the cost-benefit analysis. All costs must be considered including opportunity costs because when a decision is made to do something, other alternatives are sacrificed. For example, an increase in inventory requires extra cash. The cash used will not be available for use somewhere else in

EXAMPLE OF COST-BENEFIT ANALYSIS

Although cancer treatment may be available at a tertiary medical center 100 miles away, the dollar costs related to the benefit of not having to travel such a long distance are included in the analysis. An example of one goal of the project might be less travel time for patients in need of cancer treatment. The benefits of cancer treatment, however, are not included in the analysis because they are already available. An example of a consideration in cost is the facility may have to forgo a transplant program to finance the cancer treatment program. This opportunity cost should be estimated. These calculations include the time value of money, too.

the organization (another opportunity). This is a critical consideration in cost-benefit analysis (Finkler, 2001).

To complete the decision analysis, estimated costs and benefits are compared with each other in the form of a ratio—benefits divided by costs. If the resulting metric is greater than 1, the benefits exceed the costs and the project is desirable. The greater the benefit-to-cost ratio, the more advantageous the project (Finkler, 2001).

Break-Even Analysis

Healthcare leaders must seek out projects or ventures to improve financial stability or to subsidize loss leaders, services that lose money but provide a community need. *Break-even analysis (BEA)* determines the minimum volume of services that a program must provide to be financially self-sufficient. This tool is useful for determining the profitability of a new venture. BEA is used in situations in which there is a specific price associated with the service (Finkler, 2001). A BEA is an essential part of a business *pro forma*.

This seems like a simple endeavor—if the reimbursement per unit of service is greater than the cost, the new endeavor would be expected to make a profit. On the other hand, if the expected reimbursement is less than the cost, the new endeavor will lose money. However, cost per unit depends on volume. When volume is low, the cost per unit will be higher. As volumes increase, the venture may become profitable. Thus, it is imperative that the organization understand at what point *revenues (money expected to be received)* will be equal to *expenses (cost to provide the service)*. This is the break-even point.

To grasp the steps in calculating the break-even-point equation, key terminology must be understood:

- *Total revenue* is the average price multiplied by the number of units.
- *Total expenses* include FC and VC.

- *Fixed costs (FC)* are costs that do not change as volume changes within the relevant range (range of activity that would be reasonably expected to occur in the budget period).
- *Variable costs (VC)* vary in direct proportion to volume. When calculating expenses, VC is expressed in VC per unit.

Finkler (2001, p. 107) described the following calculation to find that break-even point. In this example, 1,000 cesarean deliveries, at a total cost of $2,500 per cesarean delivery, generate $2,500,000 in total revenue. The break-even point (at a cost of $2,500 per case) is 450 cesarean deliveries—the point at which total revenue equals total expenses. **FIGURE 9.2** provides a visual example of the break-even point for cesarean deliveries.

Recall that the break-even point occurs when the total revenues equal the total expenses. Thus, the break-even point is calculated as follows:

$$Total\ revenue = P\ (price) \times Q\ (volume)$$

$$Total\ expenses = V\ (Variable\ costs\ [VC] \times Volume\ [Q]) + Fixed\ costs\ (FC)$$

$$P \times Q = (VC \times Q) + FC$$

$$\$1,125,000 \times 450\ cases = \$625,000 \div 450\ (recall\ that\ VC\ is\ per\ case) \times 450\ cases + \$500,000$$

$$(\$1,125,000 = 450\ cases\ at\ \$2,500/case)$$

$$(\$625,000,\ the\ VC = \$1,125,000\ total\ cost - \$500,000\ fixed\ cost)$$

The next step is to subtract (VC × Q) from both sides of the equation:

$$(P \times Q) - (VC \times Q) = FC$$

$$\$1,125,000 \times 450\ cases - (\$625,000 \div 450 \times 450\ cases) = \$500,000$$

Next, factor out the Q from the left side of the equation:

$$Q \times (P - VC) = FC$$

$$450\ cases \times (\$1,125,000 - \$625,000 \div 450\ cases) = \$500,000$$

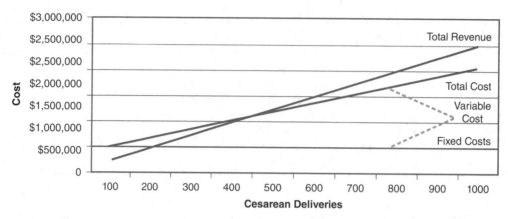

FIGURE 9.2 Break-even point

The resulting formula is as follows:

$$Q = FC \div P - VC$$

Q is the quantity needed to break even.

$$450 \text{ cases} = \$500,000 \div \$1,125,000$$
$$- \$625,000 \div 450 \text{ cases}$$
$$Q = 450 \text{ cases}$$

To summarize, BEA is used to determine the volume at which a service neither makes nor loses money. Volume is vital to profitability because healthcare prices are often fixed, whereas average cost is not fixed (Finkler, Jones, & Kovner, 2013).

Regression Analysis

Understanding regression analysis is imperative for successful budgeting and strategic planning. Nurse managers must understand how to effectively predict a variable (for example, cost) based on an independent variable (for example, patient days). Without this knowledge, nurse managers are merely guessing as to whether their nursing unit can remain financially viable. *Regression analysis* is a statistical technique available in computer software used to forecast the relationship between two variables. The independent variable is typically plotted on the *x*-axis of a scatter graph and the dependent variable is plotted on the *y*-axis. The computer software requires the user to enter the data for the *x* and *y* values. After entering these

data, little more than a command to compute the regression is required. It is important that nurse managers not be intimidated by this technique but rather become familiar with its use in the planning process. Guessing is not suitable for professionals charged with meeting the needs of suffering society.

Regression measures the linear association between a dependent (criterion) and an independent variable (predictor). Regression assumes that the dependent variable is predictively linked to the independent variable. Regression analysis is particularly valuable for forecasting because it attempts to predict the values of a continuous, interval-scaled, dependent variable from the independent variable. For example, the number of full-time equivalent (FTE) team members (the dependent variable) might be predicted on the basis of patient days (the independent variable). Forecasting in this manner is crucial to anticipate staffing needs as volumes fluctuate. Nurse managers may seek input from the finance department related to regression analysis.

▶ Role of the Nurse Leader

Nurse leaders are situated in a unique position to recognize the need for change in the organization.

Sandwiched between the front-line staff and senior leaders, nurse managers may be the first to recognize the need for changes in strategy. Nurse managers stimulate their team members by cultivating a positive culture of performance excellence and a corresponding reward system. The challenge is to define the parameters within which team members can experiment and be innovative. Nurse managers uphold the organization's value system and maintain systems that focus on the core business of patient care. Managers ensure that strategies are in tune with the current needs of customers and are balanced so that one strategy does not suffer at the expense of another. They must be sensitive to important changes and continuously inquire of all their customers as to whether their needs are being met. Of key importance is that nurse managers maintain the system by ensuring issues get picked up quickly and senior leaders are made aware before issues escalate into a crisis. Effective nurse managers do not just herald problems but offer solutions as well. Nurse managers bind the organization together within the *internal environment* so that team members are galvanized into action. Managing a nursing unit is not an easy task and is certainly not for the faint of heart.

Gelatt (1993) defined the skills needed to continually adapt, innovate, and change. "This 'flexpert' is open-minded, comfortable with uncertainty, delighted with change, and capable of unfreezing and refreezing beliefs, knowledge, and attitudes" (pp. 11–12). *Flexperts* understand that the inability to shift paradigms not only restricts flexibility but causes the individual to become out-of-date, inaccurate, and in need of revision. Culture, communities, experiences, and healthcare organizations change constantly and make old paradigms dysfunctional.

As nurse managers look toward the future, strategic planning fosters a sense of positive uncertainty that assists team members in the acceptance of change, ambiguity, uncertainty, and inconsistency. As Chapman (2003) stated in *Radical Loving Care*, "Our Vision statements need to be engraved in our hearts, not just on plaques" (p. 110). Committed leadership begins with those who make up the majority of caregivers in health care: nurses.

Summary

Nurse leaders are situated in a unique position to recognize the need for change in the organization. Sandwiched between the front-line staff and senior leaders, nurse managers may be the first to recognize the need for changes in strategy. Nurse leaders stimulate their team members by cultivating a positive culture of performance excellence and a corresponding reward system. The challenge is to define the parameters within which team members can experiment and be innovative. Nurse leaders uphold the organization's value system and maintain systems that focus on the core business of patient care. Managers ensure that strategies are in tune with the current needs of customers and are balanced so that one strategy does not suffer at the expense of another. They must be sensitive to important changes and continuously inquire of all their customers as to whether their needs are being met. Of key importance is that the nurse leaders maintain the system by ensuring issues get picked up quickly and senior leaders are made aware before issues escalate into a crisis. Effective nurse leaders do not just herald problems but offer solutions as well. Nurse leaders bind the organization together within the internal environment so that team members are galvanized into action. Managing a nurse unit is not an easy task and is certainly not for the faint of heart.

As nurse leaders look toward the future, strategic planning fosters a sense of positive uncertainty that assists team members in the acceptance of change, ambiguity, uncertainty, and inconsistency. As Chapman (2003) stated in *Radical Loving Care*, "Our Vision statements need to be engraved in our hearts, not just up on plaques" (p. 110). Committed leadership begins with those who make up the majority of caregivers in health care: nurses.

Discussion Questions

1. Because visioning and effective decision making are primary tasks of leaders, discuss mechanisms that nurse managers can use to ensure that they make the best decisions.

2. Describe positive and negative aspects of abandoning traditional healthcare strategic planning processes and adopting a contemporary approach.

3. Discuss the process of external and internal environmental analyses, and then speculate on scenarios that may result if these steps in strategic planning are omitted or are not done well.

4. Reflect on the mission, vision, values, and goals of a healthcare organization and provide examples of how individual employees, departments, and work units support all four of these as a foundation for directional strategies.

5. Describe how leaders can positively affect organizational and unit culture in the current healthcare environment, and then consider how the culture affects relationships, learning, change, and innovation.

6. Consider a healthcare organization and discuss measures that might be selected for a BSC. Explain the rationale for selection of each measure and describe how leaders could ensure a balance of measures. Next, discuss how leaders can remain informed regarding the current status of the organization considering at a minimum volume, financial, quality, and satisfaction measures.

7. Using the measures selected in discussion question 6, explain tools and techniques that could be used to display and analyze the data.

8. Qualitative tools and techniques are often dismissed in healthcare organizations. Select one qualitative method and discuss how the technique could be used to drive improvements.

9. Describe how nurse leaders and managers could contribute to evidence-based practice related to healthcare strategic planning.

10. Think about the role of the nurse manager, and discuss the importance of the role to employees and the overall organization.

Glossary of Terms

Acquisition Entry Strategy when healthcare organizations purchase an existing organization, organizational unit, or a product or service.

Adaptive Strategies how the organization will expand, contract, or maintain their scope of services (the means). They include expansion strategies, contraction strategies, and maintenance-of-scope strategies.

Alliance Strategies arrangements among existing organizations to achieve a strategic purpose not possible by any single organization.

Appreciative Inquiry (AI) the art and practice of asking questions that strengthen a system's capacity to apprehend, anticipate, and heighten positive potential.

Balanced Scorecard (BSC) measurement of key financial, quality, market, and operational indicators that provides management with an understanding of performance in relation to established strategic goals and graphically displays a snapshot of the institution's overall health.

Brainstorming a thinking process used to understand an issue and/or the impact the issue may have on the organization; also done to generate ideas for strategic alternatives.

Break-Even Analysis (BEA) determination of the minimum volume of services that a program or service must provide to be financially self-sufficient.

Contraction Strategies strategies that decrease the size or scope of operations.

Cooperation Strategies where the organization enters into mergers, alliances, and joint ventures.

Cost-Benefit Analysis comparison of the benefits and costs of a proposed endeavor.

Culture the shared assumptions, values, and behavioral norms of the group or organization.

Delphi Technique a structured group decision-making technique based on repeated use of rating scales to obtain opinions about a decision.

Directional Strategies initial direction for the organization and guidance when making key organizational decisions. They include mission, vision, values, goals, and objectives (the end).

Diversification at the corporate level, when markets outside the organization's core business offer potential for significant growth. Related diversification (concentric) includes related products and services. Unrelated diversification (conglomerate) includes businesses in the general environment.

Divestiture when one leaves a market and sells an operating unit.

Divisional Structures attempt to break down larger, diverse organizations into more manageable and focused sections.

Emergent Strategic Management relies on intuitive thinking, leadership, and learning, which correspond with contemporary strategic management processes.

Enhancement Strategies when the organization is progressing toward its vision yet improvements are still needed.

Expansion Strategies strategies to expand services.

External Customers in health care, these consist of suppliers (insurance companies, physicians not employed by the organization, labor markets, and donors), consumers (the general public and research community), and interfacing organizations (medical profession, teaching hospitals, boards of directors, health insurances, and drug and supply companies). Additional external influences include licensing, governmental, and regulatory agencies, in addition to other healthcare facilities.

External Environment the issues outside an organization's boundaries that represent opportunities and threats and that after analysis assist in identifying what the organization should do.

Focus Groups groups convened to reach conclusions regarding environmental issues.

Functional Organizational Structures structures that organize activities around mission-critical functions or processes.

Gantt Charts graphics that display activities or goals in a matrix format.

Goals statements that specify the major direction of the organization and provide actionable linkage to the mission.

Harvesting when the market has entered long-term decline or there is a need for short-term cash.

Horizontal Integration when the business grows by acquiring or affiliating with competitors, such as multihospital systems.

Internal Customers in health care, these include patients and families, physicians (when employed by the organization), visitors, team members, and volunteers.

Internal Development a development strategy for products or services closely related to existing products or services.

Internal Environment internal processes, culture, structure, and technology that, when reviewed and analyzed, reveal strengths and weaknesses.

Internal Ventures when products or services that are unrelated to current products or services are started within the organization.

Joint Ventures when two or more organizations combine resources to accomplish a designated task; a strategy used when risks are too high or the project is too large or too expensive to be done by a single organization.

Licensing Strategy a strategy of paying for use of proprietary technology that is not purchased; therefore, the organization is dependent on the licensor for support and upgrade.

Line Graphs/Multiple-Line Graphs charts that aid in assessment of trends or changes in performance (quantitative).

Liquidation selling of organizational assets.

Maintenance-of-Scope Strategies when current strategies are appropriate and few changes are needed, the organization may elect to maintain the existing strategies.

Market Development entering new markets with existing products or services.

Market Entry Strategies adaptive strategies used to bring market strategies to fruition. The three major strategies to enter a market are purchase, cooperation, and development (internal development and internal ventures).

Matrix a type of chart used to show combinations of data.

Matrix Structures structures that organize activities around problems to be solved rather than functions, products, or geography.

Merger when two organizations combine through a mutual agreement to form a single new organization.

Mission the articulation of the external opportunities of an organization, and the threats to it, as well as its internal strengths and weaknesses.

Nominal Group Technique (NGT) when team members independently generate a written list of ideas regarding an issue. After members have been given sufficient time to generate their list, each member takes turns reporting one idea at a time to the entire group.

Objectives descriptions of the results to be achieved, when and by whom, that are measurable.

Penetration Strategies strategies that focus on increasing volumes and market share.

Performance Improvement (PI) a systematic, organization-wide approach to improving the processes and outcomes of the healthcare system.

Product Development the introduction of new products or services to existing markets.

Purchase Strategies when healthcare organizations purchase an existing organization, organizational unit, or a product or service.

Regression Analysis a statistical technique available in computer software used to forecast the relationship between two variables. Multiple regression allows for the simultaneous investigation of two or more independent variables on a single interval-scaled or ratio-scaled dependent variable.

Retrenchment when the market has become too diverse and there is a decline in profitability as a result of increasing costs.

Scenario Development a technique used to implement an identified strategy where tree diagrams are used to break broad goals graphically into increasing levels of detailed actions so that a stated goal can be accomplished.

Situation Analysis the initial stage of strategic planning; the process of determining the current state of the organization. This is accomplished through three interrelated processes: external environmental analysis, internal environmental analysis, and the development of the organization's mission, vision, values, and goals.

Status Quo the assumption of a mature market when growth has ceased. The goal is to maintain the market share.

Strategic Management a process that fulfills the need for knowledge of the organization, the market, and the competitive situations healthcare leaders face, and provides for ongoing, dynamic changes in the strategic plan as needed.

Strategic Planning to devise a systematic, well-balanced process that allows the organization to fit in the environment. It stresses patient-focused quality and operational PI. It is a continuous process of revisiting the system and restoring balance.

Strategy Deployment implementing the strategic objectives. This includes culture, structure, and resources.

Strategy Formation gathering data and using these data for decision making. There are four types of strategies: directional, adaptive, market entry, and competitive.

Values the fundamental truths that the organization holds dear and that reflect the philosophy of the organization.

Venture Capital Investment a low-risk option where organizations purchase minority investment in a developing enterprise.

Vertical Integration grows the business along the channel of distribution of core process, such as an acute facility adding home care or long-term care.

Vision the view of the future based on the understanding of the environmental forces.

References

American Hospital Association, 2011 Committee on Performance Improvement. (2011, September). *Hospitals and care systems of the future.* Chicago, IL: Author.

Bennis, W., & Nanus, B. (1985). *Leaders: The strategies for taking charge.* New York, NY: Harper & Row.

Blatstein, I. M. (2012). Strategic planning: Predicting or shaping the future? *Organizational Development Journal, 30*(2), 31–38.

Boev, C. (2012). The relationship between nurses' perception of work environment and patient satisfaction in adult critical care. *Journal of Nursing Scholarship, 44*(4), 368–375.

Centers for Medicare & Medicaid Services. (2011, November). *Hospital value-based purchasing program.* Retrieved from http://www.cms.gov/Outreach-and-Education/Medicare-Learning-Network-MLN/MLNProducts/downloads/Hospital_VBPurchasing_Fact_Sheet_ICN907664.pdf

Chapman, E. (2003). *Radical loving care.* Nashville, TN: Vaughn.

Clancy, T. R. (2007). What we can learn from complex systems science. *Journal of Nursing Administration, 37*(10), 436–439.

Creative Quotations. (2009). *Artemus Ward.* Retrieved from http://www.creativequotations.com/one/1839.htm

Crowell, D. M. (2011). *Complexity leadership: Nursing's role in health care delivery.* Philadelphia, PA: F. A. Davis.

DeSilets, L., & Dickerson, P. (2008). SWOT is useful in your tool kit. *Journal of Continuing Education in Nursing, 39*(5), 196–197.

Dibrell, C., Down, J., & Bull, L. (2007). Dynamic strategic planning: Achieving strategic flexibility through formalization. *Journal of Business and Management, 13*(1), 21–35.

Drenkard, K. (2001). Creating a future worth experiencing: Nursing strategic planning in an integrated healthcare delivery system. *Journal of Nursing Administration, 31*(7–8), 364–375.

Finkler, S. (2001). *Financial management for public, health, and not-for-profit organizations.* Upper Saddle River, NJ: Prentice Hall.

Finkler, S. A., Jones, C. B., & Kovner, C. T. (2013). *Financial management for nurse managers and executives* (4th ed.). St. Louis, MO: Elsevier Saunders.

Gelatt, H. B. (1993, September–October). Future sense: Creating the future. *Futurist, 27*(5), 9–13.

Ginter, P., Swayne, L., & Duncan, W. (2002). *Strategic management of health care organizations* (4th ed.). Malden, MA: Blackwell.

Ginter, P. M., & Swayne, L. E. (2006). Moving toward strategic planning unique to healthcare. *Frontiers of Health Services Management, 23*(2), 33–37.

Ginter, P. M., Swayne, L. E., & Duncan, W. J. (2013). *The strategic management of health care organizations* (7th ed.). San Francisco, CA: Jossey-Bass.

Greene, J. (2009, November). The new pace of strategic planning. *H&HN: Hospitals & Health Networks, 83*(11), 31–32, 34.

Health Care Advisory Board. (1999). *Balanced scorecards.* Retrieved from http://www.advisory.com

Hrebiniak, L. G. (2005). *Making strategy work: Leading effective execution and change.* Upper Saddle River, NJ: Wharton School.

Kaplan, R., & Norton, D. P. (1996). *Translating strategy into action: The balanced scorecard.* Boston, MA: Harvard Business School.

Kim, W., & Mauborgne, R. (2002). Charting your company's future. *Harvard Business Review, 80*(6), 76–83.

Krueger, R. (1988). *Focus groups: A practical guide for applied research.* Newbury Park, CA: Sage.

Lazarus, I. R. (2011, March/April). What will it take? Exploiting trends in strategic planning to prepare for reform. *Journal of Healthcare Management, 56*(2), 89–93.

Lencioni, P. (2006). *Silos, politics, and turf wars: A leadership fable.* San Francisco, CA: Jossey-Bass.

Lindberg, C., & Clancey, T. R. (2010, April). Positive Deviance: An elegant solution to a complex problem. *Journal of Nursing Administration, 40*(4), 150–153.

MacPhee, M. (2007). Strategies and tools for managing change. *Journal of Nursing Administration, 37*(9), 405–413.

Martin, R. L. (2010). The execution trap. *Harvard Business Review, 88*(10), 64–71.

Mintzberg, H., & Markides, C. (2000). Commentary on the Henry Mintzberg interview. *Academy of Management Executive,* 39–42.

Morgan, D. (1993). *Successful focus groups: Advancing the state of the art.* Newbury Park, CA: Sage.

Patnaik, R. (2012). Strategic planning through complexity: Overcoming impediments to forecast and schedule. *IUP Journal of Business Strategy, IX*(1), 27–36.

Quotations Page. (2013a). *Marcel Proust.* Retrieved from http://www.quotationspage.com/search.php3?Search=&startsearch=Search&Author=proust&C=mgm&C=motivate&C=classic&C=coles&C=poorc&C=lindsly

Quotations Page. (2013b). *Yogi Berra.* Retrieved from http://www.quotationspage.com/search.php3?Search=&startsearch=Search&Author=Yogi+Berra&C=mgm&C=motivate&C=classic&C=coles&C=poorc&C=lindsly

Reed, K., & May, R. (2011, March). *HealthGrades patient safety in American hospitals study.* HealthGrades. Retrieved from https://www.cpmhealthgrades.com/CPM/assets/File/HealthGradesPatientSafetyInAmericanHospitalsStudy2011.pdf

Shirey, M. R. (2011). Brainstorming for breakthrough thinking. *Journal of Nursing Administration, 41*(12), 497–500.

Solovy, A. (2002). The paradox of planning. *Healthcare & Healthcare Network, 76*(9), 32.

Yoder-Wise, P. S. (Ed.). (2010). *Leading and managing in nursing* (5th ed.). St. Louis, MO: Elsevier Health Sciences.

Zikmund, W. (2003). *Business research methods* (7th ed.). Mason, OH: South-Western.

Zuckerman, A. M. (1998). *Healthcare strategic planning: Approaches for the 21st century*. Chicago, IL: Health Administration.

Zuckerman, A. M. (2006). Advancing the state of the art in healthcare strategic planning. *Frontiers of Health Services Management, 23*(2), 3–15.

CHAPTER 10

Financial Strategies

J. Michael Leger, PhD, MBA, RN, and **Janne Dunham-Taylor**, PhD, RN

OBJECTIVES

- Identify financial strategies for survival in the value-based environment.
- Appropriately identify and deal with financial issues and processes that impede effectiveness.

Nurse leaders need to be equal partners in the financial and budgeting process and develop financial and budget strategies—*attaching numbers and monetary amounts to strategies*. Identifying strategies is part of the administrative *and* leader roles, always supporting the basic value of giving patients what they desire with available dollars. Financial strategies are interconnected with all other strategies and decisions in the organization. Obviously, the best strategies are developed when all stakeholders are involved in the process. Although some strategies must be identified by the executive group (including a nurse executive) or other departments, nursing can identify and carry out many strategies that not only help the organization, but also better serve the patient. Everyone in the organization must continually identify financial strategies, and then implement, evaluate, and make improvements to them as successes and failures occur.

We are moving into the second-curve, value-based environment from the old volume-based reimbursement environment (first curve) that was only concerned with the number of insured patients being treated. Now this focus is no longer enough because *reimbursement can be lost if certain quality measures are not met. In addition, a percentage of reimbursement for the next year is lost if a facility's performance ratings decline.* The following environmental factors are driving this change:

- Demand-altering demographic changes
- Employer, government, and consumer pressure to curb the unsustainable increase in healthcare spending
- Shift in financial incentives away from fee-for-service reimbursement in favor of value-based payments that reward positive outcomes and efficiency
- Rise in provider accountability for the cost and quality of health care
- Consistent demand to reduce care fragmentation by redesigning care delivery
- Increased transparency of financial, quality, and community benefit data

- Projected shortages of nurses, primary care physicians, and other healthcare providers in regard to population demand
- Persistent introduction of high-cost medical technology and pharmaceutical advances
- Difficulty in raising capital to meet the strategic needs for new facilities, medical technology, and information systems
- Uncertainty about federal and state healthcare reform legislation and regulation
- Overall decline in reimbursement
- Recognition and challenge to variations in care provision and, as a result, cost (American Hospital Association [AHA], 2011, p. 8)
- Viability of the U.S. economy

As these events occur, health systems can ignore them and keep on doing things the same way, or they can prepare for the second curve (which is already occurring) to ensure success in the new environment. The present belief is that hospitals "will evolve to become part of 'care systems' or 'integrated networks,' encompassing everything from home-based chronic care management to inpatient acute treatment" (AHA, 2011, p. 10).

Thus, to survive in this new second-curve environment, we need to make major changes in the way we do business. "The second curve is concerned with value: the cost and quantity of care necessary to produce desired health outcomes within a particular population" (AHA, 2011, p. 8). According to the AHA Committee on Performance Improvement and the Health Research and Educational Trust (HRET), it is imperative we modify "core models for business and service delivery" (2013, p. 3). This is exciting because they recommend valuing nurse leaders (as well as physicians) at the point of care.

The AHA (2011) identified 10 "must-do" strategies to be successful in the second-curve environment.

1. Aligning hospitals, physicians, and other providers across the continuum of care
2. Utilizing evidenced-based practices to improve quality and patient safety

3. Improving efficiency through productivity and financial management
4. Developing integrated information systems
5. Joining and growing integrated provider networks and care systems
6. Educating and engaging employees and physicians to create leaders
7. Strengthening finances to facilitate reinvestment and innovation
8. Partnering with payers
9. Advancing an organization through scenario-based strategic, financial, and operational planning
10. Seeking population health improvement through pursuit of the triple aim (p. 11). (The Institute for Healthcare Improvement [2007] identified the triple aim "to encourage hospitals to simultaneously focus on population health, increased quality, and reduction in health care cost per capita" [p. 22])

These 10 strategies provide clues to all healthcare administrators, as well as nurses, on how to ensure success in this present unstable environment. This entire text has been designed to help nurse leaders better achieve the second curve. The goal is for the outcomes of financial strategies to achieve cost savings or reorganize available monies in a more effective way. But they also may cost additional dollars. Technology is a good example of this. Financial strategies need to be carefully crafted to achieve financial success in the second-curve environment.

In this new environment, ***our best resources for needed strategies are the patients and the leaders at the point of care***. This is a new perspective that many administrators have not presently adopted. It will take a lot of work from the board down to change for success to be achieved.

There is an infinite number of possible strategies. This chapter discusses some, but please add to this list. Certain strategies work more effectively in one setting but not as well in another because all facilities have particular quirks or differences.

▶ Complexity Issues

Growth in organizational complexity is more than a perception; it is a reality with sound theoretical underpinnings. The ramifications of growing complexity are immense. Beyond a certain level, organizational complexity can decrease both the quality and financial performance of a health system. (Clancy, 2010, p. 248)

Clancy suggests keeping four strategies in mind as we deal with complexity issues:

1. Be prepared.
2. Limit combinatorial complexity.
3. Use creative destruction.
4. Don't give up.

One example of complexity is unexpected events. The first strategy is to "be prepared for the unexpected" (Clancy, 2010, p. 248). This is why it is important to have "highly reliable systems, standardized protocols, and checklists" and make sure these are tightly controlled to prevent errors.

The second strategy is to "limit combinatorial complexity." Healthcare organizations are already too complex. Then, when something happens, we add to the complexity by using quick fixes, which only worsen the situation and make it more complex. It is so important to use systems thinking and involve all stakeholders in solutions that decrease complexity. The idea is to *simplify*. Each of our actions and those of staff leaders need to decrease complexity as much as possible. For instance, organizational processes should be simplified. Otherwise, as complexity increases, it becomes exponential, creating even more serious problems (errors, reimbursement loss, etc.)—and lower bottom lines.

The third strategy is to "use creative destruction—the systematic evaluation and elimination of nonessential activities" (Clancy, 2010, p. 249). This is why hospitals are getting into the Lean movement. The problem here is that we cannot just do this in a meeting with a group of administrators present. Staff actually doing the work need to be involved. Patients need to be involved. Physicians and other departments need to be involved. These are all important stakeholders in strategy development. Otherwise, the Lean movement just creates more complexity because someone does not realize that what he or she is changing has other harmful side effects that were not considered in the process. The same thing happens when quick decisions are made to deal with budget crises instead of carefully planning ahead for these events.

The fourth strategy is "don't give up" (Clancy, 2010, p. 249). For instance, the exponential growth of technology can be overwhelming. The good news is that technology helps us do our work better. The bad news is that it makes things more complex. It may be best not to purchase a new technology that has just been developed, but to wait until it has been used a bit and some of the initial glitches have been resolved. The idea is not to give up on expensive technology but to let it progress a bit before purchasing and to make a careful decision to determine the expense, time, and effort needed to implement the technology.

▶ Providing What the Patient Values

The most important strategy is to be sure that *everyone listens to the patient, making the patient the leader in choosing what will happen*. Often, patients need our expertise before they can make decisions about their care, so regular dialogue with front-line staff and physicians is critical.

Because the first and fifth "must-do" strategies from the AHA's list are concerned with the continuum of care, let's think about this from the nursing perspective. Presently, a first-curve volume issue is the cost strategy where *the patient is moved to the least expensive setting*. For instance, we move a surgical

patient quickly from the recovery room, to the intensive care unit, to stepdown or the general care unit, to the skilled nursing unit, and to home with home care. This saves money, but continuity is lost and errors happen because the patient has different people caring for him or her in each setting. We need to *reexamine this practice*. Surely there is a better solution. Often, caregivers in one setting do not think about, and prepare the patient for, continuing care in the next setting or in the home. How can we better achieve this?

In the second curve, *achieving the continuum of care with as little duplication as possible* has great value to the patient, saves costs and staff time, increases quality, and achieves better patient outcomes. Healthcare providers need to become more aware of the entire continuum (not get stuck in the silo that only includes the present location) and perceive how their patients might be affected by the home environment. Insurers are attempting to force the issue by not reimbursing for readmission within 30 days of discharge.

There is another continuum issue. Because so many healthcare dollars are spent on elderly adults with chronic conditions, providers need to figure out better ways to treat people at home, or in the least expensive environment, and to *teach patients and families how to deal more effectively with chronic conditions that will prevent the need for more expensive care.*

As providers, we need to find out what the patient values (eliminating many unnecessary procedures patients do not want) and figure out better ways to provide treatment in the home rather than in more expensive settings. Note that this will also help patients financially. A "Mount Sinai School of Medicine study found that out-of-pocket expenses for Medicare recipients during the five years before their death averaged about $39,000 for individuals, $51,000 for couples, and up to $66,000 for people with long-term illnesses like Alzheimer's" (Wang, 2012). Also, we know that currently 25% of Medicare dollars is spent on services for 5% of beneficiaries in their last year of life.

▶ Ensuring Quality and Safety

Another must-do strategy is concerned with *using evidenced-based practices to improve quality and patient safety.* Finding needed evidence and using it to identify best clinical, administrative, and educational practices is a continual process. As we find new knowledge, we need to change our behaviors accordingly. The information is worthless unless we use it. This means we need to be constantly looking for evidence pertaining to all areas of our practice (clinical, administrative, and educational). *All staff, including administrators, need to be proficient in finding and using pertinent information to improve work outcomes.*

The next step is to *incorporate the information that is useful into our work.* "Translation science is the process of incorporating research findings into practice" (Russell-Babin, 2009, pp. 29–30). This second step is critical (Cadmus et al., 2008). Yet studies show:

> Nurses do not consistently implement evidence-based best practices [EBP]…. Although nurses believe in evidence-based care, barriers remain prevalent, including resistance from colleagues, nurse leaders, and managers. Differences existed in responses of nurses from Magnet versus non-Magnet institutions as well as nurses with master's versus nonmaster's degrees. Nurse leaders and educators must provide learning opportunities regarding EBP and facilitate supportive cultures to achieve the Institute of Medicine's 2020 goal that 90% of clinical decisions be evidence-based. (Melnyk, Fineout-Overholt, Gallagher-Ford, & Kaplan, 2012, p. 410)

Within organizations, one of our responsibilities as nurse administrators is to achieve both steps ourselves, as well as to encourage staff to do the same. Research supports that evidence-based best practice (EBP) reduces morbidities, mortality, and medical errors. Gale and Shaffer (2009) found the following:

> Top reasons to adopt EBP [evidence-based practice] were having personal interest in the practice change, avoiding risk of negative consequences to the patient, and personally valuing the evidence. Top barriers to EBP were insufficient time, lack of staff, and not having the right equipment and supplies. (p. 91)

Other barriers were "a lack of EBP knowledge and skills, a perception that EBP is time [consuming], a belief that EBP is burdensome, and organizational cultures that [do not] support evidence-based care" (Melnyk et al., 2012, p. 411).

Systems problems that cause quality and safety issues must be fixed and are best resolved by involving *all* the stakeholders in identifying incremental changes (including the costs of these changes) to improve a situation. The idea is to decrease complexity, to find *a simpler way.* Stakeholders try each small incremental change, celebrating the successes. Or, as glitches or other unintended events happen (often this is a sign that complexity has been increased—something was not identified in the strategy), they go back to the drawing board and try another solution.

The idea is that everything we do in health care is a series of processes. These processes include time wasters that do not improve giving patients what they value (and that increase complexity). Some procedures completed are not what patients actually wanted done. And there are so many errors occurring. Bureaucracies only create additional complexity where more errors will occur, and this is what has happened in health care. We desperately need to simplify processes and question every step. Is each step necessary? Are there other simpler ways we could accomplish the work, yet still achieve what the patient values? Little by little we can fix the system.

Another quality and safety issue is *missed care,* first identified by Kalisch (2009). Missed care is when we skip doing basic nursing care and patients get infections, bedsores, and other problems. This occurs when RNs and aides do not value their work enough to ensure that this care is completed, and when staff nurses are not working carefully with aides or do not have the time because staffing is inadequate. Aides take pride in their work, too, and should be valued and involved in fixing the problem. Otherwise, it really hurts our patients and affects the bottom line.

Another problem is *duplication*. For example, we may have five or six people all taking histories from and performing physicals on the same patient. In addition, we do not use the history and physical—as well as other information—already completed by the facility that just transferred the patient to us. Or transfer information is lacking.

Interruptions are another issue in need of new strategies. Interruptions are common in health care and detract from critical thinking, causing errors. We need to implement strategies that decrease interruptions or that employ technology to better deal with communicating about patient issues.

Along with interruptions, *finding caregivers* is a big time waster. For instance, sometimes a nurse calls or pages a physician who is unavailable. Then, the physician calls the nurse and finds it hard to track down the nurse.

Quality and safety are enhanced by having *adequate numbers of staff* to do the work. If this is not so, it is an important issue to deal with. Cite the evidence: Adequate staffing makes a difference in patient outcomes and reimbursement.

Evidence shows that hiring a higher number of registered nurses (RNs) is actually *less expensive* than hiring a higher number of nursing assistants or licensed practical nurses (LPNs). (We tend to think the opposite because RN salaries are higher than the salaries of nursing assistants and LPNs, but the evidence shows this is not so.) For those with a bottom-line mentality, this may be hard to fathom. You will hear, "But nursing assistant salaries are less than an RN salary. How can this be true?" Expenses are lower when there is a higher RN ratio and there is enough support

staff present to facilitate the RN function. This is true across the healthcare continuum.

Another factor with quality and safety is making sure that the *staff is there when needed* and not there when there is less to do. For instance, perhaps certain staff members are very busy at peak times but do not have enough to do at other times. Yet we continue to schedule them in the same way. It is better to schedule someone to come in only for the peak times.

In nursing, we need to examine whether *12-hour shifts* should be used. Many errors are caused because nurses are not alert, are sleep deprived, and so forth when they work 12-hour shifts. On the other hand, nurses like these longer shifts because they get more days off—or more days to work prn at another facility—which only makes them more error prone.

Another strategy is to either provide a wellness program or obtain employee discounts at local facilities that **enhance employee health and well-being**. This can also be achieved by supporting leaders at the point of care using specific strategies identified elsewhere in this discussion.

Workarounds are another issue that can indicate certain processes or technology routines are cumbersome. Staff figure out ways to work around the issues. Some workarounds are positive, where staff are trying to help patients get the care they need in cumbersome environments. Other workarounds are negative—for instance, avoiding safety guidelines when staffing is inadequate. Strategies—both in the identification of issues and in ways to better deal with these issues—are needed.

These are fixable issues but must become important from the top down in an organization. Many of these are more appropriately fixed using a shared governance structure. Everyone needs to walk the talk and support the basic value(s) in every strategy or action that is taken.

This may also involve *environmental changes*: for example, when elderly adults have to walk long distances to the lab or x-ray, having or building or remodeling services so they are close to parking areas can be ideal. Sometimes services need to be updated and the available space changed. A current change for nurses involves ways to get more materials/supplies/technology at the bedside to reduce the walking time of nursing staff.

▶ Improving Efficiency Through Productivity and Financial Management

The fourth AHA must-do strategy concerns efficiency in productivity and financial management, which are interwoven with the seventh strategy, strengthening finances to facilitate reinvestment and innovation. Although part of accomplishing these strategies is the role of the finance department, nurses can contribute to both efforts.

One identified financial issue is RNs being pulled away from patients for more than 50% of their time, in order to perform work not related to patients—known as *non-value added time*. This costs millions of dollars per unit each year. It is a prime example of processes gone awry. Nurses want to spend more time with patients; patients value time with their nurses. So, why do nurses have to waste time on the non-value added activities? This is where practice councils can be very helpful. If operating correctly, they can identify and make changes at the bedside that are immediate, that provide what patients value, that provide higher-quality care and safety, and that meet reimbursement mandates.

In financial management, we need to move out of the old linear, ineffective, outmoded, authoritarian model where finance and nursing personnel do not discuss issues together and where finance personnel give nurse managers the same budget amounts with a bit more added for inflation or a percentage taken out for budget cuts. The nurse managers should question everything. To meet second-curve reimbursement

demands, this is *not* an acceptable way of dealing with financial issues.

It is better to identify a fixed annual budget, but with the caveat that it will continue to be tweaked as changes occur so that the organization can best meet environmental challenges. In the second curve, it is important for *financial information to be transparent and shared with all staff*. In this environment, *all staff need to be cost conscious*. It is important to take into account which departments are already more cost conscious, so that they are *not penalized* when budget cuts are necessary. Having all equally share across-the-board cuts—that often happen in more authoritarian, linear systems—is not the best way to meet budget challenges in the second curve.

Budget cuts happen regularly in health care as reimbursement amounts continue to decline. For instance, government reimbursement for Medicaid and Medicare services gives back only cents on the dollar. This means that the reimbursed amount is less than half (and even less with Medicaid) of that expended by the healthcare facility. Other insurance plans follow suit, taking similar measures, and asking for larger discounts each year.

Budget cuts also result from not meeting performance measures and making poor business decisions, such as giving too great a discount to insurance carriers, losing contracts with insurance companies, rescuing physician offices running at a deficit, providing poor leadership, or operating consistently at a loss yet never taking any measures to improve the situation. As healthcare organizations have increased in complexity there are more costs, but the outcomes do not reflect the expenditures. Strategies identified need to decrease complexity, not add to it.

An important budget strategy needs to include a *plan for how to handle different financial scenarios*, such as being at 100% occupancy when only budgeted for 80%, being 20% under the anticipated occupancy rate, or having to decrease costs by 5% or 10%. We know that these situations occur, so involving all stakeholders in developing a plan to handle these situations

TABLE 10.1 World View Financial Beliefs

Traditional Beliefs	*Quantum View*
■ Resources are scarce.	■ Resources are abundant.
■ Do things the way we have always done them.	■ Change will always happen. We cannot escape it.
■ Use bottom-line thinking.	■ The bottom line comes second, behind what the patient values.
■ Financial decisions are separate from the rest of the organization.	■ Financial decisions need to be made within the context of the total organization.

before they occur is wise management. This is a much more thoughtful way of making decisions and results in better outcomes: a second-curve strategy. When nothing is done until everyone is in the middle of the crisis, poor outcomes result.

In the budget process, *nursing needs to be a majority player* with other departments. When all stakeholders are involved in the process, staff can identify ways to save money that administrators never thought about, and this results in more effective plans.

As we work with budgets, our worldview—our silos (**TABLE 10.1**)—influences our choices and, perhaps unintentionally, inhibits the potential reality. Let's examine some examples.

One silo is that *resources are scarce*. This is not surprising because, as discussed elsewhere, *accounting and financial theories are based on scarcity*:

> Accounting and finance are applied areas of microeconomics. The theory of economics forms the foundations upon which all financial management is ultimately built. The essence of economics is that society has *a limited amount of resources*, with competing demands for them. The economic system attempts to allocate those resources in an optimal fashion. (Finkler & Kovner, 2007, p. 3)

Compare this way of thinking with the quantum view, where the world is composed of energy fields. In the quantum view, we need

to be careful about our thoughts because they create our reality. Wouldn't it be better to choose *abundance* rather than *scarcity*? Perhaps our present cost-cutting dilemmas have been caused by too many people thinking there are limited resources! We probably would make different decisions if we thought resources were abundant. In this book, we choose abundance. *Many financial people will have difficulty with this concept because their education and their work environment have always emphasized scarcity.*

Another silo is *doing things the way we have always done them*. Because the environment is always changing, this is actually the kiss of death. We cannot avoid change.

A third silo is *bottom-line thinking*. We advocate the importance of providing what the patient values first to stay viable. The bottom line is always second if we want to survive as an organization. If this is the mentality in an organization, *this will need to be changed to achieve adequate reimbursement*.

In the quantum view, we are all interconnected. Thus, we cannot *separate financial decisions from other organizational decisions*. Any action we take affects everyone else. This means that everyone in the organization needs to be aware of and involved in working with budgets/finances, as well as using and discovering financial strategies.

Each of these issues is a basis for discussion and, if resolved, will achieve better outcomes for everyone, including the bottom line.

The importance of interdisciplinary groups composed of staff, administrators, physicians,

BOX 10.1 Possible Budget Strategies

- Providing care the patient values
- Fixing organizational processes that decrease complexity—i.e., non-value added time, missed care, workarounds, duplication, interruptions, finding caregivers, having adequate staffing consistently
- Educating each staff member on importance of pay for performance issues
- Educating each staff member on new reimbursement requirements
- Providing more budget transparency
- Fixing the budget process
- Providing more effective bottom-up leadership
- Having everyone do regular rounds as top priority
- Supporting nurse managers
- Having adequate staffing
- Encouraging staff to be leaders
- Having shared governance councils
- Increasing interdisciplinary collaboration
- Improving case management by involving all staff
- Improving communication everywhere
- Using best evidence—clinical, leadership, and organizational
- Appropriately using technology
- Fixing environmental issues
- Creating a cost-conscious environment
- Getting everyone involved in spotting changes and new trends
- Employing advanced practices nurses
- Eliminating disruptive/abusive behaviors
- Identifying issues causing moral distress for clinicians and deal with them

and patients working together to identify and implement financial strategies cannot be over-emphasized, because each of us possesses only a partial answer. **BOX 10.1** identifies some possible strategies. The more we can work as a team and as equal players, the more effective our strategies will be. This is why it is so important for all administrators and staff to do regular rounds, support nurse leaders and physicians at the point of care, and only provide what the patient values because they provide a more accurate picture of what is actually happening in the trenches.

What Not to Do

Let's turn to some things to avoid because they increase complexity unnecessarily. First, many of the slash-and-burn strategies presently used are *not* advocated here. People who advocate *slash-and-burn cost cutting* would do well to

heed some research published in the *Harvard Business Review*: **"Companies with few or no layoffs performed significantly better than those with large numbers of layoffs"** (Rigby, 2002). In addition, research shows that **companies with similar growth rates that did not downsize consistently outperformed those that did downsize**. In addition, costs are associated with layoffs:

- Severance packages
- Temporary declines in productivity or quality
- Rehiring and retraining costs

Thoughtless approaches are implemented without considering future consequences. This research shows that *greater cost savings are realized by dealing with the more knotty organizational and leadership problems* and that downsizing and layoffs can actually be more expensive in the long run.

Another strategy we do *not* advocate is to resort to *quick-fix solutions,* such as suddenly reorganizing or reengineering/restructuring when in a budget crunch or when faced with personnel problems, problem departments, or systems issues. Two common ways to restructure and reorganize are inpatient bed consolidation by reaggregation of the patient population with increased outpatient or freestanding facility solutions, and downsizing and cutting present staff positions.

Making quick-fix decisions that restructure the organization most often result in increased complexity, layoffs, people in new jobs not understanding their additional responsibilities, missed care, errors, decreased patient satisfaction, and survivor issues with those left. They have drastic effects on both the remaining workforce and on efficiency in general. Most often, the result is inefficiency, realized in elevated costs and other expensive short-term and long-term effects—not to mention patient harm.

A short-term effect of redesign is that the *survivors* need to be oriented to assume the duties of displaced personnel. This means that a less effective, less efficient staff are not only dealing with the acquisition of new duties—and the resultant creation of more patient safety issues—but are also experiencing *survivor sickness.* Burke (2002) describes survival sickness as having the following characteristics: "low morale, decreased commitment, and increased cynicism, mistrust, and anger. Affected caregivers may question the effectiveness of their facility's functioning, describe their work environment as deteriorated, and believe that this deterioration threatens patient's well-being" (p. 41). They also make more errors, miss care, and exhibit other characteristics of low-quality care. These are the short-term effects, but it does not stop there.

How well the organization supports staff during times of restructuring directly affects retention of the remaining staff. A long-term effect, along with additional costs, may be a subsequent increase in staff turnover rates, resulting from restructuring. Sometimes it is easier to be the person who is displaced than to be one of the remaining staff on a unit or in a department. Based on these facts, it is very important for the nurse administrator and other healthcare organization officials to provide support for the survivors.

Actually providing survivor support is a tall order. It is best if administrators continually communicate with staff about the changes that will take place, as well as why the changes are necessary. *Once staff trust is lost, it is very difficult to regain.* In addition, staff morale suffers when layoffs or restructuring occurs, and teamwork probably is affected within and between departments. Burke (2002) advocates taking the following steps to improve staff involvement that deal more effectively with survivor issues:

- Create focus groups or hold employee meetings to discuss the restructuring, particularly what went right and solutions for what went wrong. (Note here that it would have been better to do focus groups and employee meetings as part of the planning process for redesign in the first place.)
- Develop education programs to help employees adjust.
- Identify employee concerns through surveys (or have everyone start doing rounds!).
- Formulate new communication strategies for better transparency.
- Reevaluate jobs to better reflect new responsibilities.

Both reorganization and reengineering were meant to happen in a carefully crafted way, following dialogue and careful planning by all stakeholders involved. Instead, they have actually been used to provide quick fixes that then create further problems. Meanwhile, the original issues were not resolved, complexity is increased, and the situation actually worsens. Is it any wonder that in this frenzy there are additional costs incurred that were not considered?

▶ The Budget Process: Is It Flawed or Effective?

Another strategy is the budget process itself. In our interconnected world, the best budget process involves *everyone* in the organization—including patients, families, and physicians. The budget is *transparent* and shared with staff. The budget process is *participative* but extends beyond just participation. The process is most effective when all involved are *equal partners* and use dialogue (both sharing information and listening to others). This approach is much more effective than an authoritarian, or top-down, method of communication. Therefore, everyone from the housekeeper or nursing assistant through the physician and the board chair is involved in the decision-making process (this includes the strategic plan)—with the patients and their families being the pivotal, or most important, part of this process. Physicians have to be included because physician practice patterns can have a direct effect on increasing or decreasing the budget. Nurses need to be involved in this all along the way.

We recommend being *honest* about budgets. The problem with dishonesty is that lies beget more lies, and once you have been found out, your believability is **gone**. Trust, once lost, is extremely difficult to regain or, realistically, is probably never regained! Integrity is essential.

Historically, a *flawed budget process* has been used. This process started in the 1920s when large companies used the process "as a tool for managing costs and cash flows" (Hope & Fraser, 2003, p. 113). Then, in the 1960s:

> Companies used accounting results not just to keep score but also to dictate the actions of people at all levels of the company. By the early 1970s, a new generation of leaders schooled in the finer arts of financial planning had begun to rely on financial targets and incentives—in lieu of such benchmarks as productivity and marketing effectiveness—to drive performance improvement. (p. 113)

This caused serious problems in the 1980s and 1990s when companies started paying more attention to sales targets than to satisfying customers. Suddenly, money was running the game rather than supporting it.[1] Unfortunately, some healthcare organizations continue to use this flawed process today.

Another game that is played with budgets is the *spend it or lose it* mentality that goes on at the end of the budget year. In this game, a manager knows that any money left in the budget will be lost at the end of the fiscal year, so the manager decides to find things to spend the money on just before the fiscal year closes.

Today, hopefully, we are using more participative, customer-oriented processes. This results in flatter structures and rapid responses to market changes and stays closer to the customer—emphasizing public relations, empowering workers to make appropriate decisions as they do their work, and sharing information, including information about budget expenses and revenues. All this enhances our systems so that employees have all the tools present to do their work more effectively. Yet, if we still use the cumbersome, flawed, historic budget process, we do not achieve any of these objectives.

That is why we advocate different, newer processes that include dialogue, honesty, and transparency.

Creating a Cost-Conscious Environment

Materials and supply costs, rising daily in health care, need to be examined. These costs are second only to the cost of staffing. One way to decrease supply costs is by exercising more reasonable use of supplies by nursing staff. Nurse managers who are responsible for creating and maintaining their unit's fiscal budgets can provide substantial decreases in costs by controlling supply expenditures. An overall decrease in the organization's fiscal budget may be realized as each individual unit's supply budget is trimmed for efficiency. Staff need to understand the importance of charging patients appropriately for supplies. Missed charges mean less money. Budget transparency is the key here. Trimming and charging are happening using a process involving staff who directly use the supplies. In fact, in a positive environment where staff are empowered, they will think of better ways to save costs than supervisors or finance can achieve.

As we become more conscious of supply costs as managers, it is important to *involve staff* in this issue.

> We must also communicate to patients, nurses, and physicians that [healthcare organizations] no longer can afford to give things away. Someone always ends up paying. Nurses are trained to help people, to be generous and giving. For example, a nurse may give a patient a bunch of sterile pads rather than instructing him to go to the local pharmacy. Even those who mean well can put a [healthcare organization] out of business. (Lefever, 1999, p. 30)

Inefficiencies mount up. For unit-based cost savings to occur, staff should be involved in the formulation of the department's fiscal budget and know the overall organization's financial targets. They see monthly reports showing whether they are meeting the budget goals. Staff then have a better sense of how they are contributing to either cost inefficiencies or to cost containment without compromising quality. After all, practice behaviors can affect the cost of delivering patient care.

To maximize the efficiency of supply usage by staff, it is important to take an *educational approach* to the issue.

Often, nurses have negative attitudes toward cost-effectiveness, associating it with a *bottom-line orientation,* which consequently results in staffing reductions, pay cuts, longer work hours, and diminished resources. Because of these negative attitudes, nurses may not be as cost effective in their nursing practice.

Invisible costs for unused supplies from packs and trays, obsolete and slow-moving inventory, pilferage, giveaways, and uncontrolled usage indicate waste and are a prime target for nurse managers who wish to correct supply budget variances. First, nurse managers must determine how and where the major waste is occurring. They can do this by reviewing the unit's present inventory of supplies and determining whether there are opportunities for efficiency in areas where practice creates costly waste. For example, when physicians who no longer have patients in the department request supplies from that department, this is considered waste. Correcting this waste may be as simple as revising or providing guidelines to standardize supply usage. Decreasing types of stock that are not used frequently not only decreases the number of dollars required for the department's supply budget but also provides more space for pertinent supplies.

As the financial resources available for the purchase of supplies, linen, and equipment have dwindled due to low reimbursements, there has been more *hoarding* of supplies and equipment. Although hoarding provides staff with immediate access to the resources they need for patient care, staff do not realize that they add to their supply and equipment problems overall. *Overstocking and hoarding cost money.* Tying up financial resources for purchase of more and more supplies because of stockpiling can actually build to a point where the whole facility is not efficient in the management of materials. For example, the hoarding of IV pumps (or linen, monitors, or wheelchairs) only creates the need to purchase more IV pumps for the facility—a big, unnecessary expense. This "lost" inventory would be less costly if left in circulation throughout the healthcare organization.

In actuality, *hoarding is a symptom of a larger systems problem.* Instead of hiding and storing more inventory for the unit, it is much more cost efficient to bring together a group of stakeholders from appropriate departments to work out a better solution. The solution needs to have *the right numbers at the right times in the right place.*

This systems strategy is also a useful way to examine supply and equipment fluctuations as patient volume changes. For instance, if the patient census, or acuity, has decreased, the nurse leader, as well as other appropriate departmental managers, could check to see whether the inventory usage has also decreased. A *periodic survey and inventory* of all nursing units in a facility can help with these issues.

In addition, nurse administrators can periodically review overall monthly budget costs for linen, supplies, and equipment. Sudden variances in this budget could indicate hoarding, creating the need for purchases to counteract the decreases in certain areas. (Hoarding, if it persists a long time, may not appear as an increase in the budget but must still be dealt with to achieve cost-effectiveness.) Close interaction with departments, such as the laundry, central supply, and materials management, could shed light on areas of concern. These are process issues. Complexity is involved and the processes need to be simplified.

Educating staff about supply costs so that they can adjust inventories to meet patient demands is extremely important. The staff should realize that they have a direct responsibility to achieve efficiency and, if something is not working, to express their concerns to the appropriate managers so that problems can be fixed. Everyone, including the nurse leader, needs to be involved in achieving better efficiencies.

Standardization of supply usage can also provide cost savings. For example, the standardization of items placed in sterile trays and packs for labor and delivery procedures on obstetrical units, in emergency rooms, or in surgery departments may be warranted. Meeting with the physicians upfront to elicit their input on the design of the new trays is a must. The changes need to satisfy their needs, as well as provide efficiency. Otherwise, more waste could occur.

Because the cost of medical supplies and equipment is one of the major budget items associated with health care, it is imperative for nurse administrators to be knowledgeable in the latest trends affecting the purchasing of these supplies. Having knowledge and being able to *talk the talk* with purchasing managers are essential skills for nurse leaders to have an influence on the buying practices of their units

and the institution as a whole. This is also why it is an advantage to send nurse leaders and staff to seminars and trade shows.

▶ Developing Integrated Information Systems

Where is the wisdom we have lost in knowledge?
Where is the knowledge we have lost in information?
—Thomas Stearns Eliot*

We cannot ignore that we are in the Information Age. Complexity is growing at an exponential rate, as seen in technologies: "computer processing power and storage capacity, the number of healthcare providers using various types of medical technology in hospitals, healthcare information on the intranet, and the decline in medical devices size" (Clancy, 2010, p. 247).

Another issue in the Information Age is that there is so much information available it is not humanly possible to ever know it all. And we must not become a slave to it. As expressed in the quote at the beginning of this section, we still need wisdom, and we still need our knowledge, judgment, and experience as we do our work. The issue is that we need the wisdom and knowledge *along with* the information. The information provides us with a useful *tool*—additional evidence—to add to, or correct, our present knowledge and wisdom. Because we are involved in each administrative, educational, or patient situation, there are still individual differences we must account for before we determine what to do (Matney, Brewster, Sward, Cloyes, & Staggers, 2011). We still need to make decisions based on all these factors.

---

* Excerpt from "Choruses from 'The Rock'" from *Collected Poems*, 1909–1962 by T.S. Eliot. Copyright 1936 by Houghton Mifflin Harcourt Publishing Company. Copyright © renewed 1964 by Thomas Stearns Eliot. Reprinted by permission of Houghton Mifflin Harcourt Publishing Company. All rights reserved.

Technology creates more complexity in additional ways. Now there is usually an IT or Information Technology department (or personnel) in healthcare organizations. As more organizations added technology, issues resulted when end users did not understand or resisted technology use or the technology was not adapted to the organization in a usable way. IT programmers did not understand healthcare nuances and healthcare providers did not understand the intricacies of the technology.

This resulted in a new nursing role—an *informatics nurse specialist (INS)* who has healthcare experience and who also understands how the technology (Huryk, 2011; McLane & Turley, 2011) facilitates the integration of data "to improve the health of populations, communities, families, and individuals" (ANA, 2007, p. vii). Informatics nurse specialists are assets to the organization in how they support the use of information–processes, knowledge and technology–in both the direct provision of patient care and in supporting other providers in their decision-making roles (ANA, 2007). The INS is involved with technology decisions and purchases, implementation, and updates and changes needed in the technology and they act as a liaison between IT and the nursing staff. The American Nurses Association (ANA) provides the *Scope and Standards of Nursing Informatics Practice* (ANA, 2007).

▶ Educating and Engaging Employees and Physicians to Create Leaders

The sixth AHA must-do strategy is about creating *leaders at the point of care*. This includes physicians and nurses, as well as other employees. In the second curve, the most important place in the healthcare environment is the point of

care. We have often gotten the word *leader* confused with *administrator*. Anyone can become a *leader* when two or more people get together. An *administrator* possesses the position in the organizational chart that determines who has overall responsibility for certain areas.

Here, in the second-curve environment, **leaders at the point of care are the most important people in the organization**. Administrators *support* these leaders to give the care. This is not to say that administrators should not be leaders as well, but their role is administrative, supporting leaders at the point of care. This is an enormous change for healthcare administrators who have not been educated to behave in this manner.

Many first-curve administrators (as well as most of the U.S. population) view the chief executive officer (CEO) as the most important person in the organization. So, having leaders at the point of care is a major shift in many people's perspectives.

Just saying this is the case is not enough: Actions speak louder than words. Administrators need to live this perspective and show in all their actions that those at the point of care are the most important. This is why everyone (including administrators) needs to do regular rounds. That is where the action is. To accomplish this, administrators may need to evaluate the necessity of many of the meetings they schedule. Some are excellent and promote team functioning; others do not. *Rounds need to replace many meetings because the people in the meetings are often not in touch with what is happening at the bedside*.

Effective leadership is very important wherever it occurs, at any level in the organization, and includes the ability to value the empowerment of others.

Nurse leaders need to encourage and empower all staff to be leaders at the point of care, and they must support these leaders. For some nurse leaders, this is a new way of thinking. Their support is pivotal to the success of this second-curve strategy. They can support a positive culture and environment because this results in the best outcomes, including reimbursement.

Many times, nurse leaders are not given *adequate orientation and mentoring,* or they have too many duties to perform realistically. When this is the case, generally everyone loses.

Another issue is that sometimes there are *too many full-time equivalents (FTEs)* reporting to a nurse manager. We recommend that 35 to 50 FTEs is ideal. And the nurse manager role needs to be supported by charge nurses on every shift, as well as an assistant nurse manager or co-manager who provides more consistent coverage on a unit. Patient, nurse, and physician satisfaction result from effective leadership on the part of managers. The nurse manager—along with all the staff—need to be *valued and supported by higher levels of administration.* (Upper levels of management may need to change to achieve this goal.) Positive management results in positive outcomes—and positive bottom lines.

Other actions that support leaders at the point of care include valuing the staff nurse who needs to be in equal partnership with the physician, promoting clinical autonomy, increasing messy communication, encouraging collaboration between all disciplines at the point of care, encouraging innovation, and promoting interdisciplinary shared governance. In addition, it is helpful to give staff ways to more effectively resolve conflicts that will invariably occur. Systems thinking is preferred, with all in the organization understanding how interconnected everything is. There needs to be ongoing dialogue among everyone throughout the organization with the players having *equal* importance in the dialogue. All the players—this includes nursing and finance—have key information that, when shared, results in better decisions. The best decisions are always based on what patients value. Ultimately, better finances are realized.

Disruptive/abusive behaviors are another issue that needs attention in organizations. Everyone (including physicians) needs to give respect to others in words and actions. Differences of opinion are grist for the mill for needed changes. But disruptive or abusive behaviors should not be tolerated, with appropriate action being taken with offenders. In positive environments, positive outcomes are achieved.

When caregivers experience *moral distress,* administrators need to deal with the issue. When everyone is doing rounds, it will become evident that caregivers feel moral distress around certain issues. It helps to have an ethics committee, medical staff support, and a practice council that can examine these issues. If the distress is a result of an issue such as inadequate staffing, administration must take action to resolve the problem.

In the Institute of Medicine (IOM) and Robert Wood Johnson Foundation (RWJF) report *Future of Nursing: Leading Change, Advancing Health,* published in 2010, the second and third recommendations support the AHA must-do strategies. The second recommendation is: "Nurses should achieve higher levels of education and training through an improved education system that promotes seamless academic progression." As RNs assume leadership positions at the point of care, additional education such as achieving the BSN, MSN, DNP, and PhD degrees enhances the abilities of both nurse administrators and RNs to achieve the AHA strategies.

The third IOM/RWJF recommendation is: "Nurses should be full partners with physicians and other healthcare professionals in redesigning healthcare in the United States." This goal is important to best achieve the 10 must-do AHA strategies. In the first curve, physicians and top-level administrators often considered themselves in a one-up position with nurses. In the second curve, the best results are achieved when equal partnership is valued by all groups.

▶ Partnering with Payers

The eighth AHA must-do strategy, partnering with payers, is an important activity for the executive group and the finance department. Accountable care organizations can achieve this goal, but some healthcare organizations will choose not to be involved in this arrangement. Nursing indirectly influences reimbursement, however, because the performance standards include patient outcomes and achieving pay for performance goals.

▶ Scenario-Based Strategic, Financial, and Operational Planning

The ninth AHA must-do strategy is involved with scenario-based strategic planning. In the second curve, it is most effective when all in the organization are involved in contributing to strategic planning, understanding it, and tweaking it as needed at the point of care, even though the executive group has overall responsibility for setting the course. Because change is always happening, a strategic plan is not carved in stone but is created with the idea that it will change as the environment changes.

Scenarios are an important addition in the second curve. When those at the point of care try out various scenarios as situations occur with patients, they find that some scenarios are very successful and some are not. Keeping the successful strategies, sharing them across the organization, and implementing them at different points of care provide administration with data on what is most likely to succeed in a strategic plan. Of course, regular rounds are also a must so that executives keep in touch with patient issues.

▶ Achieving Population Health Improvement Through Pursuit of the Triple Aim

The 10th AHA must-do strategy proscribes that health providers at all levels pursue the triple aim. The triple aim, as defined by the Institute for Healthcare Improvement in 2007, is "to encourage hospitals to simultaneously focus on population health, increased quality,

and reduction in health care cost per capita" (p. 22). This includes doing more health promotion and disease prevention activities with patients, as well as being more involved in the public health of the community. All of the preceding strategies can help healthcare providers achieve the 10th strategy.

It is interesting that serving populations has recently come into focus as DNP programs discuss population health and assign capstone activities to achieve better patient and organizational outcomes. Most often, these activities increase quality and also save money.

▶ Writing a Business Plan

Because budget strategies can result in making changes, especially if they alter the way money is spent, nurse leaders must be able to effectively express needed changes in an organized, professional fashion that emphasizes not only what needs to happen but the costs involved. In light of this, we offer this section on writing a business plan or a proposal.

Business plans and proposals can be used to request a needed piece of equipment, explain a different way of implementing patient care, or design a new service. A business plan example is found in the Appendix. The plan or proposal can be given to a supervisor, the nurse executive or director of nursing, or, after consultation with the nurse executive, the finance department personnel, the executive team, or even the board.

The business plan or proposal should present *actual data and costs,* as well as provide a thoughtful rationale for the solutions. It should be readable and concise—executive team members prefer one-page executive summaries. The first step is to prepare a thoughtful business plan or proposal for the nurse executive, as discussed here.

Generally, a business plan reflects changes in the way services are delivered, and involves a shift in the way money is spent. Alternately, the plan or proposal may request that the budget reflect different monetary amounts within certain categories, based on changes in the patient population. The plan might also be more extensive and ask for several different, or more updated, pieces of equipment to provide a service—such as new cardiac monitors—or request new technology such as an electronic medical record system for the entire facility or system. Because nurses are involved with patients, the plan may even suggest providing a new, innovative service that the nursing staff and the nurse leader have identified that is not presently provided.

A business plan or proposal has more credence if it is typed neatly using word processing software and illustrated effectively with PowerPoint or other computer graphic programs. The plan needs to be carefully thought out to ensure that the reader thoroughly understands a problem, provides the reader with the proposed solution to deal with the problem, and presents the reasons why this proposed solution is the best way to solve the problem. At times, it may be best to present several solutions, each costing a different amount of money, and give the pros and cons of each solution.

Consider to whom the plan will be presented. What is their perspective on the situation to which your proposal refers? What information will they need to know? What background information might be helpful to include in the plan? Be clear about what is requested and what the impact or effect will be on the whole organization. Be organized in the delivery and present a reasonable solution to the problem. Plans should include the following:

- **Title:** Be sure to include the name of the person who wrote the proposal. Sometimes it is helpful to give additional background information about them to the reader.
- **Definition:** Define the proposed item, change, service, or program.
- **Rationale:** Why is it needed? Why is this the best item, or the best way to perform

the service? Discuss the advantages of the solution: How does this proposal save on costs or increase safety? Also mention any disadvantages. Outline other alternatives you have considered, if applicable and necessary.

- **Implementation plan:** Specify what needs to happen. Provide timelines and costs.
- **Costs/benefits:** Show the actual costs and, if appropriate, how this will change existing costs. Often, this can be presented more clearly using a spreadsheet, table, pie chart, or bar graph.
- **Evaluation plan:** How will you evaluate the effectiveness of this proposed item or service?

Note

1. For more on this subject, see the book coauthored by Tom Johnson, *Relevance Lost: The Rise and Fall of Management Accounting.*

Summary

This chapter covers a number of financial strategies. In the new value-based reimbursement environment, accompanied by the addition of technology, very different approaches are required in healthcare settings. Using the AHA's 10 "must-do" strategies, this chapter explores possible ways nurse leaders can achieve better financial success in this new environment. It is important to make financial information transparent to all in the organization so that all can contribute to both cost savings and to the best use of available monies. Chapter 10 also examines the budgeting process and makes suggestions on how to both decentralize and streamline the process: Presently, in some organizations budgeting can waste 30% of an administrator's time. In addition, it is important for a nurse leader to know how to write a business plan, or proposal, that include the financial information along with what is needed.

Discussion Questions

1. For each of the 10 must-do strategies, describe an action or change you can make in your department to better prepare for the second curve.
2. Describe the effectiveness of the budget process where you work. What is very positive about it? What needs to be improved? What could be done to improve it?
3. Name 10 financial strategies that would improve the finances at your work.
4. Select one strategy from question 1 and describe how you would introduce the action or change you propose in the workplace. Then, map out what would need to happen for it to be implemented.
5. How does complexity influence budget strategies and their implementation? Give examples.
6. Write a business plan for a change, piece of equipment, or new process needed at your work.

References

American Hospital Association, 2011 Committee on Performance Improvement. (2011, September). *Hospitals and care systems of the future.* Chicago, IL: Author.

American Nurses Association. (2007). *Scope and standards of nursing informatics practice.* Silver Spring, MD: Nursebooks.org.

Burke, R. (2002). The ripple effect. *Nursing Management, 33*(2), 41–42.

Cadmus, E., Kilgallen, M., Wynen, E., Holly, C., Chamberlain, B., Gallagher-Ford, L., & Steingall, P. (2008). Nurses' skill level and access to evidence-based practice. *Journal of Nursing Administration, 38*(11), 494–503.

Clancy, T. (2010). Technology and complexity: Trouble brewing? *Journal of Nursing Administration, 40*(6), 237–249.

Cowan, L. (2013). Literature review and risk mitigation strategy for unintended consequences of computerized physician order entry. *Nursing Economic$, 31*(1), 27–31.

Finkler, S., & Kovner, C. (2007). *Financial management for nurse managers and executives* (4th ed.). St. Louis, MO: Elsevier.

Gale, B., & Schaffer, M. (2009). Organizational readiness for evidence-based practice. *Journal of Nursing Administration, 39*(2), 91–97.

Health Research & Educational Trust. (2013, April). *Metrics for the second curve of health care.* American Hospital Association. Retrieved from http://www.hpoe.org /future-metrics-1to4

Hope, J., & Fraser, R. (2003). Who needs budgets? *Harvard Business Review, 81*(2), 108–115.

Huryk, L. (2011). Interview with an informaticist. *Nursing Management, 29*(11), 44–48.

Kalisch, B. (2009). Nursing and nurse assistant perceptions of missed nursing care: What does it tell us about teamwork? *Journal of Nursing Administration, 39*(11), 485–493.

Lefever, G. (1999). Invisible costs, visible savings. *Nursing Management, 30*(8), 29–32.

Matney, S., Brewster, P., Sward, K., Cloyes, K., & Staggers, N. (2011). Philosophical approaches to the nursing informatics data-information-knowledge-wisdom framework. *Advances in Nursing Science, 34*(1), 6–18.

McLane, S., & Turley, J. (2011). Informaticians: How they may benefit your healthcare organization. *Journal of Nursing Administration, 41*(1), 29–35.

Melnyk, B., Fineout-Overholt, E., Gallagher-Ford, L., & Kaplan, L. (2012). The state of evidence-based practice in US nurses: Critical implications for nurse leaders and educators. *Journal of Nursing Administration, 42*(9), 410–417.

Rigby, D. (2002, April). Look before you lay off. Downsizing in a downturn can do more harm than good. *Harvard Business Review,* 20–21.

Russell-Babin, K. (2009). Seeing through the clouds in evidence-based practice. *Nursing Management, 39*(11), 26–33.

Wang, P. (2012). Cutting the high cost of end-of-life care. CNNMoney. Retrieved from http://money.cnn .com/2012/12/11/pf/end-of-life-care-duplicate-2 .moneymag/index.html

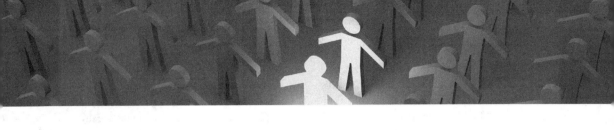

Wellmont Health System Bristol Regional Medical Center

Proposal for Neuro/Surgical Stepdown Units

Prepared by **Velvet Vanover**, MSN, RN, CCRN Clinical Manager, Wellmont Health System

December 10, 2003
Wellmont Health System
Bristol Regional Medical Center

▶ Proposal for Neuro/Surgical Stepdown Units

History: The three intensive care units (ICU, 30 beds total) are remaining full at all times. Intensive care patients often have to wait either in the emergency department or in a medical/surgical unit for a patient to be transferred out before they can be admitted to the ICU. This causes delays in patient treatment, increases nursing demands on the medical/surgical unit, and increases length of stay.

Proposal: Formation of two 4-bed Neuro/Surgical Stepdown Units to be located on the existing nursing units of 2 East and 2 West. Creation of these stepdown units would allow patients to be moved out of the ICU.

2 East

The four existing, camera-monitored, beds would be upgraded to become a full Neurological/Surgical Stepdown Unit. The primary patient would be the complex neurological/surgical patient that no longer meets the criteria of a critical care unit, but requires more intensive observation, intervention, and treatment than can be offered by a medical/surgical floor.

2 West

The four existing beds currently utilized as stepdown beds would be upgraded to become a full Surgical Stepdown Unit. The primary patient would be the complex surgical patient that no longer meets the criteria of a critical care unit, but requires more intensive observation, intervention, and treatment than can be offered by a medical/surgical floor.

The development of two stepdown units would increase both the efficiency and quality of care presently offered to patients at the hospital. Other advantages include: decreased length of stays in the SICU, smoother transitions to Medical/Surgical areas, supported "fast tracking" for discharge home, and increased patient/family satisfaction. In addition, there would be increased physician satisfaction by providing additional options and alternatives for the most appropriate patient care.

The purpose of each of the stepdown units would be to provide specialized care for neurological/surgical patients who require close clinical and technical observation with rapid interventions. Patients may require continuous monitoring of one or more of the following: Cardiac, non-invasive blood pressure (NIBP), pulse oximeter, A-line, and/or central venous catheter (CVP) line.

The stepdown units will be staffed using a nurse (registered nurse [RN])-patient ratio of 1:4.

In addition, Patient Care Technicians will be assigned to assist with patient care.

They will be responsible for assisting with the collection of vital signs to include temperature, pulse rate, respiratory rate, and blood pressure. The RN will be responsible for monitoring vital signs more frequently than every 4 hours.

Patients

Three patient types would benefit from these stepdown units.

1. Patients that are currently admitted to an intensive care unit but do not fully meet the requirements of an ICU. These patients require closer observation than a medical/surgical unit can offer.

2. Patients admitted for elective surgical procedures that require multiple care units. These patients would benefit by avoiding the surgical intensive care unit (SICU). They could be admitted and return postoperatively to the same room. This would result in increased patient satisfaction, increased communication, and ultimately may decrease the length of stay.

3. Patients that have had appropriate lengths of stay in the surgical intensive care and no longer require the same level of care. At the same time, this patient still requires more care and observation than is offered on a medical/surgical unit.

Physicians

Physicians have voiced many concerns regarding the current patient flow. Among those concerns are the following: costly delays in transfers from the SICU; the skill levels of nurses on the medical/surgical floors; and the nurse-patient ratios. Specific specialties concerns are:

1. Neurosurgeons feel additional education is needed for nursing staff to include close observation and assessment for rapid patient changes. In addition, they would like to have access for cardiac and pressure monitoring of neurosurgical patients.

2. Surgeons site concerns over delays in transfers out of the intensive care units, consistency in the nurse-patient ratio, the lack of cardiac monitoring in the current stepdown area, and the inability of staff to do basic critical drips and arterial lines.

Staff

Both nurse managers on 2 East and 2 West feel a staffing nurse-patient ratio of 1 to 4 would be possible without increasing the current full-time equivalents (FTEs) on those units. There would need to be assurance of an assigned nurse for those beds without overflowing into the other medical/surgical beds. Additional needs for staff would include:

1. Education in both cardiac and arterial line monitoring.
2. Education in critical thinking.
3. Education in assessment and observation of the neurological and surgical patient.

Benefits of Developing Stepdown Units

Improved Patient Outcomes

- Increased continuity of care due to the same caregivers and decreased transfers.
- Increased patient satisfaction and compliancy through consistent patient teaching.
- Increased observation and assessment for quick interventions.
- Increased family participation consistent with Planetree.

Improved Operating Efficiency

- Increased and appropriate use of intensive care units by eliminating admission or allowing earlier discharge from those units to stepdown units.

- Financial savings from having stepdown beds available to move patients to when an order for transfer is written.
- Increased telemetry monitoring capabilities.
- Increased rate difference on 2 East and 2 West for monitored beds.
- Increased use of the present staff at a higher level of care.

Improved Physician Relationships

- Fulfillment of requests by physicians for stepdown areas with guaranteed staffing patterns.
- Increased physician satisfaction by providing competent, quality patient care.
- Increased relations with neurosurgeons by meeting patient acuity needs.
- Increased loyalty for patient admissions to Wellmont-Bristol Regional Medical Center.

Enhanced Market Shares

Development of two, 4-bed stepdown units would increase patient flow and allow increased market shares in the neurological patient and intensive care patient. Additional stepdown beds would free up intensive care beds that are often in short supply. This would eliminate the need for possible diversion to another facility. An increase in the number of neurological surgical patients would occur because of the additional beds available, as well as increased care levels.

Financials

Initial Investment

4 Monitors	$55,712.10	
Rewiring	$1,000.00	
Education	+ $17,145.60	(16 hrs educ × $17.86 avg hourly salary ×
Subtotal	$73,857.70	60 nurses = $17,145.60)

Stepdown Charge	$607.50
Average Room Rate	−$370.00
	$237.50 increase per room per day

8 beds at	$4,860.00 per day	(Stepdown Rate)
8 beds at	−$2,960.00 per day	(Private Rm. Rate)
	$1,900.00 per day	

$1,900.00 × 365 = $69,350.00 increased revenue per year

Salary Comparison

SICU salary cost per pt. day (2:1 ratio) $857.28 per day*
SDU salary cost per pt. day (4:1 ratio) $428.64 per day
Salary Savings $428.64 per day
8 patient beds per day $857.28 per day Salary Savings

*The fixed cost of a Manager, Clinical Educator, and Unit Coordinator are approximately the same for all units. Ergo, does not influence salary cost.

Reimbursement Issues

Case Mix of Patient Population: 65% Medicare/Medicaid/TennCare
                                     35% Managed Care*

*Self pay/Worker's Comp and other payers included in Managed Care %.

A. Medicare/Medicaid/TennCare
    Pays at flat rate per stay. Savings to be achieved by providing the service at a lower cost to WBRMC would be seen in saved salary dollars.
    $857.28/day Salary Savings × 365 days × 65% Payer Mix = $203,389.68 year savings.

B. Managed Care
    Pays at per diem rate or % of charges rate. Per diem rate change would result in loss of charges to organization. Changing from ICU rate to stepdown rate equals $528.00 loss per day.
    $528.00 loss per day × 8 beds × 365 days per year × 35% payer mix = $539,616.00 loss per year *

*This would only be if all eight patients would have been in the ICU.

Impact: $539,616.00 Loss
                               − $203,389.68 Savings
                                 $336,226.32 Loss per year to Organization

Total Financial Impact   Initial Investment $73,857.77
                                 + Loss Revenue $336,226.32
                                                   $410,084.09 Loss

1st Year Increased Revenues $69,350.00
Salary Saving Per Year   + $312,907.20
                                 $382,257.20

1st Year =   Loss of $27,826.89
After 1st year =   Revenue of $23,319.12 per year

TITLE: ADMISSION AND DISCHARGE CRITERIA NEURO/SURGICAL STEPDOWN UNIT
PURPOSE: To facilitate the increased care of the complex neurosurgical patient requiring continuous observation, assessment, and intervention but not requiring intensive critical care.

OBJECTIVES: To deliver safe, effective, quality care to acutely ill neurological and/or surgical patients.

To participate in collaborative interdisciplinary healthcare teams.

To maintain a competent, highly trained nursing staff to provide acute care that utilizes the nursing process.

GUIDELINES:

Medical Staff Management

The attending physician will retain authority and responsibility for the admission, transfer, and discharge of the patient except where special problems are designated to the care of consultants.

Nursing Management

The nurse manager of the 2 East and 2 West units will have (24-hour) responsibility for each of their 4-bed stepdown units.

Admission Criteria

Admission to the surgical stepdown unit will be based on the following criteria:

a. The acuity status of the patient based upon the patient classification system.

b. The technology required for monitoring the patient.

c. The needs of the patients requiring the following:

1. Ongoing observation and assessment.

2. Monitoring of NIBP, Cardiac Rhythms, Temp, Arterial lines, and/or CVPs.

3. Frequent monitoring of vital signs.

4. Administration and monitoring of intravenous drips**:
   Dobutamine
   Low-dose Dopamine
   Lidocaine
   NTG
   Nipride
   Neosynephrine
   Cardizem
   Labetalol

**Levophed, epinephrine, and high-dose dopamine should only be used in the ICUs.

CHAPTER 11

Accounting for Healthcare Entities

J. Michael Leger, PhD, MBA, RN, and **Paul Bayes**, DBA Accounting, MS Economics, BS Accounting

OBJECTIVES

- Provide reporting of the finance side of the organization.
- Help the nurse manager to read a detailed financial statement, including a balance sheet, income statement, and cash flow operating activities.

▶ Introduction

Accounting has been called the language of business because accounting information provides direction for action. Healthcare organizations can be classified as either for-profit or not-for-profit, but much of the information is the same and requires similar decision making. Each organization has assets and liabilities. The difference occurs in the area defined as either stockholders' equity (for-profit) or unrestricted, temporarily restricted, and permanently restricted funds (not-for-profit).

The financial synopsis of management's actions is contained in the financial statements (see Appendix of this chapter for examples of profit-oriented and not-for-profit entities). Excerpts from these statements are used as examples throughout this chapter. Years ago, it was uncommon for healthcare entities to have financial problems. However, changing economic conditions and revenue-limiting measures by third-party providers (insurance companies/government) require healthcare entities to take a more proactive look at the financial condition of their business. The failure to do so may result in what has happened to many "dot-coms," as well as established companies, in recent years.

Financial statements are required every year, and publicly traded healthcare entities must also issue quarterly financial statements. These financial statements consist of the statement of financial position (balance sheet), the *income statement* (also called statement of *financial activities*—income and expenses or statement of earnings), and statement of cash flows. In recent years, more attention has focused on the statement of cash flows because cash is the lifeblood of a business. To be an informed decision maker, you must understand how to use financial statements, but you do not necessarily have to know how to prepare these financial statements. Thus, the focus of this chapter is on the understanding and use of financial information.

▶ Accounting Framework

One of the basic frameworks of for-profit accounting is the accounting equation:

$$Assets = Liabilities + Equity$$

Assets—those items that provide future cash flow or have future economic benefit; used to generate revenue for the business.

Liabilities—claims on the assets of an organization; these claims are those of creditors who have provided services such as buildings and equipment but have not been fully paid.

Equity—the difference between the assets and liabilities

In not-for-profit organizations, the result of subtracting liabilities from assets is called *net assets* or *fund balances*. Not-for-profit entities return the excess amount to the sponsoring organization if they cease to continue their stated purposes. The accounting framework for a not-for-profit organization would be Assets = Liabilities + Net assets or fund balances. Examples of these differences are illustrated as follows.

▶ Statement of Financial Position (Balance Sheet)

Assets

The *balance sheet*—consisting of the assets, liabilities, and equity—is a snapshot of the healthcare entity and is dated for a 1-day period of time. The assets, liabilities, and equity or fund balances reflect only the amounts as of a certain date. Traditional examples use December 31 as the ending day, but firms have other ending time periods. The asset portion of Hospital Anywhere USA, which is dated as of December 31, appears in **TABLE 11.1**. Complete financial statements are found in the appendix.

Assets may be classified as current versus long term or, more specifically, current assets, property and equipment (*tangible assets*), investments, and *intangible assets* such as patents. *Current assets* are those items that will be used to generate revenue in either 1 year or the operating period, whichever is longer (most often this is 1 year).

Generally, the first item listed on the statement of financial position is cash, although many

TABLE 11.1 Asset Section of Balance Sheet		
(Dollars in millions)		
Assets	**2004**	**2003**
Current assets		
Cash and cash equivalents	$314	$190
Accounts receivable, less allowance for doubtful accounts of $1,583 and $1,567	2,211	1,873
Inventories	396	383
Income taxes receivable	197	178
Other	1,335	973
Total current assets	**4,453**	**3,597**
Property and equipment at cost		
Land	793	813
Buildings	6,021	6,108
Equipment	7,045	6,721
Construction in progress	431	442
Total property and equipment	**14,290**	**14,084**
Accumulated depreciation	(5,810)	(5,594)
	8,480	8,490
Investments of insurance subsidiary	1,371	1,457
Investments in and advances to affiliates	779	654
Intangible assets, net of accumulated amortization of $785 and $644	2,155	2,319
Other	330	368
Total assets	**$17,568**	**$16,885**

times it is combined with temporary investments, which are considered *cash equivalents*. Temporary investments are cash equivalents because they can be sold quickly with little or no loss in value. This is the reserve needed to meet the operational needs of the organization, such as salaries, and to meet other obligations as they arise.

An important source of future cash is generically identified as *accounts (patients) receivable*. These may be represented by amounts owed by either patients to which the organization has provided services, or by claims filed with third-party providers, such as insurance companies. These provide future cash flows, and therefore it is imperative these insurance claims are filed quickly and accurately. Reducing the collection period provides cash more quickly for operations. This amount is often reported as a "net" number, reflecting amounts that will not be collected or as reductions from third-party providers.

Other current assets of the organization consist of *inventory* items such as drugs in the pharmacy, surgical supplies, items maintained at nursing stations, and drinks and/or food in the cafeteria. The alternative inventory cost measures are not discussed in this text. The income taxes receivable account is the equivalent of receiving a tax refund but waiting for the check.

Property and Equipment

The largest item on a for-profit healthcare entity's balance sheet is probably *buildings* and *equipment*. This may also be defined as *tangible assets*. *Land* on which a healthcare facility is located is one item included in this section. Land is not written off, unless there is something that impairs value, such as pollution of the land site. Other tangible assets, such as buildings and equipment, have skyrocketing costs because of the complexity of equipment and more rigorous building codes and regulations. Buildings are the physical facilities in which patient services are provided. Equipment may be items such as x-ray and computed tomography (CT) machines or less complex items such as patient beds. The increased costs require either the availability of

large amounts of funds for purchases (cash) or credit-granting sources.

Construction in progress is an account indicating buildings that have not been completed but are being built. The account indicates progress toward completion. *Depreciation* is an accounting charge wherein the balance of the equipment and buildings is systematically written off over a period of time. *Accumulated depreciation*, which is the sum of the annual depreciation charges, is then subtracted from the plant and equipment balance, providing a net figure. This number does not relate to current market value but rather is book value only, which is the original cost minus accumulated depreciation.

Investments

Investments are classified as long term in nature in that they are held for income purposes. These may be a result of using excess cash to either invest in items such as other organizations, joint ventures, purchase the stocks or bonds of other organizations, or the donations received from external parties. As in the case of Hospital Anywhere USA, they are investments in other organizations (affiliates of Hospital Anywhere USA) or loans made to affiliate organizations.

Intangible Assets

Intangible assets generally are those items that have no physical presence but do have value in the form of legal rights to use or sell an asset. One example is patents that have been developed by employees of the organization. Use of a patent may provide a strategic advantage over competing facilities or may reduce your firm's costs below that of competitors. One item that is harder to define as an intangible asset is *goodwill*. Goodwill occurs when an entity purchases another organization and there is an excess amount paid for the net assets of the purchased entity that exceeds market value. This excess amount is goodwill.

Most intangible assets are also systematically written off over a period of time like that of depreciation, but the process is called *amortization*.

Goodwill must be evaluated each year, and a determination must be made for impairment of value. If value declines, goodwill must be reduced ("written down") by this amount.

Liabilities

To begin our discussion of liabilities, please refer to **TABLE 11.2**.

Current Liabilities

Accounts payables are claims on assets. These are short term in nature and are generally expected to be paid in 30 to 120 days based on the type of claim but can be unpaid up to 1 year. The purchase of operating supplies such as surgical staples and food items are examples.

Accrued liabilities (i.e., salaries) are those that have been incurred in the course of business but have not yet been paid. For example, if employees are paid on the fifth of the month for their efforts in the previous month, then it is an accrued expense. Employers owe employees for services provided but have not yet made payment. Accounting recognizes expenses when incurred, not necessarily when paid. Other accrued expenses could include interest

TABLE 11.2 Liabilities Section of Balance Sheet		
(Dollars in millions, except for per share amount)		
Liabilities	**2004**	**2003**
Current liabilities		
Accounts payable	693	657
Accrued salaries	352	403
Other accrued expenses	1,135	897
Government settlement accrual	840	
Long-term debt due within 1 year	1,121	1,160
Total current liabilities	**4,141**	**3,117**
Long-term debt	5,631	5,284
Professional liability risks, deferred taxes and other liabilities	2,050	2,104
Minority interests in equity of consolidated entities	572	763
Forward purchase contracts and put options	769	
Total liabilities	**13,163**	**11,268**

incurred on debt but not paid, or taxes owed to government entities.

Most organizations finance equipment or a building that requires a large outlay of resources over a long period of time, with some financing arrangements lasting up to 40 years. Each year, as that portion of the debt becomes due in the current year, it is considered a current liability.

Long-Term Liabilities (Debt)

Long-term debt examples include such items as mortgages and bonds issued to borrow money. This debt is not paid in the current year or operating period. Other items identified as long-term debt could include professional liability risks such as unsettled lawsuits resulting from malpractice claims and employee work-related injuries. *Deferred taxes* are the differences between income reported in financial statements and that paid to the U.S. Treasury.

Stockholders' Equity

For-profit corporate firms raise funds by issuing either *preferred or common stock*. **TABLE 11.3** provides an example. These stocks represent ownership shares in an organization. Both stocks generally have a par value and sell for more than this base amount (capital in excess of par value). The *par value* is arbitrarily established as a low amount and is used for accounting records.

Preferred stock is not used as extensively as common stock but is one possible source of funds. The stock gets its name from the preference over common stock in either payments of dividends or distribution of liquidation proceeds in case of the firm ceasing business. Three additional financial items are found in the stockholders' equity section of Hospital Anywhere USA.

The final item found on the statement of financial position is *retained earnings*. The name is misleading because there is no actual money

---

TABLE 11.3 Stockholders' Equity Section of Balance Sheet

(Dollars in millions)		
Stockholders' equity:		
Common stock $0.01 par; authorized 1,600,000,000 voting shares 50,000,000 nonvoting shares; outstanding 521,991,700 voting shares and 21,000,000 shares and 21,000,000 nonvoting shares—2004; and 543,272,900 voting shares and 21,000,000 nonvoting shares—2003	5	6
Capital in excess of par value		951
Other	9	8
Accumulated other comprehensive income	52	53
Retained earnings	4,339	4,599
Total stockholders' equity	4,405	5,617
Total liabilities and stockholders' equity	**$17,568**	**$16,885**

in this account. Retained earnings is an account used by the accounting function to balance the books at the end of the year. The amount carried to retained earnings is the difference between all revenue sources, expenses and costs, and dividends paid. The equivalent section of the stockholders' equity of a not-for-profit is called a fund balance.

Income Statement

The *income statement* is a financial statement that captures information about revenue sources, expenses, and costs of doing business during a period of time. For example, a yearly income statement would be labeled for the year ended. Hospital Anywhere USA shows years ended December 31, 2004, 2003, and 2002 (**TABLE 11.4**).

Most revenue sources come from providing patient services. The problem with these sources is that the amount billed is not the amount received. For example, using the prospective payment system established in the early 1990s, many of the major insurance companies pay only between 50% and 60% of the amount billed. For

TABLE 11.4 Income Statement			
(Dollars in millions)			
	2004	**2003**	**2002**
Revenues	**$16,670**	**$16,657**	**$18,681**
Salaries and benefits	6,639	6,694	7,766
Supplies	2,640	2,645	2,901
Other operating expenses	3,085	3,251	3,816
Provision for doubtful accounts	1,255	1,269	1,442
Depreciation and amortization	1,033	1,094	1,247
Interest expense	559	471	561
Equity in earnings of affiliates	(126)	(90)	(112)
Settlement with federal government	840	0	0
Gains on sales of facilities	(34)	(297)	(744)
Impairment of long-lived assets	117	220	542
Restructuring of operations and investigation-related costs	62	116	111
Total expenses	**16,070**	**15,373**	**17,530**

Medicare and state health plans, such as Medicaid, this amount is even lower—it could be as low as 25%. This has led to major changes in the accounting of healthcare providers, such as more accuracy in billing. If a claim is filed with a third-party provider, payment must be received as soon as possible. Many healthcare providers found that claims collection was taking as many as 90 days. This means services were provided, resulting in expenditures, but the healthcare provider has only a piece of paper representing a claim. Many providers have improved their claims collection through improved accuracy of coding and by using electronic filing. The sooner the payment is received, the sooner the healthcare entity can use the funds to pay its own claims for services provided by creditors and purchase new equipment or replacement equipment for improved diagnosis.

Additional revenue may take the form of providing services for other healthcare facilities or through the investment of funds. One example of additional services is that of a healthcare facility, such as Healthy Hospital, doing laundry service for other hospitals. One section of the Hospital Anywhere USA asset section illustrated the category called investments. Revenues from invested funds in the form of interest or dividends can also supplement basic operations.

Reductions in payments by third-party providers, including government entities, have forced many healthcare facilities to establish an active foundation so that additional funds are directed to the foundation. These additional sources of funds can be used to either cover shortfalls in revenues or they can be invested to provide interest or other forms of additional revenue.

Costs and Expenses

Deductions from the revenue sources take the form of either costs or expenses. *Costs and expenses*, in the income statement, are those items used up or incurred in the generation of revenues. For Hospital Anywhere USA, the largest of these expenses is generally salaries and benefits paid to employees.

The second largest category of expenses is *supplies and services*, as shown in Table 11.4. Each patient for whom services are rendered requires some use of supplies (i.e., forms for patient information, swabs for testing, testing supplies, or food and beverages provided through food services).

The third largest item is the *provision for doubtful accounts* (bad debt expense/provision for bad debts), which is the adjustment for patient services that are expected not to be collected. Bad debt expense is the charge for not being able to collect patient accounts. Charges filed with third-party payers are reduced according to payment schedules established by these firms. This reduces the amount of revenue from the gross (full) amount billed to the net amount. The amount over that paid by the third-party payers is expected to be collected from the patient to whom services were provided. This refers to deductibles and copayments, which are amounts the patient pays over the reasonable and customary charges. However, with Medicare and Medicaid patients, it is illegal to go back and bill the patients for whatever Medicare and Medicaid doesn't pay. In some cases, the patient will not be able to make payments. These must be taken as further charges in the form of bad debts.

Depreciation is a deduction allowed by the Internal Revenue Service. This is a paper and pencil amount (accounting) and is not an actual use of cash sources. Once a building or piece of equipment is acquired, it may be "written off" over a designated period of time. The cost of the equipment is allocated to a specific time period and is used to reduce the net revenue and thus reduce taxes. For example, if a piece of diagnostic equipment having a 10-year life span is purchased for 5 million dollars, using one of the many methods allowed for the calculation of depreciation (straight-line), the depreciation amount per year would be $500,000 ($5,000,000 ÷ 10 years = $500,000 depreciation per year). As stated previously, this reduces income and will lead to fewer taxes being paid.

Depending on the size of the healthcare facility, additional costs may be incurred.

Cash Flow

As stated previously, cash is the lifeblood of a business. The *cash flow statement* shows one part of the financial stability of a firm. If all transactions were cash-based, then this statement would be easy to prepare and interpret. For-profit entities are required by generally accepted accounting principles (GAAP) to report on an accrual basis. This means that revenue must be reported when earned, not necessarily when payment is received, and expenses are recognized when incurred, not paid. This requires several estimates during the reporting period. For example, if a service has been provided and a healthcare entity has a reasonable expectation of collection and can identify the amount to be collected, then it must be reported as revenue. Cash for the service may not be received until the next period.

If employees are paid every Friday and the reporting period ends on Thursday, then salaries must be accrued. For simplicity, let us assume those salaries are $100,000 per week and no one works on the weekends. Each week, the healthcare entity makes cash payments of $100,000 until the final week of the year. Because the reporting period ends on Thursday, the firm owes the employees $80,000 (4 days of pay) for services rendered. This amount must be recorded as an expense in the current period but does not require cash expenditure until the next reporting period.

The *bad debt expense* must likewise be estimated at the end of the year. The total amount of bad debts will not be known until all efforts to collect an account have been exhausted. This requires recognition of the bad debt expense for the reporting period (quarterly or yearly). The estimate is based on past experience in collection of accounts receivable, necessitated by adjustments for economic conditions. If 2% of the accounts receivable have been identified as bad in previous years and there was a major plant closing in the current reporting period, it could be expected that the amount collected would decrease and the bad debt expense would increase.

Preparation of the cash flow statement requires a thorough knowledge of the financial statements. Taking the cash balance at the beginning of the period and subtracting the ending cash balance provides the change in cash. The cash flow statement provides information explaining why cash changed. Financial statement items causing changes in cash are identified as operating, financing, and investing activities.

Operating Activities

Operating activities focus on the current portion of financial statements. They are the most important part of the cash flow analysis. Operating activities focus on the cash inflows and outflows from events that occur in the current operating period (**TABLE 11.5**). Financing and investing activities can provide funds but are limited to the extent of the time to which they can provide cash flow. There are upper limits on the amount of debt that can be issued (borrowed) on stock that can be sold. Likewise, there is a limited amount of investments that can be sold to provide cash inflow. There is also a limit on the number of long-term assets that can be sold, and much like personal debt, there is a limit to the amount of money that can be borrowed.

Cash flow can be calculated in two ways, but the one preferred by most entities starts with the net income or loss from the income statement. All current assets and liabilities from the balance sheet must be analyzed to determine the impact on cash flow. If accounts receivable increases, how is cash impacted? Cash would decrease. If the amount of current assets represented by accounts receivable increases, you now have more paper and less cash coming in. From the perspective of the income statement, when services were provided you recorded the item as income. Net income is therefore higher than the cash generated from revenue, leading to the adjustment in net income on the cash flow statement. The same is true for all other current assets. There is an inverse relationship between the change in current assets and the impact on

TABLE 11.5 Cash Flow Operating Activities Section

(Dollars in millions)			
Cash flows from continuing activities	**2004**	**2003**	**2002**
Net income	$219	$657	$379
Adjustments to reconcile net income to net cash provided by continuing operating activities			
Provision for doubtful accounts	1,255	1,269	1,442
Depreciation and amortization	1,033	1,094	1,247
Income taxes	(219)	(66)	351
Settlement with federal government	840	0	0
Gains on sales of facilities	(34)	(297)	(744)
Impairment of long-lived assets	117	220	542
Loss from discontinued operating assets	0	0	153
Increase (decrease) in cash from operating assets and liabilities			
Accounts receivable	(1,678)	(1,463)	(1,229)
Inventories and other assets	90	(119)	(39)
Accounts payable and accrued expenses	(147)	(110)	(177)
Other	71	38	(9)
Net cash provided by continuing operating activities	**$1,547**	**$1,223**	**$1,916**

cash flow. If current assets increase, they will be deducted from net income—or vice versa: If current assets decrease, they will be added back to net income.

Current liabilities have the opposite effect. If any current liability increases, this adds to the cash balance. What is the impact on cash if current liabilities increase? The firm has acquired either goods or services without having a cash outflow. The cash balance is improved by acquisition of assets without having a cash outflow. All current liabilities have a direct relationship with the impact on cash flow. Increases are added to net income, and decreases are subtracted from net income. The result of adding or deducting changes in current assets and liabilities to net income provides cash flow from operating activities.

Financing Activities

The second portion of the cash flow statement is the *financing activities*, which focuses on long-term liabilities (those having a due date of longer than 1 year) or equity in the form of common or preferred stock (**TABLE 11.6**). If long-term liabilities increase during the year, it provides cash inflow. The firm is borrowing money to use in the business. If long-term liabilities decrease, then this implies that the liabilities are being paid off, leading to a decrease in cash. Stock operates in the same manner. If either the common or preferred stock accounts increase, then the implication is that stock is used to finance firm activities. If they decrease, then stock is being repurchased and cash is leaving the firm. Likewise, the payment of dividends on stock decreases cash outflow.

Investing Activities

The last part of the cash flow statement concerns the *investing activities* of an organization, as shown in **TABLE 11.7**. This focuses mainly on the long-term assets of a business. If these assets are sold, cash inflows occur. On the other hand, if long-term assets are acquired, then cash is presumed to decrease. An increase in investments is shown as having a decrease in cash.

Adding each category, continuing operating, financing, and investing provides the change in cash and cash equivalents. Added to or subtracted from (if cash flow is negative, as in 2003) cash and cash equivalents at the beginning of the period provides the amounts found on the balance sheet. The cash and cash equivalents account increased in both 2004 and 2002 and decreased in 2003, as shown in **TABLE 11.8**, which provides a summary of all activities.

Schedule of Changes in Equity

The *Schedule of Changes in Equity* is required for all publicly reporting companies (governed by stock markets, such as those sold on the New York Stock Exchange) and presents information for the reader to evaluate all changes in the owner's portion of the balance sheet.

TABLE 11.6 Cash Flow Financing Activities Section

(Dollars in millions)			
Cash flows from financing activities	**2004**	**2003**	**2002**
Issuance of long-term debt	$2,980	$1,037	$3
Net change in bank borrowing	(500)	200	(2,514)
Repayment of long-term debt	(2,058)	(1,572)	(147)
Issuance (repurchase) of common stock, net	(677)	(1,884)	8
Payment of cash dividends	(44)	(44)	(52)
Other	(37)	8	3
Net cash used in financing activities	**($336)**	**($2,255)**	**($2,699)**

TABLE 11.7 Cash Flow Investing Activities Section

(Dollars in millions)			
Cash flows from investing activities	2004	2003	2002
Purchase of property and equipment	($1,155)	($1,287)	($1,255)
Acquisitions of hospitals and healthcare entities	(350)	0	(215)
Spin-off of facilities to stockholders	0	886	0
Disposal of hospitals and healthcare entities	327	805	2,060
Change in investments	106	565	(294)
Investment in discontinued operations, net	0	0	677
Other	(15)	(44)	(3)
Net cash provided by (used in) investing activities	**($1,087)**	**$925**	**$970**

TABLE 11.8 Summary of Cash Flows and Changes in Cash and Cash Equivalents

(Dollars in millions)			
	2004	2003	2002
Net cash provided by continuing operating activities	**$1,547**	**$1,223**	**$1,916**
Net cash provided by (used in) investing activities	**($1,087)**	**$925**	**$970**
Net cash used in financing activities	**($336)**	**($2,255)**	**($2,699)**
Change in cash and cash equivalents	124	(107)	187
Cash and cash equivalents at beginning of period	190	297	110
Cash and cash equivalents at end of period	$314	$190	$297

▸ Internal Accounting Information

Cost/Managerial Accounting

Although public-reporting, for-profit healthcare entities must issue financial statements to external users, not-for-profit entities are not required to report to the general public. Accounting information used for internal or management decisions is not available to the general public but is used by management and others working within an organization. This information may be as specific as the pay rate for individual employees or the costs to operate a function of the firm, such as laboratories. For many healthcare workers, this is the area where management asks for employee input. This information is also used to evaluate the current operations of the organization and to solicit employee input to improve future operations. As previously mentioned, the amount of payments from third-party payers has declined in recent years. Healthcare facilities used to receive reimbursements based on costs of operation. However, with the advent of prospective payment systems, these amounts have generally been reduced. Thus, input from employees is needed to reduce costs and to improve customer services. As one nurse stated to the author, "I know the technical part of my job, but I am being asked to serve on committees that are looking at changing and improving business operations." Thus, the nurse needs to understand accounting information and how it can be used to support these changes.

Costs

Costs to be considered in making management decisions include differentiating between fixed and variable, direct and indirect, and marginal costs. Included in the discussion of costs is the term *relevant range*. To most, relevant range refers to the likely operating activity level expected to be incurred by a healthcare entity. For example, current staff can handle between 100 and 150 patients per day, which is the average use of the facilities. If the number of patients is either higher or lower than these numbers, costs must be reconsidered (i.e., reduce or add employees to provide services).

From a revenue perspective, previous discussion centered on correct coding and use of diagnosis-related groups and resource utilization groups. Discussion also centered on the collection of these revenue items and the impact on financial statements. When healthcare facilities were forced to more carefully evaluate their operations, they found many services offered were losing money. Because revenues were capped, cost containment became the issue.

Fixed Versus Variable Costs

Evaluating operations begins with the evaluation of the costs involved. First is the distinction between fixed and variable costs. *Fixed costs* do not change with levels of services. If you are dealing with a facility that has 100 beds, building costs such as depreciation will be the same regardless of whether there is 1 patient or 100 patients occupying a bed or beds. *Variable costs* do change with the increase of facility use. As more patients occupy the facility, costs such as food, medicines, and staff increase. These costs are variable because they change as the volume (number of patients or procedures) changes.

Direct Versus Indirect Costs

The second cost distinction is indirect versus direct costs. For an example, let's use the costs of laboratory services. The cost of the lab assistant who draws blood for analysis is a direct cost. Likewise, needles and other supplies are *direct costs*. The staff person, who manages the facility, handles the paperwork for the patient upon arrival, or files the claim, is an *indirect cost*.

Marginal costs are those costs related to providing additional services. Again, using the laboratory example, assume that the lab can handle 20 patients a day. If the lab is currently offering services to 15 patients, how much will it cost to provide additional services to one more patient? There will be no additional costs for the person drawing the blood sample; thus, there is no marginal cost associated with this service. There will be additional costs associated with the use of needles, bandages, and testing supplies. These are marginal costs. As long as revenue for these services increases more than the costs, services should be expanded.

Average costs are those costs divided by the total number of services provided. Let us assume that it costs $500 per day to maintain the lab. If the lab performs only one test on this day, then the average cost will be $500. However, if the lab performs five tests today, the average cost will be $100 per test. You can operate up to a certain point without expanding facilities, personnel, or equipment. As the number of tests increases, the average cost decreases (this is the relevant range). Let us assume that the facility expands these services to reach 40 tests per day but can process only 20 per day with the current number of employees. The relevant range would be up to 20 tests. More than 20 tests would require the addition of personnel or equipment.

Activity-Based Costing

Once the types of costs are identified, they need to be allocated to the specific services performed. With the limitations on cost recovery (revenue) imposed by third-party payers, healthcare entities must be aware of the costs to provide these services. Why should a facility pay $1.5 million for a magnetic resonance imaging machine and incur the other costs to maintain and staff the center when the revenues will not cover the costs? Recently, one area of thought in accounting has been introduced to help users of accounting information focus on the specific costs of providing services. This is called *activity-based costing (ABC)*.

ABC requires that you identify the cost drivers behind an activity. It requires that you break all services into specific functions and identify the costs associated with each activity. Assume you work in a physician's office and you

need to determine the costs of a patient visit for a general exam. What activities are associated with the cost of providing these services? Let us assume the following, which is not a comprehensive example, for purposes of illustration:

■ A general practitioner is paid $80,000 per year and spends, on average, 15 minutes with each patient, seeing 24 patients per day. The physician works 45 weeks per year.
■ A nurse is paid $35,000 per year and also spends 15 minutes with the patient.
■ The receptionist is paid $24,000 and spends 5 minutes per patient in taking appointment calls and answering patient questions in the reception area.
■ The cashier is paid $24,000 and spends 5 minutes per patient recording doctor information and verifying information for billing.
■ All claims are entered electronically, and it takes a data recorder 10 minutes to fill out the electronic filing version. This person is paid $20,000.
■ A bookkeeper is paid $25,000 per year to capture accounting information for the facility. The bookkeeper spends 10 minutes per patient, on average, collecting and reporting data for management of the facility.
■ A stethoscope costs $100 and lasts 2 years.
■ Each tongue depressor costs $0.01.
■ Each pair of latex gloves costs $0.01.
■ Each of the previously mentioned individuals in the physician's office has a computer that costs $2,000 and is used for 2 years.
■ Utility service per patient is $1.00.
■ The cost per patient for building (facility) in the form of depreciation is $1.50.

Based on this information, the following provides an analysis of the cost of providing patient services for a general physical examination. In the example shown in **TABLE 11.9**, the patient is the cost driver.

The diagnosis-related group code for medium intervention activity is billed at $50.00. A third-party payer remits, on average, 56% of the billed amount, yielding a payment of $35.60. Additional amounts may be collected from the patient, but

TABLE 11.9 Activity-Based Costing Example

(Dollars in millions)

Cost Driver	Cost	Cost Per Patient	Comments
Physician	$80,000	$14.81	15 minutes per patient/ 24 patients per day/45 weeks
Nurse	$35,000	$6.48	15 minutes per patient/ 24 patients per day/45 weeks
Receptionist	$24,000	$4.44	5 minutes per patient/ 24 patients per day/45 weeks
Cashier	$24,000	$4.44	5 minutes per patient/ 24 patients per day/45 weeks
Data recorder	$20,000	$3.70	10 minutes per patient/ 24 patients per day/45 weeks
Bookkeeper	$25,000	$4.62	10 minutes per patient/ 24 patients per day/45 weeks
Utility services		$1.00	
Computers	$12,000	$0.19	6 computers/$2,000 per computer cost/life of 2 years
Gloves		0.01	
Tongue depressor		0.01	
Building depreciation		$1.50	
Stethoscope	$100	0.01	$100/lasts 2 years
Total		**$41.21**	

that is not assumed in this case. (As mentioned earlier, this is true for coinsurance, deductibles, and what is above the reasonable and customary costs with regular insurance. However, with Medicaid and with Medicare, other than billing the deductible and coinsurance, it is illegal to bill the patient for the amount of reimbursement not paid by the government.) Given the cost of the service at $41.21, there is a loss of $5.61 for each patient seen by the physician. This is where decision making using accounting data can improve the profitability of services, whether this is done by a single physician, nursing home, or hospital. What would you suggest to reduce the costs or improve the revenue? The physician and nurse spend 15 minutes per patient, but the others spend less time. Could the time the physician spends with each patient be reduced to increase the number of patients examined per year? Could there be additional physicians or nurse practitioners employed to increase the workload of others, such as the receptionist and bookkeeper, thus reducing the costs of others, such as the receptionist and cashier? If the number of patients seen increases, the building and computer cost per patient would be decreased. Another alternative is to either expand the nurse's responsibilities or to hire additional nurses to reduce the physician's time with patients.

One solution would be to evaluate the use of each part of the cost structure. In the previous example, the physician was limited to seeing 5,400 patients per year. This is also the limitation for each of the other members of the physician's organization and is the cost driver. If the time spent with patients can be reduced to 10 minutes per patient, then the number of patients the physician can examine will be increased to 36 patients per day, or 8,100 per year. This causes a decrease in the physician cost per patient to $9.88, and receptionist cost per patient to $2.96. The overall effect causes cost to be reduced to a level below the third-party payment that now exceeds cost.

Previously, different types of costs were defined. Using the example, we can now illustrate the costs. Fixed costs are those that do not change in total as volume (number of patients) increases. All costs except utilities, gloves, and tongue depressors are fixed. These costs are variable in that they change as the number of patients increases. As seen in the revenue and cost comparison, the physician's salary is fixed, and as the number of patients increased, the physician's cost per patient decreased (average cost decreases). As with any fixed costs, you want to maximize the use and lower the costs to the lowest level.

Direct costs are those related to the generation of revenues. In this case, the physician and nurse are considered direct costs of providing services, as are the gloves and tongue depressors. The other costs are considered indirect because they are not directly related to production of revenue. Why is this distinction needed? If you are trying to determine whether or not to expand services, you might want to look at the direct costs. Can you cover the direct costs of providing services? If so, then each patient or procedure will add to the profitability of the healthcare entity. For example, in the original illustration, if you can cover the direct costs (physician, nurse, gloves, and tongue depressor—$21.31), then additional amounts received can be applied to the indirect costs. The fixed costs will remain if a facility operates or closes for the weekend or vacations. If you can cover the direct cost, then any excess amount would be used to help cover fixed costs.

Marginal costs are those that increase as additional services are provided. Which costs in the illustration change as additional patients are added? Only the costs of the gloves and tongue depressor are marginal costs. What will it cost to provide service for one additional patient? When evaluating whether or not to accept additional patients, you need to consider the impact on the organization. If no new costs are added for providing additional services, as long as the additional revenue exceeds the additional cost, then the service should be provided. To clarify this point, assume that a third-party insurer approaches your organization offering a new client base consisting of local county employees. However, the insurer will pay a lower amount than that provided by other insurers. If you can determine the marginal costs of the services to be provided, the marginal costs may be less than the revenue received, increasing the contribution to firm profitability. This would benefit the organization.

Summary

Employees of healthcare facilities are being asked to improve patient services by generating additional revenue and becoming valuable members of the management team. Correctly identifying services before filing claims with third parties can improve revenue collection. Additionally, making recommendations for more efficient use of services to minimize costs of these services is important for continuing organizational success. Can the healthcare entity substitute services for those currently being offered? Can someone in an organization provide the same quality services as others? For example, can I use a licensed practical nurse (LPN) in place of a registered nurse? (This decision would be best only if the work performed by the person was appropriate at the LPN level.) This is one of the major issues affecting health care today.

Discussion Questions

1. Why should you be familiar with the balance sheet? Why is it important to the organization? And what area of the balance sheet would you consider the most critical?
2. Comparing costs in this chapter, which costs do you have little control over and why? Which costs would be most important if you are expanding your services?
3. How would you know if the organization is a for-profit or a not-for-profit based on the information available from the balance sheet and the income statement?
4. Goodwill and patents are considered what types of assets?
5. Which asset is considered the lifeblood of the organization, and why?

Glossary of Terms

Accounts (Patients) Receivable these may be represented by amounts owed by either patients to whom the organization has provided services or by claims filed with third-party providers, such as insurance companies.

Accounts Payables claims on assets. These are short term in nature and are generally expected to be paid in 30–120 days based on the type of claim, but can be unpaid up to 1 year.

Accumulated Depreciation the sum of the annual depreciation charges subtracted from the plant and equipment balance providing a net figure.

Activity-Based Costing (ABC) a costing system that requires that you break all services into specific functions and identify the cost drivers associated with each activity.

Assets those items that provide future cash flow or have future economic benefit.

Average Costs those costs divided by the total number of services provided.

Balance Sheet a form that consists of the assets, liabilities, and equity.

Buildings the physical facilities in which patient services are provided.

Cash Flow Statement a form that provides information explaining why cash changed. Financial statement items causing changes in cash are identified as operating, financing, and investing activities.

Construction in Progress an account indicating buildings that have not been completed but are being built. The account indicates progress toward completion.

Costs and Expenses in the income statement, those items used up or incurred in the generation of revenues.

Current Assets those items that will be used to generate revenue in either 1 year or the operating period, whichever is longer (most often this is 1 year).

Deferred Taxes the differences between income reported in financial statements and that paid to the U.S. Treasury.

Depreciation an accounting charge wherein the balance of the equipment and buildings is systematically written off over a period of time.

Equipment may be items such as x-ray or CT machines, or less complex items such as patient beds.

Financial Activities long-term liabilities (obligations have a due date of longer than 1 year) or equity in the form of common or preferred stock.

Fund Balance section of the stockholders' equity of a not-for-profit organization.

Goodwill when an entity purchases another organization and there is an excess amount paid for the net assets of the purchased entity that exceeds market value. This excess amount is goodwill.

Income Statement a financial statement that captures information about revenue sources, expenses, and costs of doing business during a period of time.

Intangible Assets generally, those items that have no physical presence but do have value in the form of legal rights to use or sell an asset.

Inventory items such as drugs in the pharmacy, surgical supplies, items maintained in nursing stations, and drinks and/or food in the cafeteria.

Investment Activities the long-term assets of an organization.

Investments classified as long term in nature in that they are held for income purposes. These may be a result of using excess cash to invest in items such as other organizations, joint ventures, stocks or bonds of other organizations, or donations received from external parties.

Liabilities claims on the assets of an organization. The claims are those of creditors who have provided resources, such as buildings and equipment, but have not been fully paid.

Long-Term Debt such items as mortgages and bonds issued to borrow money. This debt will not be paid in the current year or operating period.

Marginal Costs costs related to providing additional services.

Net Assets in not-for-profit organizations, the result of subtracting liabilities from assets.

Net Worth the difference between the assets and liabilities of an organization is the equity, or in the personal loan application example, net worth.

Operating Activities the cash inflows and outflows from events that occur in the current operating period.

Preferred or Common Stock for-profit corporate firms raise funds by issuing these stocks. These stocks represent ownership shares in an organization.

Provision for Doubtful Accounts the adjustment for patient services that are expected not to be collected.

Relevant Range the likely operating activity level expected to be incurred by a healthcare entity.

Retained Earnings an account used by the accounting function to balance the books at the end of the year.

Schedule of Changes in Equity required for all publicly reporting companies, information for the reader to evaluate all changes in the owner's portion of the balance sheet.

Tangible Assets the largest item on a for-profit healthcare entity's balance sheet, probably buildings and equipment.

Temporary Investments cash equivalents because they can be sold quickly with little or no loss in value.

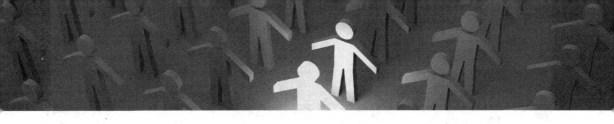

APPENDIX

(All amounts are dollars in millions, except per share amounts.)

Hospital Anywhere USA Consolidated Balance Sheets, December 31, 2004 and 2003		
Assets	**2004**	**2003**
Current assets:		
Cash and cash equivalents	$314	$190
Accounts receivable, less allowance for doubtful accounts of $1,583 and $1,567	2,211	1,873
Inventories	396	383
Income taxes receivable	197	178
Other	1,335	973
Total current assets	**4,453**	**3,597**
Property and equipment at cost:		
Land	793	813
Buildings	6,021	6,108
Equipment	7,045	6,721
Construction in progress	431	442
Total property and equipment	**14,290**	**14,084**
Accumulated depreciation	(5,810)	(5,594)

(continues)

Hospital Anywhere USA Consolidated Balance Sheets, December 31, 2004 and 2003		
Assets	**2004**	**2003**
	8,480	8,490
Investments of insurance subsidiary	1,371	1,457
Instruments in and advances to affiliates	779	654
Intangible assets, net of accumulated amortization of $785 and $644	2,155	2,319
Other	330	368
Total assets	**$17,568**	**$16,885**
Liabilities	2004	2003
Current liabilities:		
Accounts payable	693	657
Accrued salaries	352	403
Other accrued expenses	1,135	897
Government settlement accrual	840	
Long-term debt due within one year	1,121	1,160
Total current liabilities	4,141	3,117
Long-term debt	5,631	5,284
Professional liability risks, deferred taxes, and other liabilities	2,050	2,104
Minority interests in equity of consolidated entities	572	763
Forward purchase contracts and put options	769	
Total liabilities	**13,163**	**11,268**

Assets	2004	2003
Stockholders' equity:		
Common stock $0.01 par; authorized 1,600,000,000 voting shares, 50,000,000 nonvoting shares; outstanding 521,991,700 voting shares, and 21,000,000 nonvoting shares—2004 and 543,272,900 voting shares and 21,000,000 nonvoting shares—2003	5	6
Capital in excess of par value		951
Other	9	8
Accumulated other comprehensive income	52	53
Retained earnings	4,339	4,599
Total stockholders' equity	**4,405**	**5,617**
Total liabilities and stockholders' equity	**$17,568**	**$16,885**

Hospital Anywhere USA Consolidated Statement of Cash Flow for the Years Ended December 31, 2004, 2003, and 2002			
Cash flows from continuing activities	**2004**	**2003**	**2002**
Net income	$219	$657	$379
Adjustments to reconcile net income to net cash provided by continuing operating activities:			
Provision for doubtful accounts	1,255	1,269	1,442
Depreciation and amortization	1,033	1,094	1,247
Income taxes	(219)	(66)	351
Settlement with federal government	840	0	0
Gains on sales of facilities	(34)	(297)	(744)
Impairment of long-lived assets	117	220	542

(continues)

Hospital Anywhere USA Consolidated Statement of Cash Flow for the Years Ended December 31, 2004, 2003, and 2002			
Cash flows from continuing activities	**2004**	**2003**	**2002**
Loss from discontinued operating assets	0	0	153
Increase (decrease) in cash from operating assets and liabilities:			
Accounts receivable	(1,678)	(1,463)	(1,229)
Inventories and other assets	90	(119)	(39)
Accounts payable and accrued expenses	(147)	(110)	(177)
Other	71	38	(9)
Net cash provided by continuing operating activities	**$1,547**	**$1,223**	**$1,916**
Cash flows from financing activities:	**2004**	**2003**	**2002**
Issuance of long-term debt	$2,980	$1,037	$3
Net change in bank borrowing	(500)	200	(2,514)
Repayment of long-term debt	(2,058)	(1,572)	(147)
Issuance (repurchase) of common stock, net	(677)	(1,884)	8
Payment of cash dividends	(44)	(44)	(52)
Other	(37)	8	3
Net cash used in financing activities	**($336)**	**($2,255)**	**($2,699)**
Cash flows from investing activities:	**2004**	**2003**	**2002**
Purchase of property and equipment	($1,155)	($1,287)	($1,255)
Acquisitions of hospitals and healthcare entities	(350)	0	(215)
Spin-off of facilities to stockholders	0	886	0

Cash flows from continuing activities	2004	2003	2002
Disposal of hospitals and healthcare entities	327	805	2,060
Change in investments	106	565	(294)
Investment in discontinued operations, net	0	0	677
Other	(15)	(44)	(3)
Net cash provided by (used in) investing activities	**($1,087)**	**$925**	**$970**

	2004	2003	2002
Net cash provided by continuing operating activities	1,547	1,223	1,916
Net cash provided by (used in) investing activities	(1,087)	925	970
Net cash used in financing activities	(336)	(2,255)	(2,699)
Change in cash and cash equivalents	124	(107)	187
Cash and cash equivalents at beginning of period	190	297	110
Cash and cash equivalents at end of period	**$314**	**$190**	**$297**
Interest payments	$489	$475	$566
Income tax payments, net of refunds	$516	$634	($139)

Hospital Anywhere USA Consolidated Income Statement for the Years Ended December 31, 2004, 2003, and 2002			
	2004	2003	2002
Revenues	$16,670	$16,657	$18,681
Salaries and benefits	6,639	6,694	7,766

(continues)

Hospital Anywhere USA Consolidated Income Statement for the Years Ended December 31, 2004, 2003, and 2002	2004	2003	2002
Supplies	2,640	2,645	2,901
Other operating expenses	3,085	3,251	3,816
Provision for doubtful accounts	1,255	1,269	1,442
Depreciation and amortization	1,033	1,094	1,247
Interest expense	559	471	561
Equity in earnings of affiliates	(126)	(90)	(112)
Settlement with federal government	840	0	0
Gains on sales of facilities	(34)	(297)	(744)
Impairment of long-lived assets	117	220	542
Restructuring of operations and investigation-related costs	62	116	111
Total expenses	**16,070**	**15,373**	**17,530**
Income from continuing operations before minority interests and income taxes	66	1,284	1,151
Minority interests in earnings of consolidated entities	84	57	70
Income from continuing operations before income taxes	516	1,227	1,081
Provision for income taxes	297	570	549
Income from continuing operations	219	657	532
Discontinued operations:			
Loss from operations of discontinued businesses, net of income tax benefit of $26			(80)
Loss of disposals of discontinued businesses			(73)

	2004	2003	2002
Net income	$219	$657	$379
Basic earnings per share:			
Income from continuing operations	$0.39	$1.12	$0.82
Discontinued operations:			
Loss from operations of discontinued businesses			(0.12)
Loss on disposals of discontinued businesses			(0.11)
Net income	**$0.39**	**$1.12**	**$0.59**
Diluted earnings per share:			
Income from continuing operations	$0.39	$1.12	$0.82
Discontinued operations:			
Loss from operations of discontinued businesses			(0.12)
Loss on disposals of discontinued businesses			(0.11)
Net income	**$0.39**	**$1.12**	**$0.59**

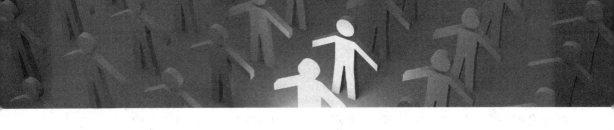

CHAPTER 12

Financial Analysis: Improving Your Decision Making

J. Michael Leger, PhD, MBA, RN, and **Paul Bayes**, DBA Accounting, MS Economics, BS Accounting

OBJECTIVES

- Provide qualitative analysis examples using the financial statements.
- Identify key financial ratios used to improve your decision-making process.
- Explain major ratio categories, including liquidity, activity, leverage, profitability, and net trade cycle.
- Discuss ratio categories, why they provide useful information for the organization, and how they affect the company's financial performance.

Numbers by themselves are data, not information. To be an informed and effective decision maker, you must be able to convert raw data (numbers) into information. Putting financial data in a format that allows comparisons, whether within your organization or between firms, makes the information meaningful.

Benchmarking is a process that provides comparisons with the best practices of other organizations. These firms do not have to be within the same industry; however, traditionally, comparisons are based within specific industries. This is a limiting factor in identifying best practices but simplifies the comparisons.

The purpose of this chapter is to introduce you to financial analysis and improve your understanding of the accounting information presented earlier. An improved understanding of financial information leads to better future policies and strategic plans. Analysis may be either qualitative (nonfinancial) or quantitative (financial). Most of this chapter focuses on quantitative analysis because this information is more readily available. Qualitative analysis examples are provided within the text of quantitative examples. All examples use the financial statements of Hospital Anywhere USA, a for-profit entity. Selected information from Children's Hospital, a not-for-profit entity, is provided as a contrast to that of Hospital Anywhere USA. The financial statements of the Retirement Homes, Inc. facility, a not-for-profit firm, are also provided as an example of a different type of not-for-profit facility. Differences in operating not-for-profit entities versus for-profit are noted.

Qualitative analysis requires a search of not only information in financial statements but also information from external sources. Stockholders' annual reports, not included in this text, along with financial statements, provide information. For example, the section on Management Discussion and Analysis provides information not found elsewhere in the financial statements, including strategic impetus and changes in the market structure. Other parts of the annual reports yield information as to accounting practices (footnotes), segment information, and risk. If an organization has subsidiaries (parts of the firm

either partially or wholly owned by the parent company), the data on segment information reveals the reliance on operations of certain products, services, or geographic areas.

The Securities and Exchange Commission (SEC) for publicly traded stock companies requires supplementary information. Additional information at the SEC Edgar Database can be found at www.sec.gov/edgarhp.htm. Information in Form 10-K and Form 10-Q reports is more comprehensive than the annual reports. In 10-Q (quarterly) reports, you can find information reported for each quarter of a firm. Rather than waiting until annual reports are issued, analysts can better track a firm's progress using these quarterly reports. Although the financial statements are the main focus of annual reports, they only make up a small portion. To illustrate, the annual report of Hospital Anywhere USA totals 51 pages, of which the basic financial statements, including summaries, equal 7 pages.

▶ Common Size Balance Sheets

Most of the focus in this chapter is quantitative and based on financial statements and the standard ratios found in both accounting and finance literature. One example of financial analysis is the use of *common size financial statements*. In the balance sheet and income statement, analysts select one number and then divide into all other numbers in the statement. Total assets (balance sheets) are used as the baseline figure in balance sheets. Either gross revenue (sales) or net revenue (sales) (income statement) is used as the basis for income statements. Gross revenue is the total sales made by a firm. The difference with the net figure is deductions, such as discounts, and returns have been removed. Dividing all items in this set of financial statements and comparing several years provide a quick method to evaluate trends (changes). The caveat is that a 2-year time frame may not be long enough to fully evaluate changes in operations (**TABLE 12.1**).

TABLE 12.1 Hospital Anywhere USA Consolidated Balance Sheets, December 31, 2004 and 2003

Dollars in Millions				
Assets	**2004**		**2003**	
Current assets				
Cash and cash equivalents	$314	1.79%	$190	1.13%
Accounts receivable, less allowance for doubtful accounts of $1,583 and $1,567	2,211	12.59%	1,873	11.09%
Inventories	396	2.25%	383	2.27%
Income taxes receivable	197	1.12%	178	1.05%
Other	1,335	7.6%	973	5.76%
Total current assets	**4,453**	**25.35%**	**3,597**	**21.30%**
Property and equipment at cost:				
Land	793	4.51%	813	4.81%
Buildings	6,021	34.27%	6,108	36.17%
Equipment	7,045	40.10%	6,721	39.80%
Construction in progress	431	2.45%	442	2.62%
Total property and equipment	**14,290**	**81.34%**	**14,084**	**83.41%**
Accumulated depreciation	−5,810	−33.07%	−5,594	−33.13%
	8,480	48.27%	8,490	50.28%
Investments of insurance subsidiary	1,371	7.8%	1,457	8.63%
Investments in and advances to affiliates	779	4.43%	654	3.87%
Intangible assets, net of accumulated amortization of $785 and $644	2,155	12.27%	2,319	13.73%

(continues)

TABLE 12.1 Hospital Anywhere USA Consolidated Balance Sheets, December 31, 2004 and 2003 *(continued)*

Dollars in Millions				
Assets	**2004**		**2003**	
Other	330	1.88%	368	2.18%
Total assets	**$17,568**	**100%**	**$16,885**	**100%**
Liabilities				
Current liabilities				
Accounts payable	693	3.94%	657	3.89%
Accrued salaries	352	2.00%	403	2.39%
Other accrued expenses	1,135	6.46%	897	5.31%
Government settlement accrual	840	4.78%		
Long-term debt due within one year	1,121	6.38%	1,160	6.87%
Total current liabilities	**4,141**	**23.57%**	**3,117**	**18.46%**
Long-term debt	5,631	32.05%	5,284	31.29%
Professional liability risks, deferred taxes, and other liabilities	2,050	11.67%	2,104	12.46%
Minority interests in equity of consolidated entities	572	3.26%	763	4.92%
Forward purchase contracts and put options	769	4.38%		0%
Total liabilities	**13,163**	**74.93%**	**11,268**	**66.73%**
Stockholders' equity:				
Common stock $0.01 par; authorized 1,600,000,000 voting shares; 50,000,000 nonvoting shares; outstanding 521,991,700 voting shares and 21,000,000 nonvoting shares—2004; and 543,272,900 voting shares and 21,000,000 nonvoting shares—2003	5	0.03%	6	0.04%

(continues)

TABLE 12.1 Hospital Anywhere USA Consolidated Balance Sheets, December 31, 2004 and 2003 *(continued)*

Assets	Dollars in Millions			
	2004		2003	
Capital in excess of par value			951	5.63%
Other	9	0%	8	0%
Accumulated other comprehensive income	52	0.30%	53	0.31%
Retained earnings	4,339	24.07%	4,599	27.24%
Total stockholders' equity	4,405	25.07%	5,617	33.27%
Total liabilities and stockholders' equity	**$17,568**	**100%·**	**$16,885**	**100%**

Table 12.1 illustrates some minor changes in the assets, liabilities, and stockholders' equity from 2003 to 2004. The cash and cash equivalents increased from 1.13% in 2003 to 1.79% in 2004. This trend indicates that Hospital Anywhere USA had more cash and cash equivalents as a percentage of total assets in 2004 than it had in 2003. This increase may be the result of management anticipation of a need for more cash or a better job of collecting patient accounts. Management may have also reduced expenses, thus improving cash flow. However, the accounts receivable percentages increased from 11.09% to 12.59%, indicating an increase in the amount of "paper" held and collection slowed. This point illustrates that the person doing the financial analysis may have to perform further evaluations rather than look at one piece of information. Total current assets also increased as a percentage of total assets, indicating that Hospital Anywhere USA was holding more liquid assets (ones that can be converted into cash quickly) in 2004 than in 2003.

Three changes occurred in the items defined as long-term assets. First, the buildings account decreased from 36.17% to 34.27% of total assets, which indicates that Hospital Anywhere USA may have sold off some of its buildings. As this account illustrates, the dollar value of buildings in fact declined from $6,108 to $6,021. Footnotes accompanying the financial statements state that three properties were sold. The second change indicates construction in progress decreased slightly, which might provide evidence of some building projects either being completed or abandoned. The third change in these assets occurred in intangible assets, which showed a decrease of 1.46% from the previous year. This could be the result of the following:

- Selling off parts of the organization, thereby reducing goodwill
- Selling off some patents
- Expired patent rights
- A more aggressive manner used to write off existing patents or other intangible assets

One item that appears in conjunction with this account is that the amortization, the systematic writing off of intangible assets, increased from $644 to $785. This explains, at least in part, the decrease in intangible assets but does not provide evidence as to the reason for the increase in write-offs. This would come with additional research in the schedules and notes accompanying the statements.

Current liabilities show one item changing drastically. The government settlement accrual went from $0 in 2003 to $840 in 2004, indicating the settlement with the government over billing charges that cost the firm $840. The percentage change was from 0% to 4.78%. Long-term debt, forward purchase contracts, and put options also went from $0 to $769, making a percentage change from 0% to 4.38%. A *forward purchase contract* is where one party agrees to buy a commodity at a specific price on a specific future date and the other party agrees to make the sale. In this case, the agreement was for the repurchase of a limited number of common shares of Hospital Anywhere USA. A *put option* provides the right to sell stock at a specified price in the future. This again was related to the repurchase of the stock from a third party. In both instances, a third party purchased shares of Hospital Anywhere USA stock in the market, and the hospital entered into a contract to purchase a set number of shares at a specified price from this third-party entity. Total liabilities also increased from 66.73% to 74.93%, indicating that a larger proportion of the business was financed using debt.

Analysis of stockholders' equity indicates that the capital in excess of par values declined from $951 to $0, going from 5.63% to 0%. Although no information is directly available, a schedule that accompanies the financial statements provides information concerning this issue. Hospital Anywhere USA repurchased 21,281,200 shares of stock. Part of that repurchase plan would eliminate this account. A second item that negatively impacted the capital in excess of par values account was the reclassification of forward purchase contracts and put options to temporary equity. This was a result of action taken by the Financial Accounting Standards Board, which regulates

reporting practices. Retained earnings declined from 27.24% to 24.70% as a result, partially, of the aforementioned reclassification.

▶ Common Size Income Statements

Information in income statements is calculated in the same manner. The baseline number for analysis is either the gross revenue or net revenue. All items in the income statement are divided by this base figure, which converts the information into a common basis to detect trends (changes) in operations (**TABLE 12.2**).

Salaries and benefits decreased slightly, which indicates that Hospital Anywhere USA may have undertaken some cost control or containment measures during the 2004 reporting period. Other operating expenses also decreased from 19.52% to 18.51%. These would include items, such as utilities, property taxes, professional fees (legal and accounting), maintenance, rent, and lease expenses. Interest expense and settlement with the federal government increased during this time period. With the aforementioned increase in debt financing, from the balance sheet analysis, there may be an increase in interest expenses. Unless a firm can negotiate a lower rate than that used in previous financing arrangements, the increased use of debt raises the risk to creditors, which causes the interest rate to increase. A simple explanation is that as more debt is issued, even at the same rate, there will be an increase in interest cost. The settlement with the federal government went from 0% to 5.04%. This had a major impact on the profitability of the firm. The only remaining item that had a major change, other than summative categories, such as income from continuing operations before taxes and income from continuing operations, was provision for income taxes. This amount decreased from 3.42% to 1.78%. This may be a result of lower income or having either tax credits or deferred taxes that can be used to reduce the current year's taxable income. Tax credits are provided in the tax laws and allow firms to carry

TABLE 12.2 Hospital Anywhere USA Consolidated Income Statements for the Years Ended December 31, 2004, and 2003

Dollars in Millions				
	2004		**2003**	
Revenues	$16,670	100.00%	$16,657	100.00%
Salaries and benefits	6,639	39.83%	6,694	40.19%
Supplies	2,640	15.84%	2,645	15.88%
Other operating expenses	3,085	18.51%	3,251	19.52%
Provision for doubtful accounts	1,255	7.53%	1,269	7.62%
Depreciation and amortization	1,033	6.20%	1,094	6.57%
Interest expense	559	3.35%	471	2.83%
Equity in earnings of affiliates	−126	−0.76%	−90	−0.54%
Settlement with federal government	840	5.04%	0	0.00%
Gains on sales of facilities	−34	−0.20%	−297	−1.78%
Impairment of long-lived assets	117	0.70%	220	1.32%
Restructuring of operations and investigation-related costs	62	0.37%	116	0.70%
Total expenses	**16,070**	**96.40%**	**15,373**	**92.29%**
Income from continuing operations before minority interests and income taxes	66	0.40%	1,284	7.71%
Minority interests in earnings of consolidated entities	84	0.50%	57	0.34%
Income from continuing operations before income taxes	516	3.10%	1,227	7.37%
Provision for income taxes	297	1.78%	570	3.42%
Income from continuing operations	219	1.31%	657	3.94%

(continues)

TABLE 12.2 Hospital Anywhere USA Consolidated Income Statements for the Years Ended December 31, 2004, and 2003   *(continued)*

Dollars in Millions				
	2004		**2003**	
Discontinued operations				
Loss from operations of discontinued businesses, net of income tax benefit of $26				
Loss of disposals of discontinued businesses		0.00%		
Net income	$219	1.31%	$657	3.94%
Basic earnings per share				
Income from continuing operations	$0.39	0.00%	$1.12	0.01%
Discontinued operations				
Loss from operations of discontinued businesses				
Loss on disposals of discontinued businesses				
Net income	**$0.39**	**0.00%**	**$1.12**	**0.01%**
Diluted earnings per share				
Income from continuing operations	$0.39	0.00%	$1.12	0.01%
Discontinued operations				
Loss from operations of discontinued businesses				
Loss on disposals of discontinued businesses				
Net income	**$0.39**	**0.00%**	**$1.12**	**0.01%**

losses incurred in any year back for 2 years and forward for 20 years. Deferred taxes are a result of differences between financial reporting tax requirements and those used for reporting taxes to local, state, and federal government units. In some cases, alternative inventory and depreciation may be used for reporting, thus creating a difference in the amounts owed, and the payments may be deferred (postponed).

▶ Financial Ratio Analysis

Key financial ratios can be classified into five categories:

1. Liquidity ratios
2. Activity ratios
3. Leverage ratios
4. Profitability ratios
5. Net trade cycle

Each category provides an analysis of different aspects of the organization and indicates how well the firm is managed. The following ratios are limited in number, and use varies by type of organization. The ones presented here are considered the more standard ratios for most businesses. Industry-specific ratios would be used to provide additional information. The names used are the standard ones, and those used by different firms and professional organizations may be different. To provide a more complete analysis, the calculated ratios should be compared with industry averages.

Several services provide this information on a for-fee basis. When making the comparisons, you must evaluate each firm by both size and type. For hospitals, the data are provided by size and geographic regions. The information can be obtained from sources for other types of not-for-profit organizations.

Liquidity Ratios

Liquidity ratios are concerned with short-term (current) items. The two most frequently used liquidity ratios are the current ratio and quick or acid-test ratio. The *current ratio* divides the current assets by current liabilities. This provides one measure of a firm's ability to pay short-term obligations, which arise in the course of operations or within one operating cycle (usually 1 year). For example, if the calculated ratio is two, this is interpreted to mean that you have 2 dollars in current assets for every 1 dollar in current liabilities. The limitation is that this ratio does not measure the true ability to pay obligations. A skewed example might be useful for improved understanding of this limitation. If current assets are $2 million and current liabilities are $1 million, then there are twice as many dollars in assets as there are in liabilities. However, let us assume that the current assets consist of $1 in cash and that inventories make up the remainder. All current liabilities are due tomorrow. The original answer shows that obligations can be met, but, as the skewed example shows, the current debt cannot be met.

Now let's figure the actual liquidity ratio:

Ratio	How Calculated	2004	2003
Current ratio	Current assets/Current liabilities	$4,453/$4141 = 1.08	$3,597/$3,117 = 1.15
Quick ratio	Current assets – Inventories/Current liabilities	$4,057/$4141 = 0.98	$3,214/$3,117 = 1.03

The current ratio declined from 1.15 to 1.08 in the preceding results, indicating the ability to pay short-term obligations has weakened since 2003. Either current liabilities grew faster than current assets or current assets declined more rapidly than current liabilities. The common size balance sheet shows that current liabilities increased faster than current assets did.

The *quick or acid-test ratio* provides additional information to evaluate the ability to meet short-term obligations. To compute this ratio, inventory must be subtracted from current assets. Sometimes items defined as "prepaid" may also be subtracted. The reason for the elimination of inventory from the numerator is that these items cannot be converted into cash quickly without a loss in value.

In the previous example, the current and quick ratio both decreased. However, most current assets of Hospital Anywhere USA can be defined as quick assets (91.1% and 89.3%, respectively, for 2004 and 2003), so the current assets are highly liquid. If items other than cash and cash equivalents plus accounts receivable are eliminated, the quick ratio becomes 0.61 and 0.67, respectively, for 2004 and 2003. Two years is not enough time to make a completely informed judgment about the trends, but the trend is showing a decline. This is one indication of a decline in the ability of the hospital to meet its current obligations.

Activity Ratios

Activity ratios measure the liquidity and efficiency of asset management. The *accounts receivable collection period* measures the average time it takes a firm to collect its accounts (patient/insurance) receivables. The quicker a firm can convert the receivables to cash, the quicker it can pay its obligations or have cash for opportunities that may arise. This ratio is calculated by dividing the accounts receivable by the average daily revenue. Average daily revenue is calculated by dividing the revenue from the income statement by 365. This measures, on average, how many times the organization has converted the receivables into cash.

Inventory turnover is found by dividing the cost of goods sold by inventory (accounting) or revenue by inventory (finance). This measures how quickly inventory is sold, which is important for firms with products that deteriorate or have a short shelf life (drugs, surgical supplies).

Ratio	How Calculated	2004	2003
Accounts	Accounts receivable/ Receivable collection period	$2,211/($16,670/ 365) = (Revenue/ 365) = 45.67 days	$1,873/ ($16,657/365) = 45.63 days
Inventory	Cost of goods sold/ Turnover inventory or Revenue/Inventory	$16,670/$396 = 42.09	$16,657/$383 = 43.49

The preceding ratios for Hospital Anywhere USA indicate that the collection of accounts receivable takes an average of approximately 45 days. Once a patient leaves a facility after receiving medical services, the hospital is waiting for money from either the patient or a third-party payer 45 days before the claim is settled. Inventory turnover, from an accounting perspective, cannot be calculated for this hospital because cost of goods sold is not separately reported and cannot be calculated. This ratio is usually provided as supplemental information to the financial statements. If it had a subsidiary that sold medical items, or the information was provided in the income statements, then the accounting ratio could be calculated. This is a standard ratio in all accounting literature. Finance literature supports a different calculation. As indicated previously, revenue is divided by the inventory. The turnover has increased slightly. For similar firms to Hospital Anywhere USA, this number would be quite high compared with standard manufacturing organizations.

Management's effectiveness in using assets to generate revenues can be measured by using two ratios. First, *fixed asset turnover* measures

how well management is using the long-term assets of the organization to generate revenue. As the balance sheet for this firm shows, this asset consists primarily of buildings and equipment used for providing patient services. For a healthcare organization, this is important in that supplying beds and using equipment creates billable revenue. Fixed asset turnover is found by dividing net revenues by net property, plant, and equipment (cost of property, plant, and equipment minus accumulated depreciation). *Total asset turnover* measures how management is using all assets of the organization to generate revenue. The measure is found by dividing net revenues by all assets.

Ratio	How Calculated	2004	2003
Fixed asset turnover	Net revenue/Net property, plant, and equipment	$16,670/$8480 = 1.966	$16,657/$8490 = 1.96
Total asset turnover	Net revenue/Total assets	$16,670/$17,568 = 0.949	$16,657/$16,885 = 0.986

Evaluation of the preceding indicates a minor change in the use of assets to generate revenue. Fixed asset turnover was relatively stable, whereas total asset turnover has declined slightly. However, this may be caused by the increase in current assets as previously discussed.

Leverage Ratios

Leverage ratios, also called *capital structure ratios*, are one measure of how an organization is financed. For-profit firms can either borrow funds using a debt instrument (notes payable or bonds) or sell shares of stock (equity financing). Creditors look at this important ratio to determine if they will provide more funds to an organization or if the cost of funds (interest) will be changed. Remember that A = L − K. If an organization fails to continue in business because

of financial setbacks (bankruptcy), the assets of the organization will be sold and distributed first to the creditors. If there is a remainder, the owners (those holding shares of stock) receive this amount. Thus, the more debt you have, the more risk you take on. This risk limits the amount of debt that creditors are willing to extend and raises the cost to finance projects.

However, on the positive side, debt can be used to improve the investment of stockholders (owners) of an organization. For instance, if you can borrow funds at 6% and invest at 10%, then the stockholders receive the differential. Profits are increased, and these are reinvested in the firm. For Hospital Anywhere USA, the following three ratios provide an analysis of how much debt is used to finance the organization and the amount of debt compared with equity used to fund the operations and long-term projects of the firm:

Ratio	How Calculated	2004	2003
Debt ratio	Total liabilities/Total assets	$13,163/$17,568 = 0.749	$11,268/$16,885 = 0.667
Long-term debt to total capitalization	Long-term debt/ (Long-term debt − Stockholders' equity)	$9,022/($9,022 − $4,405) = 0.672	$8,151/($8,151 − $5617) = 0.592
Debt to equity	Total liabilities/ Stockholders' equity	$13,163/4405 = 2.988	$11,268/$5617 = 2.006

The *debt ratio* measures how much of the total assets have been financed using debt (obligations to pay a future amount of funds). The trend from 2003 to 2004, up from 66.7% to 74.9%, shows an increase, which indicates that more of the operations were financed using debt, and a future outflow of funds, either in interest costs or the repayment of debt, will be required. This debt may also increase the interest rate charged on these funds based on the increased risk. Remember that analysis of the common size income statement revealed that interest costs were higher in 2004 than in 2003. The other ratios confirm this trend in that debt has increased in relation to total funding (L − K) and compared with the use of equity financing (stocks).

Long-term debt to total capitalization (long-term debt divided by long-term debt plus stockholders' equity) shows that more long-term debt is being used for financing (67.2% up from 59.2%). This number ($9,022 for 2004) is found by subtracting total current liabilities from total liabilities and dividing by long-term debt ($9,022) plus $4,405.

Debt to equity also indicates a larger use of debt financing in the business. This ratio indicates that debt was used approximately twice as often as equity in 2003, and almost three times as much in 2004. Firms with stable revenues can borrow more (increase their debt) than others with revenues that fluctuate. However, there is generally a limitation on the amount of funds that will be provided for operations.

Profitability Ratios

Profitability ratios measure how well a firm is doing in its basic operations. These ratios measure the percentage that revenues minus certain costs exceed the revenues. They also determine how well the assets of the organization and owner's investment are being used. These ratios are the gross profit margin, operating profit margin, net profit margin, return on total assets, and return on equity.

Because Hospital Anywhere USA does not engage in selling physical assets, such as beds and drugs, and these items are not reported separately, the gross profit margin is not applicable. The gross profit amount is determined by subtracting from revenues the cost of goods sold. However, there is no cost of goods sold for this hospital—thus, this amount cannot be calculated.

The *operating profit margin* is found by looking at the net revenues from the normal course of business, providing healthcare services, and subtracting all expenses of operations necessary to generate these revenues. This measure, sometimes called EBIT (earnings before interest and taxes), indicates whether the firm is covering its costs of operations. This amount is then divided by net revenues. Both 2004 and 2003 indicate a reasonable operating profit margin. For 2004, this means that Hospital Anywhere USA is covering operating costs and has approximately 12 cents on the dollar left to cover all other costs, including interest paid on debt and income taxes. The government settlement negatively impacted the earnings, but because of cost reduction measures in 2004, other costs such as salaries were reduced, helping to alleviate the impact on earnings.

The remaining three measures indicate that expenses were covered but that there was little, percentage-wise, left over to reinvest in the firm. Without knowing how others in the industry are doing, it becomes difficult to make a conclusion about the effectiveness of operations. The results presented indicate a decline in profitability of operations.

Ratio	How Calculated	2004	2003
Gross profit margin	Gross profit/Net revenue	N/A	N/A
Operating profit margin	Operating profit/Net revenue	$2,018/$16,670 = 12.1%	$1704/$16,657 = 10.2%
Net profit margin	Net earnings/Net revenue	$219/$16,670 = 1.31%	$657/$16,657 = 4.18
Return on total assets or Return on investment	Net earnings/Total assets	$219/$17,568 = 1.24%	$657/$16,885 = 3.89%
Return on equity	Net earnings/ Stockholders' equity	$219/$4405 = 4.97%	$657/$5617 = 11.69%

Trade or Cash Conversion Cycle Ratio

The final group of standard ratios, the *trade or cash conversion cycle ratio*, used to analyze a firm's operations evaluates the trade or cash conversion cycle. These ratios measure, on average, how long it takes to collect from either the patient or third-party providers or how long we are taking to pay our short-term obligations. The number of days in revenue is calculated as accounts receivable turnover previously discussed:

Ratio	How Calculated	2004	2003
Number of days revenue	Accounts receivable/ (Revenue/365)	$2,211/ ($16,670/365) = 48.41	$1,873/ ($16,670/365) = 41.01
Number of days payable	Accounts payable/ (Revenue/365)	$693/ ($16,670/365) = 15.17	$657/ ($16,657/365) = 14.38

If creditors provide 30 days in which to pay an obligation and your organization takes 40 days, a cash flow problem may exist. For Hospital Anywhere USA, the number of days in payables, accounts payable divided by average daily revenues, increased from 14.38 to 15.17, which indicates that the hospital took longer to pay current obligations. This is a minor change, and anyone doing an evaluation would have to know the terms for payment that the hospital has with its creditors. This does, however, increase cash flow in that you retain cash longer by postponing the payment (cash outflow). A variation of this ratio is current liabilities divided by operating expenses minus depreciation divided by 365.

▶ Not-for-Profit Comparisons

Not-for-profit entities have some differences that make comparisons more difficult than for for-profit

entities. Because profitability is not a mission of not-for-profit organizations, profitability ratios may not be calculated in the same manner. Healthcare organizations must provide an alternative performance indicator. This is normally in a footnote but must be clearly distinguished from other notes. It may take the form of either revenue over expenses, revenues and gains over expenses and losses, earned income, or performance income.

As the financial statements in **TABLE 12.3** illustrate, there are differences between hospitals—especially between for-profit and not-for-profit firms. First, the dates of the statements are for June rather than December. The selection of a date is arbitrary. Second, other sources of revenue

TABLE 12.3 Children's Hospital Operating Revenues and Expenses June 30, 2004 and 2003		
	2004	**2003**
Net patient services and revenue	$238,736,833	$228,094,450
Other sources of revenue		
Government research grants	45,160,159	36,757,430
Support provided to cover operating expenses	100,137,765	82,342,438
Total operating revenues	**$384,034,757**	**$347,194,318**
Operating expenses		
Salaries and benefits	$195,621,776	$172,757,651
Services, supplies, other	146,371,984	131,094,528
Depreciation	28,116,508	24,262,840
Interest	5,899,845	5,492,360
Bad debt expense	3,048,592	6,182,778
Total operating expenses	**$383,268,634**	**$339,790,157**
Income (loss) from operations	**$769,123**	**$7,404,161**

consist of government research grants and support provided to cover operating expenses. The latter is probably a result of donations by outside persons or organizations. The remaining accounts on the income statements are standard and would be expected to be found on both for-profit and not-for-profit organizations.

The balance sheet has one major difference from that of a for-profit entity. Instead of having stockholders (owners) of the firm, the accounts

become unrestricted and temporarily restricted fund balances. *Unrestricted fund balances* are provided by others to support the mission of the hospital. *Temporarily restricted fund balances* are used for projects having a specific purpose and then returned to use for unrestricted purposes (**TABLE 12.4**).

The four ratios presented in the following table are variations of those used in the analysis of Hospital Anywhere USA, but are applied to that of Children's Hospital:

Ratio	How Calculated	2004	2005
Long-term debt to total capitalization	Long-term debt/(Long-term debt + Fund balances)	$234,213,357/ $502,059,690 = 0.4665	$143,476,762/ $400,372,493 = 0.3584
Debt to fund balances	Total liabilities/Fund balances	$283,587,276/ $267,846,333 = 1.058	$191,239,673/ $256/895/731 = 0.744
Reported income index	Net income/Changes in fund balance	$786,123/ $10,950,602 = 0.072	N/A
Long-term debt to fund balances	Long-term debt/Fund balance	$234,213,357/ $267,846,333 = 0.874	$143,476,763/ $256,895,731 = 0.558

All three previously used ratios are smaller than those of Hospital Anywhere USA and declined in this time period, indicating this hospital does not use as much debt to finance operations as does Hospital Anywhere USA. The reported income index was not directly applicable to Hospital Anywhere USA but is somewhat equivalent to profitability ratios that used net earnings computed for Hospital Anywhere USA. Again, a direct comparison should not be made with Hospital Anywhere USA, but this hospital could be compared with other not-for-profit hospitals.

A further problem in comparing not-for-profit entities is the lack of standardized terminology or presentation formats. Some of these same problems exist with for-profit entities, but the differences are not as glaring as that of not-for-profits. The last consideration in analyzing different not-for-profit firms is that

information is not as readily available as that for publicly reporting firms.

The consolidated balance sheets and statement of activities (equivalent to for-profit income statements) of Retirement Homes, Inc. are introduced in **TABLES 12.5** and **12.6**. Selected financial ratios follow the financial statements.

Retirement Homes, Inc. shows several differences between the previously reported organizations. In addition to being a smaller entity, it has permanently restricted funds; Children's Hospital does not. It also has gift fees and long-term obligations from advance payments from persons entering the facility. Patients may pay in advance, but until the retirement facility provides the services, the income is not earned. The income statement format for Retirement Homes, Inc. also includes fund balance changes that were not included in previously presented income statements.

TABLE 12.4 Condensed Balance Sheets as of June 30, 2004 and 2003

	2004	2003
Assets		
Cash and temporary investments	$6,084,671	$3,767,117
Patient accounts receivable, net of allowances for uncollectible accounts	55,084,671	49,121,350
Other current assets	36,059,481	27,737,663
Current assets	$97,388,219	$80,626,130
Plant and equipment, net of accumulated depreciation	$261,633,535	$223,695,756
Funds held in trust	82,118,866	42,568,303
Long-term in trust	110,292,993	101,245,215
Total assets	**$551,433,613**	**$448,135,404**
Liabilities and fund balance		
Accounts payable and accrued expenses	$44,489,716	$43,222,493
Current portion of long-term debt	4,884,203	4,540,418
Current liabilities	**$49,373,919**	**$47,762,911**
Long-term debt	$212,548,645	$119,007,882
Other long-term liabilities	21,664,716	24,468,880
Unrestricted fund balance	213,986,611	207,562,498
Temporarily restricted fund balance	53,859,722	49,333,233
Total liabilities and fund balances	**$551,433,613**	**$448,135,404**

TABLE 12.5 Retirement Homes, Inc. Consolidated Balance Sheet

	2000	1999
Assets		
Current assets:		
Cash and equivalents	$1,343,467	$557,494
Investments held by bond trustee	50,653	254,572
Accounts receivable, net of allowance for doubtful accounts of $166,200 and $45,200 in 2000 and 1999	444,396	371,746
Contributions and grants receivable	88,127	
Inventories	56,705	54,597
Prepaid expenses and other	62,133	90,567
Total current assets	**2,045,481**	**1,328,976**
Investments		
Held by bond trustee, net of amount requires to meet current obligations	4,845,585	4,562,685
Board designated funds	869,603	823,758
Foundation	1,832,579	1,637,170
	7,547,767	7,023,613
Property and equipment		
Land and improvements	2,630,999	2,537,686
Buildings and improvements	34,046,631	33,359,106
Equipment	1,679,668	1,513,251
Furniture and equipment	1,440,448	1,385,729
	39,797,746	38,795,772

(continues)

TABLE 12.5 Retirement Homes, Inc. Consolidated Balance Sheet		*(continued)*
	2000	**1999**
Assets		
Less accumulated depreciation	12,289,748	11,173,504
	27,507,998	27,622,268
Construction in progress	593,335	521,608
	28,101,333	28,143,876
Beneficial interest in charitable remainder trusts	72,250	
Net deferred charges:		
Marketing and consulting costs	1,568,833	1,758,238
Financing costs	2,437,811	2,774,112
Prepayment in lieu of taxes	210,000	280,000
	4,216,644	4,812,350
Other assets	21,500	21,500
Total assets	**$42,004,975**	**$41,330,315**
Current liabilities:		
Accounts payable	$308,493	$399,480
Salaries, wages, and related liabilities	164,551	130,589
Accrued compensated absences	130,843	120,501
Accrued interest	81,580	83,561
Current portion of long-term debt	904,031	854,212
Other current liabilities	12,012	49,860
Total current liabilities	1,601,510	1,638,203

(continues)

TABLE 12.5 Retirement Homes, Inc. Consolidated Balance Sheet *(continued)*

	2000	1999
Assets		
Other liabilities:		
Long-term obligations	33,247,449	34,163,586
Entrance fees received in advance and deposits	308,124	202,288
Gift annuities payable	377,079	254,184
Deferred entry fee revenue	23,022,153	22,865,940
	56,954,805	57,485,998
Net assets (deficit):		
Unrestricted	(18,014,253)	(19,176,458)
Temporarily restricted	1,415,676	1,382,572
Permanently restricted	47,237	
Total net assets (deficit)	(16,551,340)	(17,793,886)
Total liabilities and net deficit	**$42,004,975**	**$41,330,315**

TABLE 12.6 Retirement Homes, Inc. Consolidated Statements of Activities
Year Ended December 31

	2000	1999
Revenue and other support		
Resident services:		
Monthly service fees	$8,340,317	$8,111,191
Amortization of deferred revenues	3,345,893	3,075,632

(continues)

TABLE 12.6 Retirement Homes, Inc. Consolidated Statements of Activities
Year Ended December 31   *(continued)*

	2000	1999
Revenue and other support		
Patient revenue from nonresidents	2,217,990	1,629,027
Interest income	258,845	322,954
Medicare and other	804,211	615,273
Net assets released from restriction	132,171	
Total revenue and other support	**15,099,427**	**13,754,077**
Expenses:		
Salaries and wages	5,059,124	4,728,354
Employee benefits	733,960	691,892
Total employment expenses	5,793,084	5,420,246
Purchased services	1,534,747	1,082,729
Supplies	1,247,315	1,286,860
Provision for bad debts	123,404	5,000
Utilities	637,598	624,457
Rent	4,815	4,515
Insurance	204,503	42,417
Interest	2,410,079	2,426,461
Program expenses-foundation	116,924	
Foundation operating expenses	66,282	
Miscellaneous	369,046	
Depreciation and amortization	1,672,950	1,765,252
Total expenses	**14,180,747**	**13,073,233**

(continues)

TABLE 12.6 Retirement Homes, Inc. Consolidated Statements of Activities
Year Ended December 31 *(continued)*

	2000	1999
Revenue and other support		
Excess of revenue over expenses	918,680	680,844
Net asset reclassification	172,018	
Net assets released from restriction for capital	78,896	
Net unrealized holding losses on investments	(7,389)	1,817
Increase in unrestricted assets	1,162,205	682,661
Temporarily restricted net assets:		
Net asset reclassification	(187,018)	
Contributions	308,263	127,066
Net unrealized holding losses on investments	(168,582)	(54,993)
Investment income	291,508	244,550
Net assets released from restrictions	(211,067)	(50,443)
Increase in temporarily restricted net assets	33,104	266,180
Permanently restricted net assets:		
Net asset reclassification	15,000	
Contributions	32,237	
Increase in permanently restricted net assets	47,237	
Increase in net assets	1,242,546	948,841
Net deficit, beginning of year	**(17,793,886)**	**(18,742,727)**
Net deficit, end of year	**$(16,551,340)**	**$(17,793,886)**

Current Ratios

Retirement Homes, Inc. shows an improvement in its ability to meet current obligations. In 2003, both ratios were below 1, whereas both improved to above 1 in 2004. How does this compare with the ratios presented for Hospital Anywhere USA?

The ratios for Hospital Anywhere USA deteriorated, whereas those of Retirement Homes, Inc. improved. The trends can be compared, but a direct comparison cannot be made because the firms are in two different industries and operate as two different types of organizations (for-profit versus not-for-profit).

Ratio	How Calculated	2004	2003
Current ratio	Current assets/Current liabilities	$2,045,481/ $1,601,510 = 1.28	$1,328,976/ $1,638,203 = 0.81
Quick ratio	Current assets – Inventories/Current liabilities	$1,926,643/ $1,601,510 = 1.20	$1,183,812/ $1,683,203 = 0.70

Activity Ratios

Notice in the following table that the number of days in the accounts receivable collection period increased, as did the inventory turnover. This indicates that the firm has slowed the time to make collections, whereas inventory was being used faster. Again, a direct comparison cannot be made with Hospital Anywhere USA data. However, you can purchase industry comparison data (*benchmarking*) from either national services or associations and determine how well you are doing compared with others.

Ratio	How Calculated	2004	2003
Accounts receivable collection period	Accounts Receivable/ [(Revenue)/365]	$444,396/ [($15,099,427)/365] = 10.7 Days	$371,746/ [($13,754,077)/365] = 9.86 Days
Inventory turnover	Cost of Goods Sold/Inventory or Revenue Inventory	$15,099,427/$56,705 = 266.3	$13,754,077/$54,597 = 251.9

Notice again that both ratios improved, but assets are not used as well to generate revenue for Retirement Homes, Inc. as they were for Hospital Anywhere USA. You are cautioned again not to make direct comparisons.

Ratio	How Calculated	2004	2003
Fixed asset turnover	Net revenue/Net property, plant, and equipment	$15,099,427/ $28,101,333 = 0.587	$13,754,077/ $28,143,876 = 0.488
Total asset turnover	Net revenue/Total assets	$15,099,427/ $42,004,975 = 0.359	$13,754,077/ $41,330,315 = 0.382

Leverage Ratios

In each case, the amount of debt—long-term and total—is greater than total assets and long-term debt plus net assets. Net assets—equivalent to for-profits' stockholders' equity—are negative. This negative figure is probably a result of losses in previous years of operation. As a result of this negative figure, the calculation is not applicable.

Ratio	How Calculated	2004	2003
Debt ratio	Total liabilities/Total assets	$56,954,805/ $42,004,975 = 1.356	$57,485,998/ $41,330,315 = 1.39
Long-term debt to total capitalization	Long-term debt/ (Long-term debt + Net assets)	$55,353,295/ $38,801,955 = 1.43	$55,847,795/ $38,053,909 = 1.47
Debt to equity	Total liabilities/Net assets	$56,954,805/ ($16,551,340) = N/A	$57,485,999/ ($17,793,886) = N/A

Profitability Ratios

Two of the following ratios cannot be calculated either because of a lack of available data or because one part of the equation has a negative (deficit) balance. Two of the ratios (indicated with *) are variations of those presented previously for Hospital Anywhere USA. These ratios use the increase in net assets because a not-for-profit does not report profits but rather looks at increases or decreases in assets. All three ratios that were calculated improved in year 2004 over that of 2003.

Ratio	How Calculated	2004	2003
Gross profit margin	Gross profit/Net revenue	N/A	N/A
Operating profit margin*	Excess of revenue over expenses/Net revenue	$918,680/ $15,099,427 = 6%	$680,844/ $13,654,077 = 4.95%
Net profit margin*	Increase in net assets/ Net Revenue	$1,242,546/ $15,099,427 = 8.2%	$948,841/ $13,754,077 = 6.89%
Return on total assets or return on investment	Increase in net assets/Total assets	$1,242,546/ $15,099,427 = 8.22%	$948, 841/ $13,754,077 = 6.89%
Return on equity	Increase in net assets/ Total net assets	$1,242,546/ ($16,551,340) = N/A	$948, 841/ ($17,793,881) = N/A

Additional Financial Ratios

One ratio that can be applied to both not-for-profit and for-profit entities is the number of day's *cash on hand*. This is the amount of cash necessary to meet actual daily cash operating expenses. This measure excludes both bad debt and depreciation expenses from operating expenses. Remember, these are estimates and are a "paper and pencil" item only. They do not cause cash outflows. The calculation for this ratio follows:

$$Days\ of\ cash\ band = \frac{Cash + Marketable\ securities}{(Operating\ expenses - Bad\ debts - Depreciation)/365}$$

One healthcare organization maintains 200 days of cash on hand. However, this amount is probably high for most firms. The more cash on hand, the less a firm has to invest in assets that have higher returns. A variation of the preceding ratio is the cash flow coverage. This measures how well you are able to cover required payments such as interest, rent, and debt payments. Information for calculation of this ratio would be found in the cash flow statements. Calculation of this ratio follows:

$$Cash\ flow\ coverage = \frac{Cash\ from\ operations + Interest + Rent}{Interest + Rent + Debt\ payments}$$

If the previous ratio is less than 1, it indicates that you are only able to make that percentage of required payments. For example, if the ratio is 0.8, you are only able to make 80% of the required payments.

A ratio unique to not-for-profit organizations, and one that only recently has been calculated, is the *program service ratio*. This ratio is designed to determine what proportion of a firm's expenditures goes directly into its program services (core business). This ratio is calculated by dividing program service expenses by total expenses. A firm should be spending a large proportion of its cash inflows on its mission.

Programs service

$$Ratio = \frac{Programs\ service\ expenses}{Total\ expenses}$$

Other financial ratios that might be computed for either for-profit or not-for-profit entities are as follows:

- Revenue per employee: Net revenue/Number of employees
- Net income per employee: Net income/Number of employees
- Price earnings ratio: Market price of stock/Earning per common share
- Growth rate of revenue: Percentage change in revenue from previous time period

Ratios that are more applicable to not-for-profit and healthcare entities are these:

- Percentage of deductibles: Deductibles/Gross patient service revenue
- Reported income index: Net income/Changes in fund balance
- Long-term debt to fund balance: Long-term debt/Fund balance

In any of the previously calculated ratios where stockholders' equity numbers were used, the not-for-profit sector would use the fund balance as a replacement number for calculations. Deductibles are unique to the healthcare industry. The industry is affected negatively by third-party payment systems. Once a claim is filed, deductions based on contracted rates are removed from the expected payment. The actual amount received varies from amounts as low as 25 cents on the dollar to a high of around 60 cents on the dollar.

Summary

As with any comparisons that use ratios or common size financial statements, caution must be used. Comparisons must be made for a longer period than 2 years. Past results may not be indicative of future performance. Differences in management, whether risk aversive or risk taking, can affect how a firm is managed. Competition, geographic differences, and other factors can affect operations. Nonetheless, ratios and common size comparisons can provide indications of action that needs to be undertaken. Benchmarking allows a firm to judge how well it is doing in relation to other organizations in the same industry and in other industries. Recall that benchmarking is looking at best practices, not just in firms in your industry but in all firms.

Discussion Questions

1. Which ratios would you consider most important in the daily and monthly operation of the organization? Why?
2. If you were analyzing an organization's ability to borrow money, which ratios would be most helpful?
3. Why is the accounts receivable turnover ratio important to the organization?
4. What process do organizations use to compare themselves with other organizations and how effective is this process?
5. When using common size financial statements, what number do analysts use for the balance sheet and what number is used for the income statements?

Glossary of Terms

Accounts Receivable Collection Period the average time it takes an organization to collect its accounts (patient/insurance) receivable.

Activity Ratios the liquidity and efficiency of asset management.

Benchmarking a process that provides comparisons with the best practices of other organizations. These firms do not have to be within the same industry, but traditionally comparisons are based within specific industries. This is a limiting factor in identifying best practices but simplifies the comparisons.

Cash on Hand applies to both not-for-profit and for-profit entities; the number of days of cash on hand. This is the amount of cash necessary to meet actual daily cash operating expenses. This measure excludes both bad debt and depreciation expenses from operating expenses.

Common Size Financial Statements in the balance sheet and income statement, one number is selected and then divided into all other numbers in the statements.

Current Ratio the current assets divided by current liabilities. This provides one measure of a firm's ability to pay short-term obligations.

Debt Ratio how much of the total assets have been financed using debt (obligations to pay a future amount of funds).

Fixed Asset Turnover how well management is using the long-term assets of the organization to generate revenue.

Forward Purchase Contract where one party agrees to buy a commodity at a specific price on a specific future date and the other party agrees to make the sale.

Inventory Turnover how quickly inventory is sold; a measure that is important for firms with products that deteriorate or have a short shelf life (drugs, surgical supplies).

Leverage Ratios, or Capital Structure Ratios one measure of how an organization is financed.

Liquidity Ratios concerned with short-term (current items). The two most frequently used liquidity ratios are the current ratio and quick or acid-test ratio.

Operating Profit Margin found by looking at the net revenues from the normal course of business, providing healthcare services, and subtracting all expenses of operations necessary to generate these revenues. This measure, sometimes called EBIT (earnings before interest and taxes), indicates whether the firm is covering its costs of operations.

Profitability Ratios measures of how well a firm is doing in its basic operations.

Program Service Ratio a ratio unique to not-for-profit organizations and one that only recently has been calculated. This ratio is designed to determine what proportion of a firm's expenditures go directly into its program services (core business).

Put Option the right to sell stock at a specified price in the future.

Quick or Acid-Test Ratio additional information to evaluate the ability to meet short-term obligations.

Total Asset Turnover how management is using all assets of the organization to generate revenue. The measure is found by dividing net revenues by all assets.

Trade or Cash Conversion Cycle Ratio a measure of, on average, how long it takes to collect from either the patient or third-party providers or how long the organization is taking to pay short-term obligations.

Index

Note: Page numbers followed by *b*, *f*, or *t* indicate entries in boxes, figures, or tables, respectively